Sleep Surgery in a Nutshell

Liang Chye Goh • Song Tar Toh
Editors

Sleep Surgery in a Nutshell

Springer

Editors
Liang Chye Goh
Department of Otorhinolaryngology
Faculty of Medicine, Universiti Malaya
Kuala Lumpur, Malaysia

Song Tar Toh
Department of Otorhinolaryngology-Head & Neck Surgery
Singapore General Hospital
Singapore, Singapore

ISBN 978-981-95-9748-2 ISBN 978-981-95-9749-9 (eBook)
https://doi.org/10.1007/978-981-95-9749-9

This Springer imprint is published by the registered company Springer Nature Singapore Pte Ltd.
The registered company address is: 152 Beach Road, #21-01/04 Gateway East, Singapore 189721, Singapore

To my parents who never gave up on me
To my loving wife, Katherine, who supported me through thick and thin
To my daughter, Jovanne, who brings joy to my life
To my Teachers and Colleagues who inspire me to do better every day

Julius Goh LC

Foreword

Obstructive sleep apnea (OSA) is a heterogeneous disorder that affects millions of people across all ages, genders, and racial groups. It is a significant public health concern exerting a substantial burden not only on patients but also on healthcare systems and society at large. The impact of OSA extends beyond disrupted sleep and snoring; it is associated with increased risk of cardiovascular disease, neurocognitive impairment, metabolic disorders, reduced quality of life, and motor vehicle accidents.

As our understanding of the disorder continues to grow, so does the recognition that effective treatment requires a multidisciplinary and personalized approach. While nonsurgical therapies such as positive airway pressure, oral appliances, and weight loss have been shown to be effective in the management of OSA, the role of surgery has steadily expanded over the years, offering targeted solutions for patients who do not benefit from or cannot tolerate non-invasive treatments.

Sleep Surgery in a Nutshell is a timely contribution to the evolving field of sleep surgery. It provides a concise yet comprehensive overview of OSA treatment principles, addressing concepts of disease pathophysiology and most current surgical interventions. The book is carefully structured, guiding the reader from the history and etiology of OSA to the full spectrum of operative strategies and technological advances. The book not only highlights surgical anatomy and techniques; it also summarizes evidence-based concepts of decision-making to address unique causes of OSA and individual needs. The authors highlight the rationale for intervention, patient selection criteria, expected outcomes, potential complications, and perioperative considerations.

This book serves both as a surgical manual and as a practical reference for understanding when, why, and how surgery should be applied in the management of OSA. It encourages a comprehensive patient-centered approach to treatment that prioritizes long-term outcomes and individualized care. It will undoubtedly be a valuable reference for otolaryngologists, sleep surgeons, and all clinicians engaged in the care of patients with OSA.

I would like to congratulate the editors and contributors for creating a practical resource that will enhance surgical education, advance clinical practice, and ultimately improve the well-being of patients with sleep apnea.

Maria V. Suurna, MD
Professor of Clinical Otolaryngology-Head and Neck Surgery and Director of Sleep Surgery University of Miami Health System
Coral Gables, FL, USA

Preface 1

We are proud to present *Sleep Surgery in a Nutshell*, a concise yet practical guide for those seeking to understand, perform, and teach sleep surgery with greater clarity and structure. Surgical management of obstructive sleep apnea continues to evolve and is often underrepresented in mainstream literature. When performed without the appropriate training or understanding, sleep surgery can be detrimental to patients—especially when operating in the delicate anatomy of the upper airway.

The technical skills and knowledge required for sleep surgery are often scattered across a multitude of sources. Though various techniques are described in the published literature, they are seldom standardized.This lack of streamlining makes structured training in sleep surgery inconsistent and sometimes frustrating for both aspiring sleep surgeons to undestand and perform these procedures, and for seasoned consultants seeking to refine their craft and teach their students. OSA surgery is currently one of the most rapidly progressing subspecialties within otolaryngology. The discipline has moved beyond traditional soft tissue procedures to include skeletal reconstruction, robotic-assisted techniques, and neurostimulation therapies such as hypoglossal nerve stimulation. This rapid evolution is not just a testament to innovation, but also a call to arms—inviting us to rethink how we empower patients with treatment options beyond conventional PAP therapy.

This book aims to bridge the training gap by offering a focused overview that supports both trainees and practicing specialists interested in advanced sleep surgery. It does not intend to replace comprehensive reference texts or proper formal fellowship, but rather to serve as a practical, approachable update on techniques and philosophies shaping modern surgical management of OSA.

The opening chapters lay a foundation by reviewing the basics of sleep apnea, treatment decision-making, and the anatomical rationale behind various surgical strategies. Subsequent chapters are organized by anatomical region, culminating in focused discussions on cutting-edge techniques such as hypoglossal nerve stimulation and skeletal framework surgery. We are deeply grateful to our contributors—both local and international—for sharing their insights and enriching this book with their experience and expertise. We hope Sleep Surgery in a Nutshell serves not only as a resource but as an invitation for dialogue, growth, and collaboration as we continue to explore and expand this important field.

Kuala Lumpur, Malaysia Liang Chye Goh, MS(ORL-HNS)
Singapore, Singapore Song Tar Toh, MMED(ORL)

Preface 2

All praise is due to The Almighty, who has granted me the gift of drawing, especially in the field of medical illustration. It is my sincere intention that these illustrations serve as a source of benefit—helping surgeons to better understand surgical techniques and, ultimately, contributing to the improvement of patient care and healthcare delivery.

A good medical illustration is more than just a picture; it strikes a balance between realism and clarity, highlighting the details that are most essential to know. With this principle in mind, I have endeavored to ensure that every diagram in this textbook supports the understanding of critical surgical steps in sleep surgery. I am deeply grateful to my lecturers at the Faculty of Medicine, Universiti Malaya, for giving me the wonderful opportunity to contribute as an illustrator to this important book. Their trust and guidance have been invaluable throughout this journey.

At the same time, I humbly acknowledge that these illustrations may have imperfections. I warmly welcome any constructive feedback or suggestions for improvement, as refinement is the heart of both academic and artistic growth. It is my hope that the illustrations in this textbook will not only enhance your understanding of the essential steps in sleep surgery but also assist you in providing the best possible care for patients—helping them regain their quality of sleep and, with it, a better quality of life.

Kuala Lumpur, Malaysia — Muhammad Ariff bin Sobani, MBBS

Disclaimer

This book, *Sleep Surgery in a Nutshell*, is intended for educational and informational purposes only. It provides a summary of surgical principles and procedures in the field of sleep surgery and should not be considered a substitute for comprehensive surgical training, clinical judgment, or professional medical advice.

The authors and publishers have made every effort to ensure that the information presented is accurate, current, and evidence-based at the time of writing. However, medical knowledge, surgical techniques, and clinical guidelines evolve over time, and variations in practice may exist. Readers are advised to consult updated references, institutional protocols, and experienced colleagues when applying the concepts described in this book.

The contents of this book are not intended to serve as a definitive guide for patient management. Individual patient care should always be tailored based on thorough clinical evaluation, diagnostic findings, and the treating surgeon's professional expertise. The authors, editors, and publishers accept no responsibility or liability for any injury, loss, or damage incurred as a result of reliance upon the information contained in this text.

Mention of specific products, devices, instruments, or brand names does not imply endorsement or recommendation by the authors or publishers. By using this book, the reader acknowledges that surgical practice carries inherent risks, and clinical responsibility ultimately rests with the treating physician or surgeon.

The authors used ChatGPT, a large language model, for drafting assistance and language refinement. All content was reviewed, verified, and approved by the authors to ensure accuracy, originality, and compliance with professional standards.

Contents

Contributors

Mohd Zulkiflee Abu Bakar Department of Otorhinolaryngology, Faculty of Medicine, Universiti Malaya, Kuala Lumpur, Malaysia

Ahmad Izuanuddin Ismail Faculty of Medicine, Universiti Teknologi Mara (UiTM), Sungai Buloh, Malaysia

Mohd Ayzam Ahmad Department of Otorhinolaryngology, Hospital Sultanah Bahiyah, Alor Setar, Kedah, Malaysia

Chee Chean Lim Department of Otorhinolaryngology, Faculty of Medicine, Universiti Malaya, Kuala Lumpur, Malaysia

Abdul Rahim bin Md Din Department of Otorhinolaryngology, Faculty of Medicine, Universiti Malaya, Kuala Lumpur, Malaysia

Nor Anis Elini Ismail Department of Otorhinolaryngology, Faculty of Medicine, Universiti Malaya, Kuala Lumpur, Malaysia

Liang Chye Goh Department of Otorhinolaryngology, Faculty of Medicine, Universiti Malaya, Kuala Lumpur, Malaysia

Andrew Junior Charles Gomez Department of Otorhinolaryngology, Faculty of Medicine, Universiti Malaya, Kuala Lumpur, Malaysia

Firdaus Hariri Department of Oral & Maxillofacial Clinical Sciences, Faculty of Dentistry, Universiti Malaya, Kuala Lumpur, Malaysia

Muhammad Kamil Hassan Department of Oral & Maxillofacial Clinical Sciences, Faculty of Dentistry, Universiti Malaya, Kuala Lumpur, Malaysia

Clemens Heiser ENT & Sleep Center Mangfall-Inn, Bad Aibling, Germany

Hui Yan Ong Department of Otorhinolaryngology, Faculty of Medicine, Universiti Malaya, Kuala Lumpur, Malaysia

Ahmad Syahir Md Ismail Department of Otorhinolaryngology, Faculty of Medicine, Universiti Malaya, Kuala Lumpur, Malaysia

Ng Boon Han Kevin Department of Otorhinolaryngology, Faculty of Medicine & Health Sciences, Universiti Malaysia Sarawak, Kota Samarahan, Malaysia

Srinivas Kishore AIG Hospitals, Gachibowli, Hyderabad, India

Ahmad Kusyairi Khalid KPJ Healthcare University, Nilai, Negeri Sembilan, Malaysia

Rajendran Laavanya Department of Otorhinolaryngology, Faculty of Medicine, Universiti Malaya, Kuala Lumpur, Malaysia

May Nak Lau Department of Orthodontics, Paediatric and Special Care Dentistry, Faculty of Dentistry, Universiti Malaya, Kuala Lumpur, Malaysia

Prepageran Narayanan Department of Otorhinolaryngology, Faculty of Medicine, Universiti Malaya, Kuala Lumpur, Malaysia

Chu Qin Phua Department of Otorhinolaryngology, Sengkang General Hospital, Singapore, Singapore

Nurul Asma Che Ab Rahim Department of Otorhinolaryngology, Faculty of Medicine, Universiti Malaya, Kuala Lumpur, Malaysia

Kugan Raman Department of Otorhinolaryngology, Faculty of Medicine and Health Sciences, University Putra Malaysia (UPM), Seri Kembangan, Malaysia

John Ming Ren Loh Department of Otorhinolaryngology, Changi General Hospital, Singapore, Singapore

Jeyasakthy Saniasiaya Department of Otorhinolaryngology, Faculty of Medicine, Universiti Malaya, Kuala Lumpur, Malaysia

Moideen Sanu Centre for Advanced Care in ENT, Head and Neck Oncology, Muvattupuzha, India

Emelda Rose Sebastin Department of Otorhinolaryngology, Faculty of Medicine, Universiti Malaya, Kuala Lumpur, Malaysia

Muhammad Adam Mohd Shariff Department of Otorhinolaryngology, Faculty of Medicine, Universiti Malaya, Kuala Lumpur, Malaysia

Gagandeep Singh Mann Department of Otorhinolaryngology, Faculty of Medicine, Universiti Malaya, Kuala Lumpur, Malaysia

Muhamad Ariff bin Sobani Department of Otorhinolaryngology, Faculty of Medicine, Universiti Malaya, Kuala Lumpur, Malaysia

Mackay Stuart Grayson Department of ENT Head and Neck Surgery, Wollongong Hospital, Wollongong, NSW, Australia

Jeremy Sin Hun Tan Department of Anesthesiology, Faculty of Medicine, Universiti Malaya, Kuala Lumpur, Malaysia

Stephen Shih-Teng Kao Department of ENT Head and Neck Surgery, Lyell McEwin Hospital, Adelaide, South australia, Australia

Song Tar Toh Department of Otorhinolaryngology-Head & Neck Surgery, Singapore General Hospital, Singapore, Singapore

Maythad Uataya Department of Otorhinolaryngology, Faculty of Medicine, Siriraj Hospital, Mahidol University, Bangkok, Thailand

Claudio Vicini Department of Head-Neck Surgery, Otolaryngology, Head-Neck and Oral Surgery Unit, Morgagni Pierantoni Hospital, Azienda USL Della Romagna, Forlì, Italy

Chee Kuan Wong Department of Medicine, Faculty of Medicine, Universiti Malaya, Kuala Lumpur, Malaysia

Lee Keng Wong Department of Otorhinolaryngology, Faculty of Medicine, Universiti Malaya, Kuala Lumpur, Malaysia

Wei Jin Wong Department of Surgery, Faculty of Medicine, Universiti Malaya, Kuala Lumpur, Malaysia

Chun Hong Yeap Department of Anesthesiology, Faculty of Medicine, Universiti Malaya, Kuala Lumpur, Malaysia

Siti Nadzrah Yunus Department of Anesthesiology, Faculty of Medicine, Universiti Malaya, Kuala Lumpur, Malaysia

Abbreviations

AASM	American Academy of Sleep Medicine
AHI	Apnea Hypopnea Index
AI	Apnea Index
AP	Antero-Posterior
APOS	Asian Pacific Orthodontic Society
BIS	Bispectral Index
BMI	Body Mass Index
BRP	Barbed Repositioning Pharyngoplasty
BSSO	Bilateral Sagittal Split Osteotomy
CCC	Complete Circumferential Collapse
CPAP	Continuous Positive Airway Pressure
CRS	Chronic Rhinosinusitis
DISE	Drug Induced Sleep Endoscopy
DNVC	Dynamic Nasal Valve Collapse
EEG	Electroencephalogram
EMG	Electromyogram
ENT	Ear, Nose And Throat
ESP	Expansion Sphincter Pharyngoplasty
ESS	Epworth Sleepiness Score
ET	Endotracheal Tube
ETD	Eustachian Tube Dysfunction
ETT	Eustachian Tube
FESS	Functional Endoscopic Sinus Surgery
FNPLS	Flexible Nasopharyngolaryngoscopy
FOSQ	Functional Outcomes of Sleep Questionnaire
FTP	Friedman Tongue Position
GA	General Anesthesia
HNS	Hypoglossal Nerve Stimulation
HSAT	Home Sleep Apnea Test
ICU	Intensive Care Unit
IPG	Implantable Pulse Generator

IV	Intravenous
KTP	Potassium Titanyl Phosphate
LA	Local Anesthesia
LAUP	Laser-Assisted Uvulopalatoplasty
LPW	Lateral Pharyngeal Wall
MAD	Mandibular Advancement Device
MAT	Microdebrider-Assisted Turbinoplasty
mEq	Milliequivalent
MMA	Maxillo Mandibular Advancement
MRI	Magnetic Resonance Imaging
MTA	Myoclonic Twitch Activity
NIM	Nerve Integration Monitor
NIPPV	Non-Invasive Positive Pressure Ventilation
NREM	Non-Rapid Eye Movements
NSAID	Non-Steroidal Anti-Inflammatory Drugs
OAT	Oral Appliance Therapy
OHS	Obesity Hypoventilation Syndrome
OMFS	Oral Maxillofacial Surgery
OR	Operation Room
ORL	Otorhinolaryngology
OSA	Obstructive Sleep Apnea
PACU	Post Anesthesia Care Unit
PAP	Positive Airway Pressure
PNIF	Peak Nasal Inspiratory Flow
PNS	Paranasal Sinus
PPW	Posterior Pharyngeal Wall
PSG	Polysomnogram
REM	Rapid Eye Movement
RF	Radiofrequency
RFA	Radiofrequency Ablation
RFVTR	Radiofrequency Volumetric Tissue Reduction
SMILE	Submucosal Minimally Invasive Lingual Excision
TMJ	Temporomandibular Joint
TORS	Transoral Robotic Surgery
TPA	Transpalatal advancement
UAS	Upper Airway Stimulation
UPPP	Uvulopalatopharyngoplasty
VAS	Visual Analogue Scale
VPI	Velopharyngeal Insufficiency
ZPP	Z-Palatoplasty

Chapter 1
Overview of Obstructive Sleep Apnea

Liang Chye Goh, Muhammad Adam Mohd Shariff, Abdul Rahim bin Md Din, Lee Keng Wong, Ahmad Syahir Md Ismail, Rajendran Laavanya, Emelda Rose Sebastin, Nor Anis Elini Ismail, Chee Kuan Wong, Ahmad Izuanuddin Ismail, Wei Jin Wong, Ng Boon Han Kevin, Nurul Asma Che Ab Rahim, and Jeyasakthy Saniasiaya

1.1 A Brief History of Sleep Surgery

Liang Chye Goh

Sleep surgery has evolved in step with how obstructive sleep apnea (OSA) is understood, measured, and treated. Long before it had a name, the condition was recognized in literary and clinical archetypes: Charles Dickens's "Fat Boy" Joe, the perpetually drowsy servant in The Pickwick Papers (1837), became so iconic that when Burwell and colleagues described a syndrome of obesity, somnolence, and hypoventilation in 1956, they called it the Pickwickian syndrome [1]. That case report was one of the first to link excessive daytime sleepiness with disordered breathing. The operations themselves changed, but so did the questions surgeons

L. C. Goh (✉) · M. A. Mohd Shariff · Abdul Rahim bin Md Din · L. K. Wong · A. S. M. Ismail · R. Laavanya · E. R. Sebastin · N. A. Elini Ismail · N. A. Che Ab Rahim (✉) · J. Saniasiaya
Department of Otorhinolaryngology, Faculty of Medicine, Universiti Malaya, Kuala Lumpur, Malaysia
e-mail: juliusglc@um.edu.my; asma.rahim@ummc.edu.my

C. K. Wong (✉)
Department of Medicine, Faculty of Medicine, Universiti Malaya, Kuala Lumpur, Malaysia

A. I. Ismail
Faculty of Medicine, Universiti Teknologi Mara (UiTM), Sungai Buloh, Malaysia

W. J. Wong (✉)
Department of Surgery, Faculty of Medicine, Universiti Malaya, Kuala Lumpur, Malaysia
e-mail: wongweijin@um.edu.my

N. B. H. Kevin
Department of Otorhinolaryngology, Faculty of Medicine & Health Sciences, Universiti Malaysia Sarawak, Kota Samarahan, Malaysia

L. C. Goh, S. T. Toh (eds.), *Sleep Surgery in a Nutshell*,
https://doi.org/10.1007/978-981-95-9749-9_1

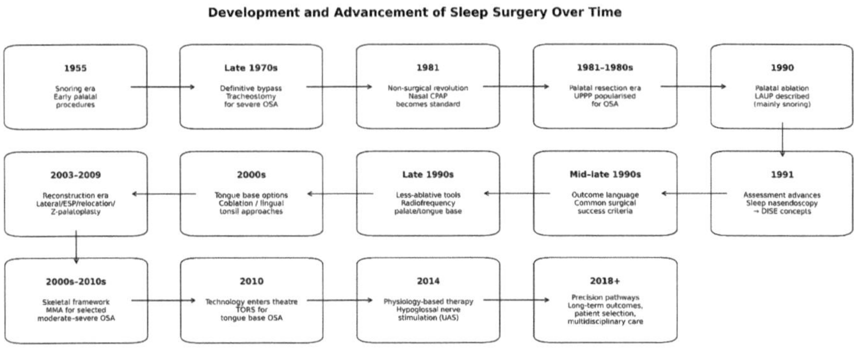

Fig. 1.1 Flow chart describing the development of the surgical management of obstructive sleep apnea over time

asked. At the beginning, the aim was often straightforward: reduce snoring, relieve obvious obstruction, and protect patients who were at immediate risk. As sleep testing became more available and outcomes could be measured, the field began to define OSA more precisely and to treat it more deliberately.

Over time, the language of sleep surgery shifted. That shift has mattered for a large number of people: conservative estimates place OSA prevalence at nearly one billion adults worldwide, many of whom remain underdiagnosed or undertreated. Early descriptions were largely anatomic and local: the palate, the tonsils, the tongue. Later, the same anatomy was framed within a broader concept of collapsible upper airway physiology. Surgeons moved from single-site procedures toward multilevel assessment, functional reconstruction of the pharynx, and, more recently, device-based therapies that aim to restore neuromuscular tone rather than remove tissue.

This chapter follows a simple timeline of milestones and the clinical ideas that shaped them. It is not meant to be exhaustive. Instead, it highlights a few turning points that explain why we do not approach the palate, tongue base, or pharyngeal walls today in the same way we did several decades ago (Fig. 1.1).

1.1.1 The Pre-PAP Era

Before positive airway pressure (PAP) therapy, the pathophysiology of OSA was poorly defined, and objective sleep testing was not widely available. Many patients were seen through the lens of snoring, daytime fatigue, or cardiopulmonary strain, without a unified diagnostic framework. In that setting, surgery reflected what clinicians could observe: noisy breathing, narrow oropharyngeal anatomy, and the practical need to secure an airway.

Some early operations focused on the soft palate. Heinberg described a palatal operation for snoring in 1955 [2]. These early reports matter less for their specific technical details than for what they represent: an early recognition that the velopharynx can be a critical point of vibration and resistance during sleep.

For severe, life-threatening obstruction, tracheostomy served as a definitive bypass of the upper airway. Motta and colleagues reported hemodynamic improvement after tracheostomy in patients with sleep-induced apnea [3]. Earlier still, Gastaut and colleagues had published polygraphic recordings of nocturnal apneic episodes in obese somnolent patients, providing some of the first objective physiologic evidence that breathing repeatedly ceased during sleep [4]. Kuhlo and colleagues then demonstrated that prolonged tracheostomy could reverse the cardiopulmonary and neurologic consequences of what was then called Pickwickian syndrome, establishing tracheostomy as the first effective—if drastic—intervention [5]. In modern practice, tracheostomy is rarely used as primary therapy for typical OSA. Historically, however, it underscored a hard truth: in the most severe forms of sleep-related obstruction, the priority was survival and physiologic stabilization, even if the solution was invasive.

This landscape changed in 1981 when Sullivan and colleagues introduced nasal continuous positive airway pressure (CPAP) [6]. The original report, published in the *Lancet*, described five patients whose severe apnea was abolished with pneumatic splinting of the airway—a remarkably elegant solution to what had been, until then, a largely surgical problem. By preventing upper airway occlusion during sleep, CPAP rapidly became first-line therapy for many patients. For surgeons, CPAP did not end the story of sleep surgery, but it redefined it. Surgery was no longer the only option for airway control, and the bar for surgical benefit rose: procedures needed to show meaningful improvements on measured indices and patient outcomes, not only subjective relief of snoring.

1.1.2 The UPPP Era

In parallel with the rise of CPAP, surgeons continued to refine palatal and oropharyngeal procedures for selected patients. In the 1980s, many surgical efforts centered on enlarging the retropalatal airway and reducing palatal flutter. The palate was accessible, familiar territory for otolaryngologists, and it was a logical early target in a condition that was still being defined.

Historical reviews describe earlier palatal operations for snoring and airway obstruction that helped set the stage for modern palatal surgery [7]. It is worth remembering that these developments occurred during an era when the boundaries between snoring, upper airway resistance, and OSA were still being clarified. Surgeons were often responding to the most visible symptoms and the most obvious anatomic constraints.

In 1981, Fujita and colleagues reported uvulopalatopharyngoplasty (UPPP) as a surgical approach for OSA, designed to enlarge the oropharyngeal airway [8]. The operation provided a structured way to address the soft palate, uvula, and lateral oropharyngeal tissues in a single procedure. Importantly, UPPP also created a common reference point in the literature: surgeons could describe what they did, what changed in the airway, and how patients responded.

Through the 1980s, several groups reported improvements in snoring and OSA symptoms after palatal and oropharyngeal surgery in selected patients [9]. These early series reinforced an intuitive idea: reducing resistance at the retropalatal level could make sleep breathing quieter and, in some patients, less obstructed. At the same time, experience also revealed the practical limitations of a palate-centered strategy. Some patients improved dramatically, while others showed little change on objective metrics despite an apparently adequate operation.

As experience grew, it became clear that palatal-only surgery has variable effectiveness, particularly when collapse occurs beyond the palate. Later reviews emphasized careful patient selection and highlighted the limits of single-site surgery in a multilevel disorder [10, 11]. In quantitative terms, pooled analyses estimated UPPP surgical success rates of roughly 40–50% when applied broadly to unselected OSA populations [12]. A later systematic review and meta-analysis by Caples and colleagues reinforced this picture, finding modest mean reductions in AHI across studies and underscoring the need for better patient selection [13]. This was a turning point in how surgeons talked about OSA. Instead of asking whether UPPP worked in general, the more useful question became: in which patients, with which collapse patterns, does a palatal procedure contribute meaningful benefit?

1.1.3 The Multilevel Concept and Airway Evaluation

OSA is now understood as a disorder in which obstruction may occur at more than one upper airway level. Common sites include the nasal cavity, retropalatal region, lateral pharyngeal walls, tongue base, and hypopharynx [11]. This multilevel view changed both diagnosis and surgical planning. It also explained why a technically successful palatal operation could still leave a patient with residual disease: the airway could remain vulnerable at a different segment.

Once multilevel obstruction was accepted as the rule rather than the exception, dynamic airway assessment became more important. Traditional awake examination can describe anatomy, but it cannot fully reproduce the muscle tone changes and collapse patterns that occur during sleep. Surgeons therefore looked for methods to observe the airway under sleep-like conditions, with enough reproducibility to guide treatment.

In 1991, Croft and Pringle described sleep nasendoscopy (a precursor to modern drug-induced sleep endoscopy (DISE) to characterize collapse patterns during sleep [14]. This approach was influential because it shifted the surgeon's attention from static narrowing to dynamic behavior. Instead of seeing the pharynx as a fixed tube, the airway could be understood as a structure that buckles, rotates, and narrows in specific ways, depending on posture, sedation level, and individual anatomy. The practical utility of DISE was further enhanced by the introduction of the VOTE classification (Velum, Oropharyngeal lateral walls, Tongue base, Epiglottis) by Kezirian and colleagues, which provided a standardized framework for describing collapse sites and patterns and has since been widely adopted in clinical practice and research [15].

Standardized outcome reporting also developed. Sher and colleagues proposed commonly used adult surgical success criteria: a 50% or greater reduction in AHI with a postoperative AHI below 20 [12]. These criteria were not perfect, but they allowed surgical results to be compared with a shared definition of improvement. Over time, they also encouraged more honest conversations with patients: the goal in many cases is meaningful reduction of risk and symptoms, not necessarily complete normalization of an index.

Multilevel assessment and standardised reporting helped the field mature. They encouraged surgeons to think in terms of patterns, predictability, and incremental benefit. They also made room for combination strategies, where palatal surgery, tongue-base therapy, and adjunctive management could be integrated into a coherent plan. One influential early example was the phased multilevel surgical protocol described by Riley, Powell, and Guilleminault at Stanford, which formalized a two-stage approach: palatal and nasal surgery first, followed by tongue base or skeletal advancement if needed [16]. This protocol demonstrated that sequential, targeted operations could achieve cumulative benefit and helped establish multilevel surgery as a systematic discipline.

1.1.4 Tissue-Preserving and Functional Reconstruction

From the 1990s onward, many techniques aimed to reduce complications seen with more ablative palatal resections, while preserving function and improving airway stability. As clinical follow-up became more systematic, the trade-offs of aggressive tissue removal became clearer. Voice change, swallowing symptoms, and scarring-related stiffness were not rare concerns. This motivated a broader shift: rather than simply enlarging the airway by excision, surgeons began to ask whether the pharynx could be made more stable by rebalancing its structures.

Laser-assisted uvulopalatoplasty (LAUP) was described for snoring by Kamami in 1990 [17]. LAUP reflected the appeal of a minimally invasive, clinic-friendly approach. However, the logic of snoring surgery does not always map neatly onto OSA physiology. In later guidance, the American Academy of Sleep Medicine concluded that LAUP is not recommended for treatment of sleep-related breathing disorders, including OSA [18]. This distinction helped clarify an important principle: reducing vibration may improve sound, but it does not necessarily address collapse.

Submucosal radiofrequency approaches were introduced to reduce soft-palate volume with less surface injury. Powell and colleagues described radiofrequency treatment of the palate in sleep-disordered breathing, and Li and colleagues reported extended follow-up [19, 20]. These techniques aimed to create controlled tissue remodeling while preserving mucosa, with the practical goal of reducing postoperative pain and minimizing functional disturbance. They also fit within a broader movement toward procedures that could be staged, combined, and tailored.

Attention also turned to the tongue base and lingual tonsils. Coblation lingual tonsillectomy was described as a technique for lingual tonsil hypertrophy, and radiofrequency tongue-base reduction was explored for sleep-disordered breathing [21, 22]. The tongue base is a challenging region: it can contribute to obstruction even when the palate is adequately addressed, and it is closely linked to airway reflexes and swallowing. Techniques that allowed safe reduction or reshaping of tongue-base bulk expanded the options for patients with persistent retrolingual collapse.

At the same time, reconstructive approaches expanded, particularly for lateral wall collapse. Examples include lateral pharyngoplasty, expansion sphincter pharyngoplasty, relocation pharyngoplasty, and Z-palatoplasty [23–26]. While each technique has its own details, the shared theme is functional. Rather than treating the pharyngeal walls as passive tissue to be removed, these operations treat them as structures that can be repositioned, tensioned, and supported. This concept aligns well with what DISE and clinical experience often show: in many patients, lateral wall collapse is a major driver of obstruction and is not reliably corrected by palatal trimming alone.

Nonresective lifting concepts were also reported (e.g., the velouvulopharyngeal lift described by Mantovani and colleagues) [27]. These procedures reflect growing confidence that repositioning and suspension can be as important as excision. In everyday practice, they also align with what patients value: preserving voice, swallowing, and the sensation of a normal throat, while still working toward better sleep breathing.

Barbed suture techniques were later described as another way to reposition the palate (e.g., barbed reposition pharyngoplasty) [28]. Barbed sutures offered a practical advantage by simplifying tissue suspension without the need for extensive knot tying.

Separately, maxillomandibular advancement (MMA) became a key skeletal operation for carefully selected patients with moderate to severe OSA. A systematic review and meta-analysis reported large reductions in AHI after MMA [29]. Postoperative airway studies have also shown airway enlargement [30]. MMA occupies a distinct place in sleep surgery because it addresses the airway framework rather than the soft tissues alone. By advancing the jaws, it can enlarge and stiffen multiple airway segments at once. At the same time, it is a major operation with orthodontic and facial considerations. Its role therefore highlights another important evolution in the field: success is not only about efficacy but also about matching invasiveness to patient goals, risk profile, and expected benefit.

1.1.5 Robotic Surgery and Implantable Therapies

In the 2010s, technology-supported approaches broadened options for tongue-base treatment and neuromuscular collapse. The motivation was partly anatomical and partly practical. The tongue base sits deep in the oropharynx, and conventional access can be limited. At the same time, a purely resective approach cannot fully address patients whose collapse is driven by loss of tone rather than bulk.

Transoral robotic surgery (TORS) was introduced as a way to access and reduce tongue-base tissue in selected patients with OSA [31]. Robotic platforms provided improved visualization and instrument control, enabling surgeons to work in a confined space with greater precision. As with other tongue-base procedures, TORS is best understood as part of a multilevel strategy: it may be helpful for patients with demonstrable retrolingual collapse, particularly when other levels are addressed or when CPAP intolerance drives the search for alternatives.

Hypoglossal nerve stimulation (HNS) emerged as an implantable therapy to improve upper airway patency by activating tongue protrusor muscles. The idea that a small implanted device could keep the airway open by timing electrical pulses to the breathing cycle was, at the time, a striking departure from the scalpel-and-suture tradition of sleep surgery. Early work described physiologic effects on airway mechanics, and later clinical studies evaluated feasibility and outcomes [32, 33]. Conceptually, HNS represented a different solution to the same problem. Instead of removing tissue to create space, it aims to restore a key stabilizing force during sleep. This approach fits well with the idea that OSA is, in many patients, a disorder of collapsibility and neuromuscular control.

The STAR trial reported outcomes of upper airway stimulation in CPAP-intolerant patients with moderate to severe OSA [34]. The Inspire upper airway stimulation system subsequently received U.S. FDA PMA approval in 2014 for a defined patient subset [35]. These milestones mattered because they placed an implantable therapy within a clear regulatory and selection framework. They also reinforced a theme that has become central in modern sleep surgery: careful selection is not a limitation but a pathway to reliable outcomes.

Longer-term follow-up has shown sustained improvements in respiratory indices and patient-reported outcomes in many treated patients [36]. For clinicians, the practical significance is that durable benefit is possible without repeated tissue removal, provided the anatomy and collapse pattern are suitable. For patients, the significance is more personal: an option that can reduce disease burden while preserving the throat's normal function.

1.1.6 Current Practice and Future Directions

Today, sleep surgery is usually delivered as part of multidisciplinary OSA care, rather than as a stand-alone pathway. That shift reflects how OSA is now framed: as a chronic condition with heterogeneous causes, varying risk profiles, and multiple effective therapies. In many clinics, the surgeon is one member of a team that includes sleep physicians, dentists, respiratory therapists, and weight management services.

Current reviews emphasize matching treatment to disease severity, symptoms, comorbidity risk, and patient preferences. Surgery may be appropriate alongside PAP, oral appliances, weight management, and positional therapy [11]. In this context, surgery is not an act of opposition to CPAP. It is often a response to real-world barriers, including intolerance, residual symptoms, or anatomic constraints that make nonsurgical therapy less effective. The therapeutic landscape has also been reshaped by pharmacologic advances. The SURMOUNT-OSA trial demonstrated that tirzepatide, a GLP-1/GIP receptor agonist, produced substantial reductions in AHI in patients with obesity-related OSA, leading to the first FDA approval of a medication for OSA [37]. While this does not eliminate the need for surgery, it introduces a powerful new tool for weight-related airway collapse and may alter the population of patients who ultimately present for surgical evaluation.

For many patients, the goal is not a single curative operation. It is a tailored plan based on anatomy, dynamic collapse pattern, and expected benefit versus risk. That plan may involve staged procedures, combination therapy, or a clear decision to avoid surgery when the likely gains are small. This is a mature way to think about intervention: not whether surgery can be done, but whether it should be done for this patient, at this time, with these alternatives available.

Looking ahead, the most important trend is better patient matching, not new tools. Better phenotyping, more consistent use of dynamic airway assessment, and clearer definitions of meaningful patient-centered outcomes can make established operations more effective by putting them in the right place. An important conceptual advance in this direction is the endotyping framework described by Eckert and colleagues, which identifies four key pathophysiologic traits underlying OSA: pharyngeal collapsibility (Pcrit), arousal threshold, loop gain, and pharyngeal muscle responsiveness [38]. By characterizing which traits drive a given patient's disease, clinicians may be able to predict who will benefit most from surgery (those with high anatomical collapsibility) versus those better served by pharmacologic or combination approaches. This precision-medicine framework is still evolving, but it represents a conceptual shift that could fundamentally reshape surgical selection criteria in the years ahead. The story of sleep surgery has always been a story of refinement. As measurement improves and collaboration widens, the field continues to move toward more predictable benefit with less unnecessary morbidity. What began with tracheostomy and an obese literary character has become a discipline of patient selection and phenotype-guided planning.

1.2 Pathophysiology of Obstructive Sleep Apnea

Muhammad Adam Mohd ShariffAbdul Rahim bin Md Din,
and Liang Chye Goh

1.2.1 Overview (Fig. 1.2)

Obstructive sleep apnea (OSA) arises when a vulnerable upper airway repeatedly collapses during sleep, producing apneas, hypopneas, and arousals that fragment sleep and induce intermittent hypoxemia. This vulnerability reflects a convergence of anatomic predisposition (narrow, compliant airway) and sleep-related changes in ventilatory control and dilator muscle tone that transform a stable waking airway into an unstable sleeping one [39–41]. OSA is a syndrome, not a single disease but as a syndrome in which multiple traits interact to determine the threshold for collapse, the severity of events, and the physiologic consequences that follow [41].

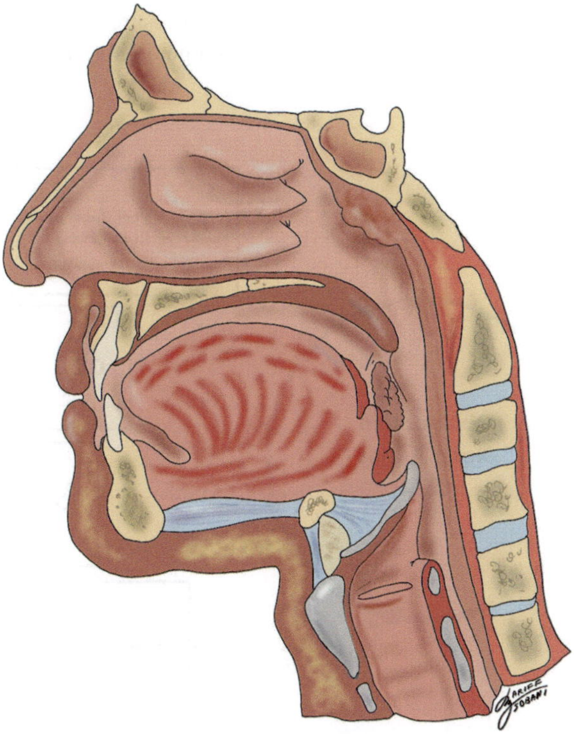

Fig. 1.2 Sagittal cross-section of the upper airway

1.2.2 Normal Upper Airway Physiology During Sleep

The upper airway—principally the velopharynx and oropharynx—is a muscular conduit without rigid support. While awake, tonic and phasic activity of key dilator muscles (e.g., the genioglossus, tensor/levator veli palatini) maintains patency against negative inspiratory pressure. During sleep, generalized reductions in neuromuscular drive and reflex gain increase airway compliance; positional factors (supine posture) and reduced lung volume further diminish longitudinal "tracheal traction," narrowing the lumen and increasing resistance. Imaging and physiologic studies have shown that the soft palate, tongue base, and lateral pharyngeal walls are the most collapse-prone structures, with interindividual variability driven by soft-tissue volume and craniofacial shape [40, 42].

1.2.3 Why the Airway Collapses: Interacting Traits (Fig. 1.3)

A unifying framework for OSA pathogenesis recognizes that multiple endotypes—some anatomic, others neurophysiologic—combine to produce collapse. The principal traits are: *upper airway anatomy and passive collapsibility*, often summarized by the pharyngeal critical closing pressure (Pcrit); *upper airway dilator muscle responsiveness* (the ability to recruit genioglossus and related muscles during rising

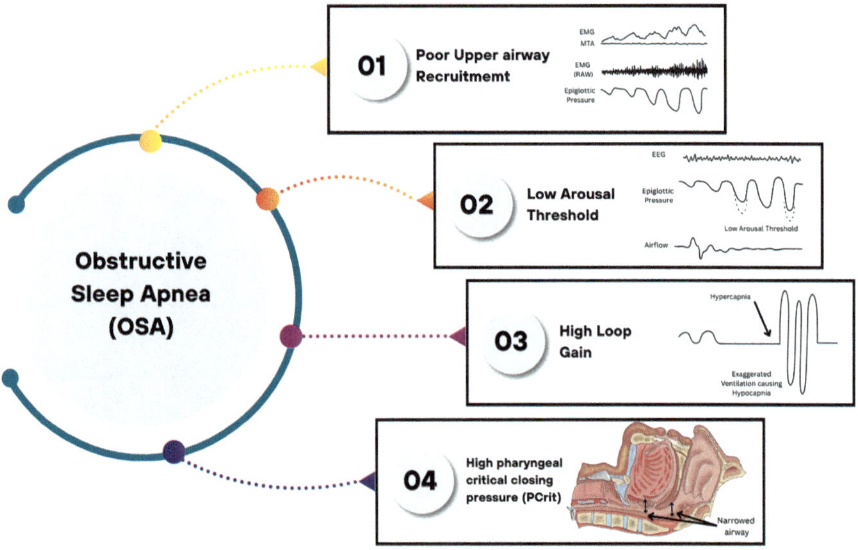

Fig. 1.3 Functional pathophysiology of obstructive sleep apnea. (Adapted from McKeown et al. [43])

ventilatory drive); *arousal threshold* (ease of sleep disruption); and *loop gain* (stability of the ventilatory control system). Individuals with a narrow, compliant airway (high Pcrit) are structurally predisposed; if, in addition, they recruit dilator muscles poorly or wake too easily, the airway will collapse earlier and more often [41, 44]. Younes emphasized how abnormal controller gain and timing—independent of anatomy—can amplify ventilatory overshoot/undershoot after an obstructive event, perpetuating cyclical apnea [44]. Later clinical syntheses integrated these traits to explain phenotypic heterogeneity (e.g., REM-predominant or positional OSA) and variable treatment responses among patients with similar body mass index (BMI) and AHI [39, 41].

1.2.4 The Suction Cascade: Negative Intrathoracic Pressure

A classic description of OSA pathogenesis is the "suction" cascade that unfolds when inspiratory effort persists against a narrowing airway. Increasingly negative intrathoracic pressure draws pharyngeal soft tissues inward (Bernoulli and Starling resistor effects), promotes further luminal collapse, and augments venous engorgement of the lateral walls and tongue, thereby worsening obstruction. The event typically ends with an arousal that restores muscle tone and airflow—but at the cost of sleep fragmentation and sympathetic surges. Over hundreds of cycles per night, these swings in pressure, oxygenation, and autonomic state impose mechanical and biochemical stress on multiple organ systems [39, 41].

1.2.5 Anatomic Contributors and Imaging Insights

Anatomic risk resides in both *soft tissues* (tongue volume, lateral wall thickness, palatal redundancy, lymphoid hypertrophy) and *skeletal shape* (retrognathia, narrow maxilla/mandible). Fast spin-echo MRI and other imaging modalities have linked OSA to increased tongue volume, thickened lateral walls, and reduced retropalatal/retroglossal caliber; importantly, lateral wall behavior emerges as a particularly influential determinant of collapse in many patients [40]. The site and pattern of failure vary: *anteroposterior* soft-palate "flap" collapse, *lateral* wall medialization in the oropharynx, *tongue-base* posterior displacement, and *epiglottic* retroflexion or lateral "book-type" behavior. These patterns often coexist in multilevel disease, with retropalatal narrowing being nearly universal and retroglossal contributions common [40]. Figure 1.2 (sagittal cross-section) situates these structures and illustrates the relationship between the soft palate, tongue base, epiglottis, and posterior pharyngeal wall.

1.2.6 Event Definitions and Scoring

OSA severity is quantified by polysomnographic scoring. An *apnea* is a near-complete cessation of airflow for ≥10 s; a *hypopnea* is a discernible reduction in airflow for ≥10 s, typically coupled with oxygen desaturation and/or cortical arousal. Event frequency is summarized by the Apnea–Hypopnea Index (AHI) to classify severity and track treatment response. Uniform criteria and signal standards—codified by the American Academy of Sleep Medicine—are essential to compare studies and to ensure that mechanistic and therapeutic research aligns with clinical outcomes [45].

1.2.7 From Collapse to Consequences: The Pathophysiologic Cascade (Fig. 1.4)

Intermittent hypoxia and reoxygenation trigger oxidative stress and activate inflammatory pathways, including endothelial dysfunction and upregulation of adhesion molecules. *Sympathetic surges* at the termination of events and with arousals elevate nocturnal and daytime catecholamines, contributing to *systemic hypertension*, increased arterial stiffness, and altered baroreflex sensitivity [39]. Large *swings in intrathoracic pressure* (−40 to −80 cm H_2O in severe events) impose afterload on the left ventricle, can precipitate atrial stretch and arrhythmia, and exacerbate heart failure physiology [42]. Repetitive *sleep fragmentation* impairs synaptic plasticity and glymphatic clearance, underpinning *neurocognitive* complaints (inattention, executive

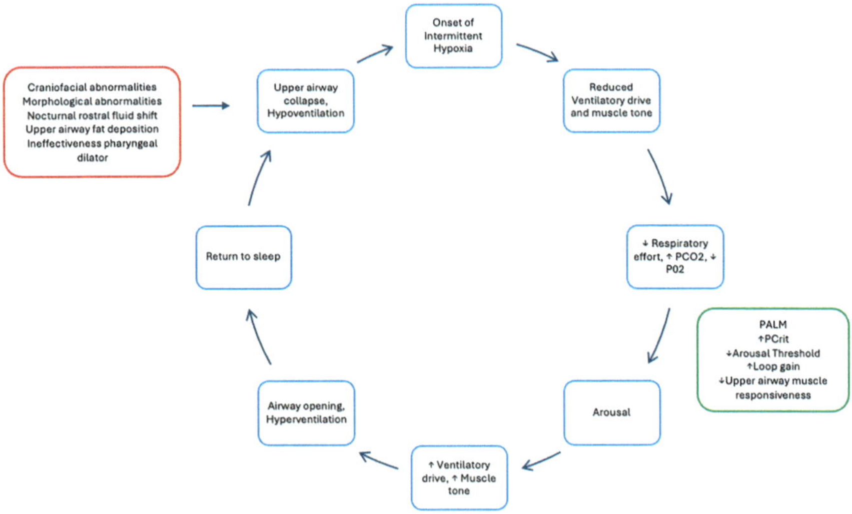

Fig. 1.4 The OSA pathophysiologic cascade

dysfunction, memory consolidation deficits) and worsening mood and pain perception [39]. Metabolically, OSA promotes *insulin resistance*, *glucose intolerance*, and *dyslipidemia*, partly via sympathetic and hypothalamic–pituitary–adrenal activation and partly via intermittent hypoxia-induced adipose tissue inflammation [39, 41]. The net result is a systemic phenotype in which cardiometabolic and neurobehavioral sequelae are disproportionately severe for a given AHI in individuals with high loop gain, low arousal threshold, or prominent REM-predominant disease [41, 44].

1.2.8 Starling Resistor Model in OSA Pathogenesis (Fig. 1.5)

The Starling resistor models the pharynx as a collapsible segment between a rigid upstream source (nasal cavity) and a downstream sink (trachea). When intraluminal pressure in this segment drops below surrounding tissue pressure, airflow becomes flow-limited and can cease when pressure falls to the critical closing pressure (Pcrit). In OSA, many patients have an elevated Pcrit, indicating a highly collapsible airway; raising intraluminal pressure with CPAP prevents collapse by keeping pressure above Pcrit [47].

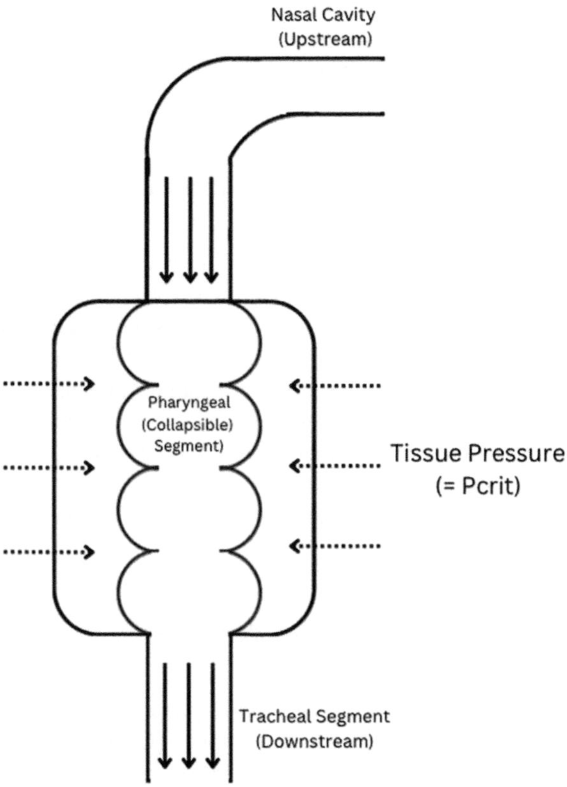

Fig. 1.5 Starling resistor model of the upper airway. The collapsibility of the pharyngeal segment represented by the Pcrit value. Collapsibility is affected by the rigid upstream segment (nasal cavity) and downstream (trachea) segment. (Adapted from Hillman et al. [46])

The classic Starling framework captures the passive mechanics of collapse but real upper airway behavior also depends on state-dependent dilator muscle activity, which can change with sleep stage; experimental and clinical work using Pcrit shows this variability. Pcrit (or proxies like therapeutic CPAP requirement) helps phenotype OSA and guide therapy selection, yet other nonanatomic traits (e.g., loop gain, arousal threshold) also matter—so contemporary models layer ventilatory-control and arousal mechanisms onto the Starling substrate [48, 49].

1.2.9 Sleep Stage, Body Position, and Lung Volume

Sleep state strongly modulates collapsibility. During *NREM*, modest reductions in dilator muscle tone are usually offset by reflex recruitment as CO_2 rises, but in *REM sleep*, cholinergic atonia suppresses genioglossus responsiveness more profoundly; Pcrit becomes less negative (i.e., the airway is more prone to close), events lengthen, and desaturations deepen [41]. Body position exerts parallel effects: the *supine* posture promotes posterior displacement of the tongue and soft palate, increases pharyngeal length, and reduces functional residual capacity (FRC), removing stabilizing caudal traction. Conversely, the *lateral* position reduces passive collapsibility and often normalizes breathing in positional OSA endotypes [41]. These gradients explain familiar clinical patterns—REM-predominant OSA, supine-only OSA—and the observed night-to-night variability in AHI [41].

1.2.10 Nasal Resistance as an Upstream Modifier

Although the nose is rarely the primary collapsible segment in adult OSA, *elevated nasal resistance* raises upstream load, promotes mouth breathing, and increases the inspiratory suction that acts on downstream segments. Structural lesions (septal deviation, turbinate hypertrophy, nasal valve compromise) and inflammatory states (allergic or nonallergic rhinitis, chronic rhinosinusitis) can therefore *magnify* OSA in predisposed patients, worsen snoring, and undermine adherence to positive airway pressure (PAP) by increasing required pressures and discomfort [39]. Optimizing nasal airflow (medical therapy or surgery when indicated) improves comfort and can reduce therapeutic pressures, even when it does not eliminate apneas outright [50].

1.2.11 Pediatric Considerations

In children, *adenotonsillar hypertrophy* remains the single most important anatomic risk factor for obstructive sleep apnea (OSA). Enlargement of the tonsils and adenoids narrows the nasopharyngeal and oropharyngeal airway, producing a critical reduction in airway caliber during sleep. The pathophysiology, however, is not simply a scaled-down version of the adult disorder. While the same broad physiologic principles apply—loss of neuromuscular tone during sleep, craniofacial restriction in certain populations, and instability of ventilatory control—the *relative weight of each factor differs in the pediatric population* [39, 41].

Adenotonsillectomy is the first-line intervention and generally produces significant improvements in airway size and collapsibility. Numerous studies have demonstrated substantial reductions in Apnea–Hypopnea Index (AHI) and improved gas exchange following surgery. Yet, the presence of *residual OSA* in a subset of children underscores that adenotonsillar hypertrophy is not the only contributor. Persistent disease may reflect *craniofacial factors* (such as midface hypoplasia, retrognathia, or syndromic anomalies), *obesity*, or *nonanatomic endotypes*, including high loop gain, low arousal threshold, or impaired pharyngeal dilator muscle responsiveness [39, 41].

Importantly, the prevalence of residual OSA is higher in children with obesity and in those with craniofacial or neuromuscular disorders, suggesting that adenotonsillectomy alone may not be curative in these groups. For such patients, adjunctive therapies—ranging from weight management and orthodontic interventions to continuous positive airway pressure (CPAP)—are often required. Recognition of these multifactorial influences is essential for tailoring therapy.

Another key consideration is that *pediatric sleep physiology differs from adults*: children often present with behavioral disturbances, learning difficulties, or growth impairment rather than excessive daytime sleepiness. This difference reinforces the need for pediatric-specific outcome measures and treatment goals.

1.2.12 Phenotype–Treatment Implications

Understanding the interacting traits in OSA clarifies *why* treatments work and *for whom* they are most effective.

- *PAP therapy* converts a collapsible airway into a pneumatic splint by abolishing the pressure gradient that would otherwise draw the walls together. Its effectiveness across endotypes reflects the dominance of mechanics in most adults; however, residual events may persist when unstable control (high loop gain) or low arousal threshold promotes repeated arousals or central events despite adequate splinting.
- *Non-PAP therapies* target anatomic or physiologic traits selectively [39, 41, 44].
- *Oral appliances* advance the mandible to enlarge the retroglossal airway and tension the velum; they work best when jaw-thrust during sleep (or DISE) demonstrably improves patency, implying adequate muscle responsiveness and favorable palatal behavior [50].

- *Upper airway surgery* reduces soft-tissue load, stiffens lateral walls, and shortens the palate; success is highest when procedures match the dominant collapse pattern identified on imaging or endoscopy [47].
- *Weight reduction* lowers tongue and lateral wall fat, improves lung volume, and reduces Pcrit, with broad benefits across mechanisms [39].
- *Positional therapy* leverages the physiology of posture to normalize breathing in positional endotypes [41].
- *Controller-focused approaches*—oxygen supplementation or acetazolamide for high loop gain; strategies to raise the arousal threshold in select patients; and breathing reeducation or myofunctional therapy to optimize route of breathing and muscle recruitment—illustrate the expanding palette of *trait-targeted* intervention [43].

1.2.13 Integrating it in Practice

A practical, physiology-guided pathway begins with *standardized event scoring* and careful phenotyping of severity, sleep stage distribution, and positional dependency [45, 48]. Next, the *anatomic substrate* is characterized via examination and imaging (when indicated) to estimate passive collapsibility and to infer likely sites and patterns of failure. Finally, *nonanatomic traits* are considered—sometimes directly measured in research settings, more often inferred from clinical patterns (e.g., marked ventilatory overshoot, REM-predominant disease, low arousal threshold suggested by frequent arousals with minimal desaturation). This layered understanding helps align first-line PAP with *adjunctive* measures that address the bottlenecks most relevant for a given patient: nasal optimization for high resistance; mandibular advancement for retroglossal susceptibility; surgical lateralization/stiffening for dominant lateral wall disease; weight loss and lung-volume augmentation strategies where obesity and reduced FRC contribute; and controller-stabilizing tactics when ventilatory oscillation predominates [43, 50].

1.3 Sites of Obstruction in Obstructive Sleep Apnea

Muhammad Adam Mohd Shariff, Abdul Rahim bin Md Din,
and Liang Chye Goh

Accurately determining *where the upper airway collapses* is central to modern, phenotype-guided management of obstructive sleep apnea (OSA). Yet, this task is rarely straightforward. Collapse is seldom confined to a single level, and most symptomatic adults exhibit *multilevel obstruction* involving the palate, tongue base, lateral walls, or epiglottis. Moreover, the dominant sites of collapse may shift depending on *body position* or *sleep stage*, making OSA a dynamic rather than static disorder.

A practical discussion of "sites of obstruction" must therefore do more than simply catalogue anatomical regions—it must *bridge anatomy with physiology* and link these insights to the *diagnostic tools* that guide treatment. In particular, *drug-induced sleep endoscopy (DISE)* and *dynamic sleep imaging* have become indispensable in visualizing and characterizing the collapse patterns that dictate whether surgical or nonsurgical interventions will succeed. (See also the chapter outline emphasizing DISE, collapsibility, and multilevel disease.)

Evidence from large DISE series underscores the importance of this approach. Roughly *three-quarters of OSA patients* demonstrate obstruction involving both the *palate and hypopharynx*, a finding that explains why single-level interventions—such as isolated uvulopalatopharyngoplasty—often fall short in unselected candidates [51]. These data have shifted surgical philosophy away from *"one-size-fits-all" strategies* and toward *multilevel or targeted procedures*, tailored to the individual's collapse pattern and physiologic vulnerabilities.

In essence, accurate site identification transforms surgery from a generic structural intervention into a *precision therapy*, matching the intervention to the patient's specific phenotype. This shift marks one of the most significant conceptual advances in the field of sleep surgery and remains the cornerstone of contemporary practice.

1.3.1 Physiology That Shapes "Where" Collapse Occurs

OSA reflects not only anatomical compromise but also the contribution of *nonanatomic endotypes*. These include a *low arousal threshold*, *high loop gain* (unstable ventilatory control), and *impaired pharyngeal dilator muscle responsiveness*. The interaction of these traits with airway narrowing determines "where" collapse occurs.

A useful physiological marker of anatomic susceptibility is the *pharyngeal critical closing pressure (Pcrit)*, the pressure at which the airway occludes. Typical OSA patients have Pcrit values near atmospheric pressure, while higher (more positive) values reflect greater collapsibility [38]. These values are not fixed: they tend to worsen in *REM sleep* and improve in the *lateral sleeping position*, explaining why many patients show stage- and position-dependent variation [48, 52, 53].

Clinically, these gradients matter. Patients with *REM-predominant OSA* or *supine-predominant OSA* often demonstrate collapse concentrated at the retropalatal and retrolingual segments. Recognizing this pattern allows clinicians to direct patients toward positional therapy, stage-specific interventions, or multilevel strategies when needed [53–55].

1.3.2 How We Localize the Sites

DISE provides real-time visualization of upper airway behavior under sedative-induced sleep. It has moderate-to-substantial reliability, especially in confirming palatal and hypopharyngeal collapse [51]. To standardize interpretation, the *VOTE system* evaluates four subsites—Velum (soft palate), Oropharyngeal lateral walls/tonsils, Tongue base, and Epiglottis—scoring both the degree (0–2) and the configuration (anteroposterior, lateral, concentric) of collapse [15]. Recent consensus papers advocate for *modified VOTE scoring*, allowing examiners to highlight site-specific drivers such as lymphoid hypertrophy [56]. This refinement is crucial for designing interventions that target the underlying pathology rather than the collapse pattern alone.

1.3.3 Dynamic Sleep MRI

Cine or dynamic sleep magnetic resonance imaging (MRI) is an increasingly valuable tool for evaluating upper airway obstruction in OSA. Unlike DISE, which relies on endoscopic visualization under pharmacologically induced sleep, sleep MRI offers a *noninvasive, radiation-free method* that captures both structural anatomy and airway motion in real time. Its strength lies in providing *dynamic, three-dimensional assessment* of the airway during simulated or natural sleep, allowing clinicians to observe not only *where* collapse occurs but also *how* different airway segments interact during respiration (Fig. 1.6).

From a diagnostic standpoint, dynamic sleep MRI complements DISE by quantifying airway narrowing and collapse patterns across the *retropalatal, retroglossal,*

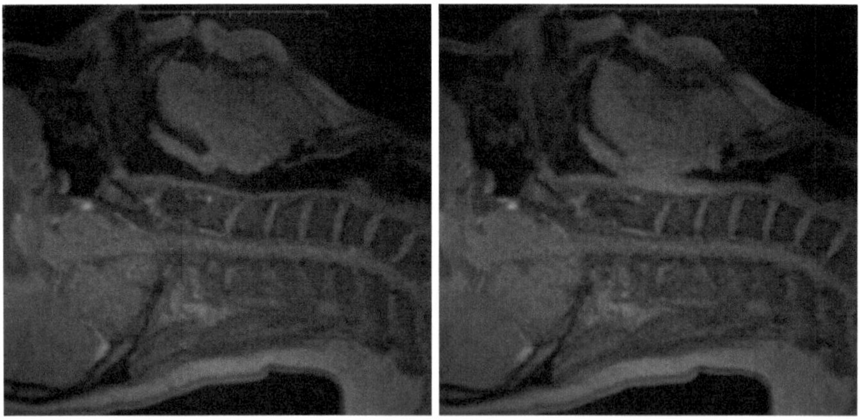

Fig. 1.6 Image showing dynamic MRI image of the same individual during sleep with normal inspiration (Left) and when the tongue base collapses (Right) during deep sleep

lateral pharyngeal, and hypopharyngeal segments. Meta-analytic data suggest that retropalatal collapse is nearly ubiquitous (~98% of OSA patients), retroglossal collapse occurs in approximately 41%, lateral wall collapse in nearly half, and hypopharyngeal collapse in about 5% [57]. These findings emphasize that OSA is rarely confined to a single structure and that a significant proportion of patients demonstrate *mixed or multilevel collapse*, highlighting the limitations of isolated surgical approaches.

A unique advantage of MRI is its ability to *characterize soft tissue contributions* to airway obstruction. For example, it can distinguish between obstruction caused by palatal elongation, lingual tonsillar hypertrophy, or lateral wall bulging. In obese patients, MRI can also delineate the impact of parapharyngeal fat pads on airway caliber, providing a more nuanced picture of obesity-related airway compromise. Furthermore, because MRI can assess adjacent structures such as the tongue, mandible, and hyoid bone, it offers insight into craniofacial dynamics that are difficult to appreciate endoscopically.

Clinically, the use of dynamic sleep MRI remains limited by availability, cost, and the need for specialized expertise in acquisition and interpretation. The procedure often requires sedation to simulate sleep, although newer protocols are exploring natural sleep imaging with motion-correction techniques. Despite these challenges, MRI continues to grow in research and specialized clinical settings, where it is used not only to guide *site-specific surgical planning* but also to evaluate responses to interventions such as mandibular advancement or hypoglossal nerve stimulation.

1.3.4 Segment-by-Segment: Where and How the Airway Fails

1. *Nasal Cavity and Nasopharynx (Ventilatory "Gatekeepers")*

While the nose is seldom the *primary* collapsible segment in OSA, elevated nasal resistance increases upstream load, destabilizes breathing in predisposed patients, and degrades CPAP or oral appliance tolerance. Nasopharyngeal narrowing can accentuate retropalatal collapse during sleep; DISE and dynamic MRI frequently reveal retropalatal narrowing even when nasal findings appear modest awake [57]. Clinically, nasal optimization is often necessary but rarely sufficient in moderate–severe OSA; it is best conceptualized as facilitating downstream airway stability and therapy adherence.

2. *Velum/Retropalatal Segment (the Most Frequent Site)*

Retropalatal obstruction is almost universal on dynamic imaging and common on DISE [57]. DISE patterns at the velum include *anteroposterior (AP)*, *lateral*, and *concentric* collapse. *Complete concentric collapse (CCC)* at the velum is phenotypically important: it predicts poor response to hypoglossal nerve stimulation (HNS) and remains a formal contraindication to HNS candidacy in contemporary guidance derived from the STAR trial and subsequent series [58, 59]. In contrast, AP palatal collapse—especially when coupled with favorable hypopharyngeal behavior—can coexist with successful HNS or oral appliance therapy when other criteria are met [60]. For palatal surgery, recognizing whether lateral wall components dominate (see below) versus a primarily AP palatal "flutter" helps select techniques (e.g., expansion/relocation sphincter pharyngoplasty vs. more midline-focused palatoplasty).

3. *Oropharyngeal Lateral Walls and Tonsils (Often the Hidden Driver)*

The lateral pharyngeal walls are pivotal determinants of airway caliber. MRI work shows that enlarged lateral wall soft tissues substantially increase OSA risk independent of tongue size and craniofacial bony constraints [61]. Surgically, acknowledging lateral wall collapse shifted palatal strategies beyond classic midline uvulopalatopharyngoplasty: *lateral pharyngoplasty* [23] and *expansion sphincter pharyngoplasty* [24] were designed to stiffen and lateralize these walls with improved outcomes in appropriately selected patients. On DISE (VOTE), dominant lateral wall collapse at the "O" level predicts weaker responses to mandibular advancement alone and encourages either combined palatal–lateral wall procedures or multilevel approaches.

4. *Tongue Base/Retroglossal Segment*

Tongue-related collapse typically occurs in an *AP* direction and is influenced by reductions in genioglossus tone during sleep. On DISE, *jaw-thrust/mandibular advancement maneuvers* serve as a physiologic test: a clearly positive response (airway opens with advancement) is associated with better oral appliance outcomes; persistent lateral oropharyngeal collapse during advancement predicts failure of oral appliances [57] For surgery, tongue-dominant phenotypes may improve with HNS (if no CCC), tongue-base reduction or skeletal expansion (maxillomandibular advancement, MMA) when multilevel disease coexists. Of note, DISE findings also bear on MMA prognosis—complete concentric palatal collapse and complete AP epiglottic collapse have both been associated with poorer MMA responses [57].

5. *Hypopharynx and Larynx (Epiglottis and Lateral Walls)*

The hypopharynx contributes via lateral wall infolding and *epiglottic* behaviors. Contemporary DISE cohorts indicate epiglottic collapse [62, 63] is more prevalent than once assumed (~16% overall; ~12% primary, ~4% secondary), with distinct patterns—"trapdoor" rigid AP, "floppy" AP, lateral "book-type," and secondary epiglottic collapse driven by upstream forces [64]. Recognizing epiglottic phenotypes matters because their management differs from tongue- or palatal-led disease: options include glossoepiglottopexy, epiglottis stiffening, partial epiglottectomy, and targeted robotic techniques, all of which show symptom and AHI improvement in selected adults, while also enabling CPAP tolerance in some.

1.3.5 *Position and Sleep Stage: Why the Site You See Is Not the Site You* Always *Get*

Upper airway collapsibility is not a static property; it shifts dynamically with *body position* and *sleep stage*, meaning the obstruction observed at one moment may not fully reflect the patient's real-world disease.

Supine Position Lying supine increases pharyngeal collapsibility and elongates the airway, favoring collapse at the *retropalatal* and *retrolingual* levels. The pharyngeal critical closing pressure (Pcrit) becomes less negative, reflecting greater vulnerability to obstruction. In contrast, moving to the *lateral position* reduces passive collapsibility (more negative Pcrit) and often shortens or abolishes respiratory events [53, 54]. Clinically, this is the basis for *positional OSA*, defined as disease substantially worse in the supine posture. By lenient definitions, positional OSA is present in nearly half of patients, particularly those with lower BMI. In these individuals, collapse tends to localize to the palate and tongue base, which are most sensitive to gravitational effects [54, 55].

REM Sleep Sleep stage also modifies airway behavior. REM sleep is characterized by a rise in Pcrit and a *reduction in upper airway dilator muscle responsiveness*, both of which make collapse more likely. As a result, REM-predominant OSA often reveals obstruction sites not apparent in non-REM (NREM) sleep. Vulnerable regions include the *epiglottis* and *lateral pharyngeal walls*, where muscular hypotonia in REM unmasks latent collapsibility [52]. Importantly, this stage-specific vulnerability explains why some patients present with minimal obstruction during NREM but experience severe disease during REM.

Clinical Implications These interactions between posture, sleep stage, and airway physiology help explain the *variability of OSA* from night to night and even across a single night. They also clarify why certain interventions—especially single-site surgeries—may achieve only partial responses. For example, a procedure that stabilizes the soft palate may be highly effective in lateral NREM sleep but less so in supine REM sleep, when collapse at the tongue base or lateral walls becomes dominant. Recognizing these dynamics highlights the need for *multilevel assessment* and sometimes *multimodal therapy*, including positional therapy, stage-targeted strategies, or staged surgical planning.

In practice, mapping OSA severity to *sleep position* and *stage distribution* is as important as identifying the anatomical sites of collapse themselves. For surgeons, this means appreciating that DISE findings under supine sedation may not capture the full complexity of disease. For clinicians, it underscores the importance of reviewing polysomnography beyond the overall Apnea–Hypopnea Index, paying attention to positional dependency and REM-related severity. Ultimately, a patient's "true" OSA phenotype emerges from the interplay of anatomy, posture, and neurophysiology—variables that shift across the night and strongly influence treatment success.

1.3.6 Putting it Together: A Site-Guided, Phenotype-Aware Workflow

1. *Define the physiologic terrain.* Use polysomnography to characterize REM vs. NREM burden, positional dependency, and arousal profile; infer likely Pcrit (e.g., severe, REM-worse disease suggests higher collapsibility).
2. *Map dynamic anatomy.* Perform DISE with standardized (modified) VOTE scoring and jaw-thrust/mandibular advancement testing; consider dynamic sleep MRI when anatomy is equivocal or when quantification of wall motion adds value.
3. *Match the site to therapy*
   - *Velum-dominant, AP*: palatal stiffening/relocation procedures; oral appliance if jaw-thrust positive.
   - *Velum CCC*: avoid HNS; consider techniques addressing circumferential collapse and lateral walls ± skeletal expansion.
   - *Lateral wall O-level*: lateral pharyngoplasty/expansion sphincter approaches ± multilevel surgery.
   - *Tongue-dominant*: HNS (if no CCC), tongue-base reduction, or MMA in multilevel collapse. Jaw-thrust-nonresponsive cases are poor oral appliance candidates.
   - *Epiglottic collapse*: phenotype the pattern; consider epiglottopexy, stiffening, or partial epiglottectomy, especially where CPAP intolerance is epiglottis-mediated.
4. *Layer positional/REM strategies.* Add positional therapy and REM-specific considerations to reduce load on vulnerable segments.

1.3.7 Conclusion

In OSA, "the site" is almost never singular. Retropalatal narrowing is nearly universal, lateral wall behavior is frequently decisive, tongue-base collapse modulates responses to mandibular or neuromodulatory therapies, and epiglottic phenotypes deserve deliberate identification. A structured, physiology-informed, site-guided approach is essential to deliver durable, individualized outcomes.

1.4 Nasal and Nasopharyngeal Obstruction

Muhammad Adam Mohd ShariffAbdul Rahim bin Md Din, and Liang Chye Goh

1.4.1 Overview and Anatomic–Physiologic Context (Fig. 1.7)

The nasal cavity and nasopharynx form the upstream segment of the upper airway and strongly influence downstream pharyngeal mechanics during sleep. When nasal resistance rises—from septal deviation, turbinate hypertrophy, nasal valve compromise, or inflammatory disease—greater inspiratory negative pressure is required to sustain flow, predisposing collapsible downstream segments (retropalatal and retroglossal) to occlude. Habitual or forced oral breathing further reduces stabilizing reflexes, alters upper airway geometry, and can worsen snoring and obstructive sleep apnea (OSA) in susceptible phenotypes. Physiologically, upper airway collapsibility can be expressed as the pharyngeal critical closing pressure (Pcrit): more positive Pcrit values indicate a more collapsible airway. Sleep stage and route of breathing modulate Pcrit; REM sleep often increases collapsibility relative to slow-wave sleep, and oral/oronasal breathing is associated with higher therapeutic CPAP pressures and greater residual events [48]. These principles explain why optimizing nasal patency improves comfort and efficacy of positive airway pressure (PAP) even when it does not "cure" OSA [65, 66].

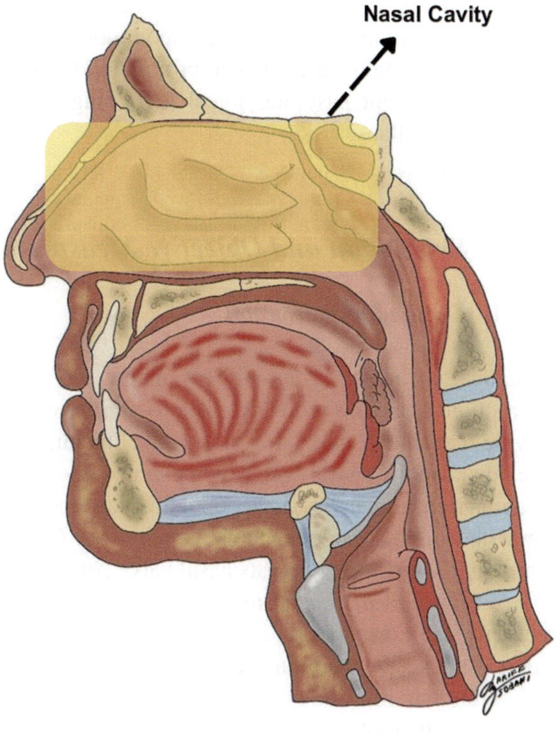

Fig. 1.7 Sagittal cross-section of the upper airway. Shaded area representing the nasal cavity and nasopharynx

1.4.2 Patterns of Obstruction and Clinical Significance

1.4.2.1 Nasal Obstruction

Deviated septum, inferior turbinate hypertrophy, and internal or external nasal valve compromise are the most common anatomic contributors. Inflammatory conditions—especially allergic and nonallergic rhinitis and chronic rhinosinusitis—produce mucosal edema and reversible congestion. Each adds series resistance to airflow; collectively they elevate inspiratory suction forces, encourage oral breathing, and aggravate snoring or apnea propensity in predisposed individuals. On average, isolated nasal surgery yields modest changes in Apnea–Hypopnea Index (AHI) but reliably improves subjective sleep quality and Epworth Sleepiness Scale (ESS) scores, and it enhances PAP tolerance in properly selected patients [67, 68].

1.4.2.2 Nasopharyngeal Obstruction

In children, adenoidal hypertrophy narrows the posterior choanae and is a dominant driver of pediatric OSA; adenotonsillectomy is the usual first-line therapy and improves symptoms, quality of life, and PSG indices (e.g., CHAT trial) [69, 70]. In adults, nasopharyngeal masses are uncommon but should be excluded with endoscopy when symptoms are atypical or unilateral; choanal stenosis/atresia is rare but relevant. Persistent nasopharyngeal narrowing sustains mouth breathing, raising downstream collapse risk.

1.4.3 Evaluation and Objective Measurements

1.4.3.1 Focused Examination

A meticulous *nasal examination* remains the cornerstone of evaluating nasal obstruction in patients with OSA. *Anterior rhinoscopy* and *flexible nasal endoscopy* provide first-line visualization, allowing clinicians to assess septal deviation, turbinate hypertrophy, nasal valve competence (both static and dynamic), mucosal inflammation, and, in pediatric populations, adenoid hypertrophy. Relief of obstruction with simple bedside maneuvers such as the *Cottle maneuver* or *manual lateralization of the sidewall* suggests nasal valve compromise.

A recent *clinical consensus statement* underscores that careful history and targeted physical examination form the *primary basis* for diagnosing nasal valve disorders. Endoscopy, while invaluable for ruling out alternate or coexisting pathology such as chronic rhinosinusitis or neoplasms, serves as a complementary rather than sole diagnostic tool [71].

1.4.3.2 Physiologic Testing

Beyond endoscopy, *objective physiologic assessments* are available to quantify nasal airway caliber and resistance:

- *Acoustic rhinometry* measures cross-sectional areas and volumes of the nasal cavity using reflected sound waves, offering a simple, reproducible assessment of anatomic narrowing.
- *Active anterior rhinomanometry* quantifies nasal resistance by measuring pressure–flow relationships during respiration.
- *Peak nasal inspiratory flow (PNIF)* provides a portable, inexpensive measure of nasal airflow that is useful for longitudinal monitoring.

These tools are especially relevant when planning CPAP or surgical therapy. For example, *supine rhinomanometry* has been shown to better predict *PAP titration pressures* compared with seated measurements, with higher supine nasal resistance correlating to higher optimal CPAP requirements [72]. Acoustic rhinometry, although correlated with rhinomanometry, demonstrates *variable associations with OSA severity on polysomnography*, suggesting that it should be viewed as a *complementary test* rather than a stand-alone diagnostic.

Emerging research highlights the possibility of a distinct *"nasal endotype"* of OSA, in which objective nasal measurements correlate with greater symptomatic burden and specific therapy needs [73]. While still investigational, this concept reinforces the importance of quantifying nasal obstruction beyond clinical impression alone.

1.4.3.3 Sleep Testing and Imaging

Formal *sleep testing* remains central to evaluating OSA in any patient with nasal obstruction. *Polysomnography (PSG)* or, in appropriate adults, *home sleep apnea testing (HSAT)* provides a baseline measure of disease severity and a means of assessing treatment effect following nasal or multilevel interventions.

Drug-induced sleep endoscopy (DISE) is seldom required purely for nasal pathology, as nasal obstruction itself rarely causes pharyngeal collapse. However, DISE is valuable in *pediatric patients with residual OSA after adenotonsillectomy* and in adults undergoing *multilevel surgical planning*, where it helps to delineate the interaction between nasal obstruction and downstream collapse at the palate or tongue base.

Adjunctive imaging plays a limited but targeted role. *Lateral neck radiographs* remain a simple and inexpensive tool for screening adenoid hypertrophy in children when endoscopy is unavailable. More advanced imaging, such as *CT or MRI*, is reserved for complex revision cases or when there is suspicion of mass lesions, sinonasal tumors, or craniofacial anomalies [74].

1.4.4 How Nasal/Nasopharyngeal Disease Modifies OSA and PAP Therapy

1.4.4.1 Route of Breathing and Mask Interface

The route of breathing—nasal versus oronasal—exerts a measurable effect on OSA physiology and CPAP therapy. *Meta-analytic and mechanistic studies* show that the use of *oronasal masks* compared with nasal interfaces is consistently associated with:

- Higher therapeutic pressures (≈ +1.5–2.5 cm H_2O).
- Higher residual AHI despite titration.
- Worse adherence over time [65, 66].

These findings align with experimental evidence that *oronasal breathing increases upper airway collapsibility*, particularly at the velopharyngeal and retropalatal levels. By contrast, exclusive nasal breathing stabilizes the airway and lowers the pressure required to maintain patency.

Clinical strategies that restore or promote nasal breathing can therefore improve PAP tolerance and efficacy. These include *medical therapy* for rhinitis, *humidification* to reduce mucosal dryness, *chinstraps* when appropriate to limit oral leak, and *targeted nasal surgery* for structural obstruction. Together, these measures can facilitate a switch back to nasal interfaces, reducing therapeutic pressures and improving comfort.

1.4.4.2 Impact on Adherence and Pressures

The effect of correcting structural nasal obstruction on PAP adherence is particularly well-documented. *Prospective cohort data* show that procedures such as septoplasty with inferior turbinoplasty can transform patients from minimal CPAP use (~0.5 h/night preoperatively) to sustained, clinically meaningful adherence (~5 h/night postoperatively) [75]. Importantly, these benefits are not just behavioral; they are often accompanied by a trend toward *lower optimal CPAP pressures*, further improving tolerability.

From a health economics perspective, *modeling studies* suggest that nasal surgery is cost-effective when the primary goal is to enhance CPAP adherence in patients with objectively documented nasal obstruction [76]. By increasing nightly use and improving therapy acceptance, nasal procedures amplify the long-term cardiovascular and neurocognitive benefits associated with PAP therapy, while also reducing healthcare costs linked to untreated OSA.

1.4.4.3 Effect on AHI and Symptoms

When considered as a *stand-alone intervention*, isolated nasal surgery produces *modest average reductions in AHI* across meta-analyses. However, these aggregate figures often obscure the more clinically important improvements in *subjective outcomes*. Robust improvements are consistently reported in the *Epworth Sleepiness Scale (ESS)*, disease-specific quality-of-life instruments, and symptom domains such as *snoring intensity, nasal breathing, and daytime function* [67, 68].

The heterogeneity in AHI response likely reflects differences in patient selection, baseline nasal disease burden, and comorbidities. Patients with isolated nasal obstruction and milder OSA may experience more substantial physiologic improvement, whereas those with multilevel collapse generally require adjunctive therapies.

1.4.5 Management Strategies

1.4.5.1 Adult Medical Therapy

Optimizing the nasal airway with *medical management* is an important adjunct in the care of adults with OSA, especially for those struggling with PAP adherence. First-line pharmacologic and supportive therapies include:

- *Intranasal corticosteroids*, which reduce mucosal inflammation and edema, thereby improving nasal airflow.
- *Antihistamines*, particularly for patients with allergic triggers, to decrease mucosal congestion and secretions.
- *Saline irrigation*, which enhances mucociliary clearance, reduces mucosal edema, and improves tolerability of PAP interfaces.

Clinical studies in adults with OSA have shown that intranasal corticosteroids primarily improve *nasal symptoms and PAP tolerance*. Their *direct impact on AHI* is generally modest, unless there is a strong inflammatory component—such as allergic rhinitis or CRS—contributing to nasal obstruction. Thus, the primary value of medical therapy in adults is to *facilitate PAP use* rather than to cure OSA directly.

For patients with *comorbid chronic rhinosinusitis (CRS)*, guideline-directed management is critical. This may include prolonged topical corticosteroid therapy, antibiotics in selected cases, and surgical intervention when medical therapy fails. Addressing CRS not only alleviates nasal congestion and improves quality of life, but also optimizes nasal airflow and enhances the likelihood of successful PAP adherence. In this sense, CRS therapy is not simply symptom control but a key enabler of broader OSA management.

1.4.5.2 Pediatric Anti-inflammatory Therapy

In children, the therapeutic role of anti-inflammatory agents is more direct. *Adenotonsillectomy remains the first-line treatment* for pediatric OSA, but pharmacologic strategies play an important role in *selected scenarios*, particularly:

1. *Bridge therapy* before adenotonsillectomy in children awaiting surgery.
2. *Mild OSA* in otherwise healthy children when surgery may not be immediately indicated.
3. *Residual disease* following adenotonsillectomy.

High-quality randomized controlled trials demonstrate that *intranasal corticosteroids* and the leukotriene receptor antagonist *montelukast* can significantly reduce AHI, improve nocturnal oxygen saturation, and alleviate symptoms in children with mild OSA. These therapies target airway inflammation and adenotonsillar hypertrophy, mechanisms that contribute strongly to pediatric airway collapsibility.

However, several caveats remain:

- Long-term efficacy and durability of anti-inflammatory therapy are uncertain, with most studies focusing on short-term (weeks to months) outcomes.
- Data on patient-centered outcomes—such as neurocognitive performance, behavior, and growth—are limited.
- The *FDA boxed warning* on montelukast regarding potential neuropsychiatric adverse effects necessitates *shared decision-making* with families. Careful counseling is essential, emphasizing that while montelukast can be effective, its risks must be weighed against its benefits [77].

1.4.6 Procedural and Surgical Therapy

1.4.6.1 Septoplasty and Turbinate Reduction

In carefully selected adults with obstructive nasal anatomy and PAP intolerance, septoplasty with turbinate surgery improves adherence, subjective obstruction (e.g., NOSE score), and may reduce required pressures. Postoperative follow-up should include both symptom instruments and objective adherence data [75].

1.4.6.2 Nasal Valve Stabilization

When dynamic or static valve compromise is the dominant lesion, targeted lateral wall/alar rim support (e.g., batten grafts, suture suspension) is indicated; medical therapy alone is insufficient for valve collapse in the absence of significant rhinitis. Selection is clinical, guided by symptom relief on manual lateralization (Cottle) and endoscopic findings [71].

1.4.6.3 Integrating Nasal Surgery in Multilevel Plans

In patients undergoing palate and/or tongue-base surgery, adding nose surgery when indicated improves overall surgical success rates and augments reductions in AHI and ESS compared with multilevel surgery alone [67, 68]. This supports viewing the nose as a facilitator of comprehensive airway surgery rather than a competing target.

1.4.6.4 Interface Optimization and Adjuncts

Prefer nasal masks when feasible; add heated humidification, chinstrap for jaw-opening/leak, and consider myofunctional strategies to promote nasal breathing. If persistent leaks or high pressures occur with oronasal masks, reevaluate nasal patency. In selected cases, mouth-seal techniques or soft vestibular shields may help—but only after optimizing nasal airflow and confirming no significant nasopharyngeal obstruction.

1.4.6.5 Practical Algorithm (Adult Focus, Adaptable to Pediatrics)

1. *Confirm symptoms and phenotype.* Document nasal obstruction (daytime and nocturnal), mouth-breathing, PAP intolerance, allergy/CRS features; examine septum, turbinates, and valves (Cottle maneuver, dynamic collapse). Track responses using NOSE and SNOT-22 (or SN-5 in pediatrics).
2. *Treat inflammation first.* Trial intranasal corticosteroid (and antihistamine for allergic rhinitis), saline irrigation, and guideline-directed CRS therapy. Reassess nasal patency and PAP comfort.
3. *Optimize PAP interface.* Favor nasal masks when possible; add humidification and chinstrap as needed. If oronasal interface is unavoidable, anticipate higher pressures and consider strategies to restore nasal breathing [65, 66].
4. *Objective testing when needed.* Supine rhinomanometry can inform expected PAP pressures and the value of nasal surgery; consider acoustic rhinometry/PNIF to document change [72, 73].
5. *Offer surgery for structural disease undermining PAP or symptomatic control.* Septoplasty/turbinoplasty for fixed obstruction; valve stabilization for dynamic collapse; reassess PAP after healing to confirm pressure/adherence gains [75, 76].
6. *Pediatrics.* Adenotonsillectomy is the first-line therapy when adenotonsillar hypertrophy is present. For mild or residual disease, consider intranasal steroids ± montelukast after shared decision-making about benefits/risks, and use DISE selectively for persistent OSA to guide targeted interventions (e.g., turbinate reduction) [69, 70, 77, 78].

1.4.7 Conclusion

- The nose and nasopharynx govern upstream resistance and influence downstream collapsibility; optimizing this segment improves PAP comfort and can bolster multilevel surgical outcomes even when isolated nasal surgery yields modest AHI changes.
- Oronasal breathing typically requires higher therapeutic pressures and leaves more residual events under CPAP than nasal breathing; prioritize nasal patency and a nasal interface whenever feasible.
- In children, adenoidal hypertrophy is central; adenotonsillectomy improves symptoms and PSG indices, and anti-inflammatory therapy offers short-term benefit in mild/residual cases with appropriate counseling and follow-up.

1.5 Oropharyngeal and Palatal Obstruction in Obstructive Sleep Apnea

Lee Keng WongAhmad Syahir Md Ismail, and Liang Chye Goh

1.5.1 Overview and Anatomic–Physiologic Context (Fig. 1.8)

The *oropharynx* represents a central site of upper airway collapse in obstructive sleep apnea (OSA), particularly in adults. Anatomically, it is bounded superiorly by the *soft palate and uvula (velopharynx)*, laterally by the *tonsillar pillars and palatine tonsils*, posteriorly by the *pharyngeal wall*, and anteriorly by the *tongue base*. This region serves as a dynamic conduit for airflow, where even small structural or functional alterations can critically affect airway patency during sleep.

The *static anatomy* of the oropharynx contributes significantly to its vulnerability. Features such as a *redundant or elongated soft palate*, *tonsillar hypertrophy*, or increased *lateral wall thickness* reduce luminal dimensions, creating a predisposition to collapse. In obese individuals, deposition of parapharyngeal fat can further narrow the airway and increase lateral wall compliance, making the oropharynx particularly sensitive to pressure fluctuations.

Superimposed on this static framework is the role of *neuromuscular tone*, which varies with vigilance state. During wakefulness, tonic activity of the pharyngeal dilator muscles—particularly the palatoglossus, palatopharyngeus, and genioglossus—maintains airway caliber. With sleep onset, and especially during rapid eye movement (REM) sleep, this muscle tone diminishes, exposing the structural vulnerabilities of the oropharynx. These sleep stage-dependent reductions in dilator activity explain why some patients demonstrate *REM-predominant OSA* or exhibit more severe obstruction in deeper stages of sleep.

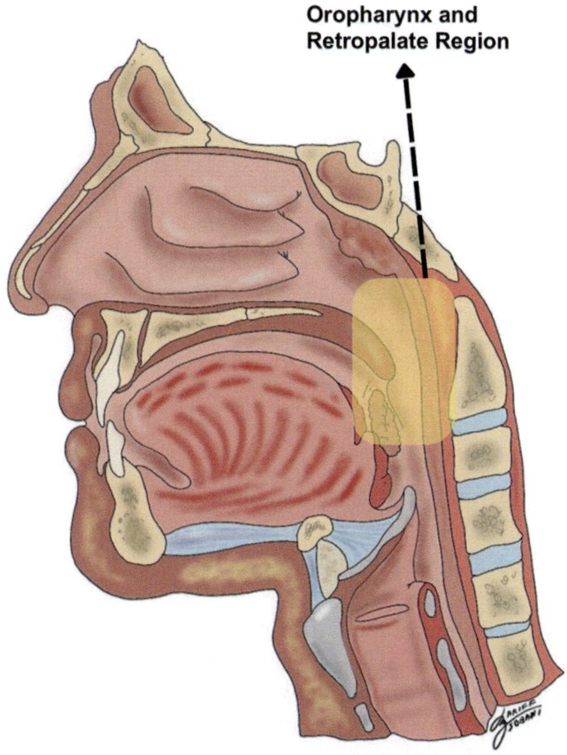

Fig. 1.8 Sagittal Cross-section of the upper airway. Shaded area representing the retropalate and oropharynx

Contemporary dynamic sleep MRI has consolidated and extended earlier physiologic insights into oropharyngeal behavior. Imaging consistently demonstrates that *retropalatal narrowing is nearly universal* among OSA patients, confirming the primacy of the palate as a collapse locus [60]. However, the same studies highlight that obstruction is rarely confined to this level. *Retroglossal collapse*, reflecting tongue-base involvement, and *lateral wall medialization* are frequently observed, often in combination. These findings underscore that OSA is typically a *multilevel disorder*, and they explain why isolated palatal procedures—though historically common—may be insufficient in patients with broader collapse patterns.

1.5.2 Patterns of Collapse and Clinical Significance

1.5.2.1 Anteroposterior (AP) Retropalatal Collapse

Posterior displacement of the soft palate onto the posterior pharyngeal wall narrows the velopharyngeal segment; elongation/redundancy of the palate/uvula and the supine position exacerbate the effect (Fig. 1.9).

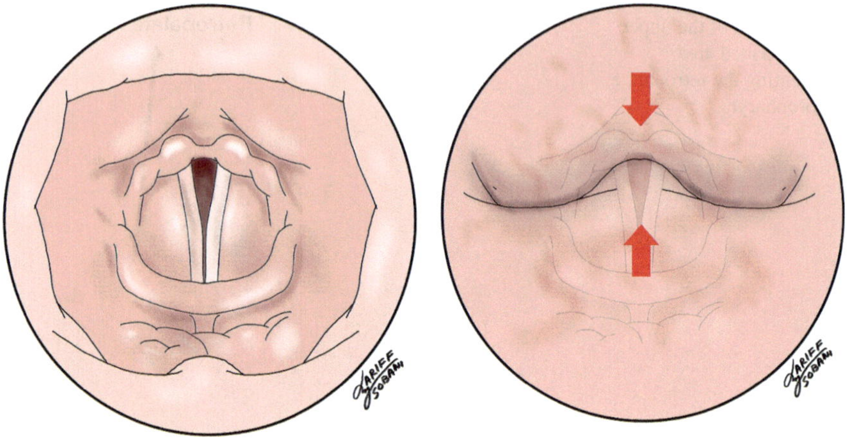

Fig. 1.9 AP Collapse of the retropalatal region

1.5.2.2 Lateral Wall Collapse

Medialization of the lateral pharyngeal walls—amplified by tonsillar hypertrophy or parapharyngeal fat—produces luminal narrowing and often coexists with AP collapse. Beyond simple crowding, multicenter DISE analyses associate oropharyngeal lateral-wall involvement with reduced surgical response if not directly addressed, reinforcing the need for techniques that tension or reposition the lateral walls [79] (Fig. 1.10).

1.5.2.3 Concentric (Circumferential) Velopharyngeal Collapse

Concomitant AP and lateral collapse yields uniform lumen narrowing; it is frequently observed on DISE in severe OSA, correlates with multilevel disease, and complicates CPAP tolerance and surgical planning. In addition to being a marker of complexity, complete concentric palatal collapse (CCC) has specific therapeutic implications (e.g., hypoglossal nerve stimulation candidacy) discussed below (Fig. 1.11).

1.5.2.4 Tonsillar Hypertrophy and Its Contribution

Tonsillar enlargement is a well-recognized contributor to upper airway obstruction and plays a central role in the pathophysiology of OSA across age groups. In children, tonsillar and adenoidal hypertrophy are the *primary drivers of lateral pharyngeal wall narrowing*, and *adenotonsillectomy* is frequently curative, restoring airway patency and normalizing sleep parameters in the majority of cases. In adults, the role of tonsillar hypertrophy is more complex but remains clinically meaningful,

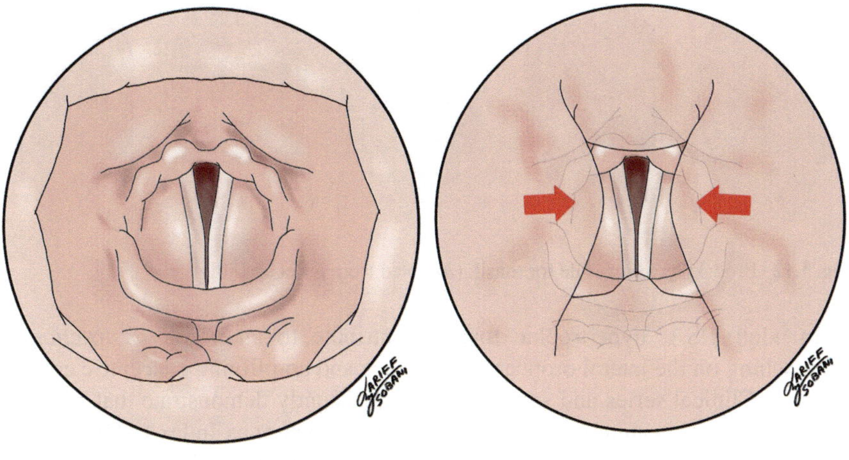

Fig. 1.10 Lateral collapse of the retropalatal region

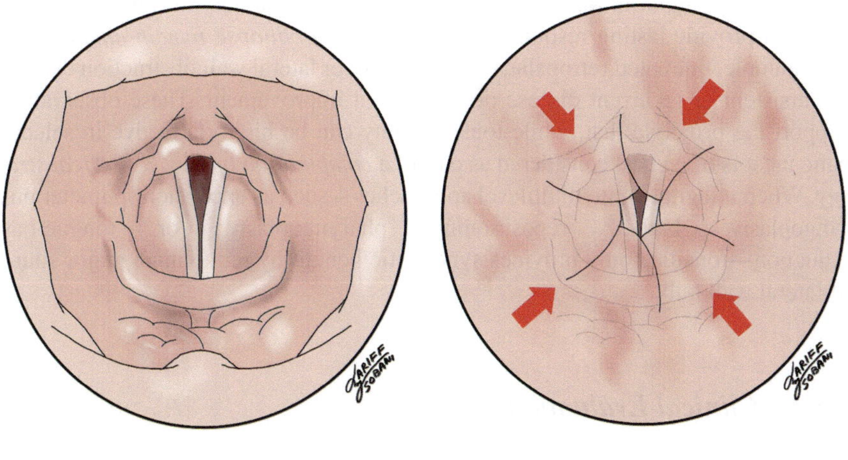

Fig. 1.11 Concentric collapse of the retropalate region

particularly when it coexists with palatal elongation, tongue-base bulk, or lateral wall collapsibility.

To facilitate clinical assessment, the *Brodsky grading scale* (Fig. 1.12) provides a standardized method for quantifying tonsillar size relative to the oropharyngeal airway. This grading system, originally developed for pediatric populations, is now widely applied in adults as well, offering a reproducible framework for correlating tonsil size with airway compromise [80]. In some contexts, *radiographic surrogates*, such as the *tonsil–oropharynx ratio* measured on imaging studies, can complement bedside grading—particularly in research settings or when surgical planning requires objective documentation of airway narrowing.

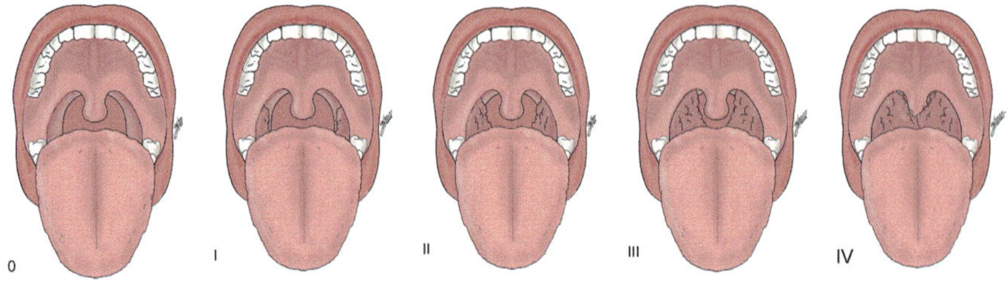

Fig. 1.12 Brodsky grading scale for tonsil. (Adapted from Lv et al. [80])

In adult OSA, hypertrophic tonsils contribute to *multilevel obstruction* by encroaching on the lateral oropharyngeal space and amplifying concentric collapse patterns. Clinical series and surgical trials consistently demonstrate that *tonsillectomy alone* can meaningfully reduce the Apnea–Hypopnea Index (AHI), particularly in adults with *mild to moderate disease* and markedly enlarged tonsils. Symptomatic improvements—including reduced snoring intensity, better sleep quality, and improved daytime function—often parallel physiologic gains.

However, long-term durability is variable. In many adults, tonsillectomy alone does not provide lasting resolution if *other sites of collapse remain unaddressed*. For example, untreated retropalatal, retroglossal, or lateral wall obstruction can lead to persistent or recurrent disease despite initial improvement. These observations support the principle that, while tonsillectomy can be highly effective in selected patients, it is often best considered as part of a *combination or staged surgical strategy*. When integrated into multilevel approaches—such as expansion sphincter pharyngoplasty, barbed repositioning pharyngoplasty, or tongue-base reduction—tonsillectomy provides synergistic benefit by removing a major source of lateral wall bulk.

1.5.3 Clinical Evaluation

Oral Examination Modified Mallampati and Friedman tongue position grades convey crowding at the tongue–palate interface and correlate with OSA risk and palatal surgical outcomes; they also inform Friedman staging when combined with tonsil size [81] (Fig. 1.13).

Awake Flexible Nasoendoscopy Endoscopic inspection during quiet breathing and Müller's maneuver surveys nasal, nasopharyngeal, oropharyngeal, and laryngeal anatomy, highlighting soft-tissue redundancy, tongue-base position, and dynamic pharyngeal behavior that may predict sleep-state collapse.

Drug-Induced Sleep Endoscopy (DISE) DISE remains the cornerstone for dynamic phenotyping of palatal and oropharyngeal collapse and for gauging jaw-

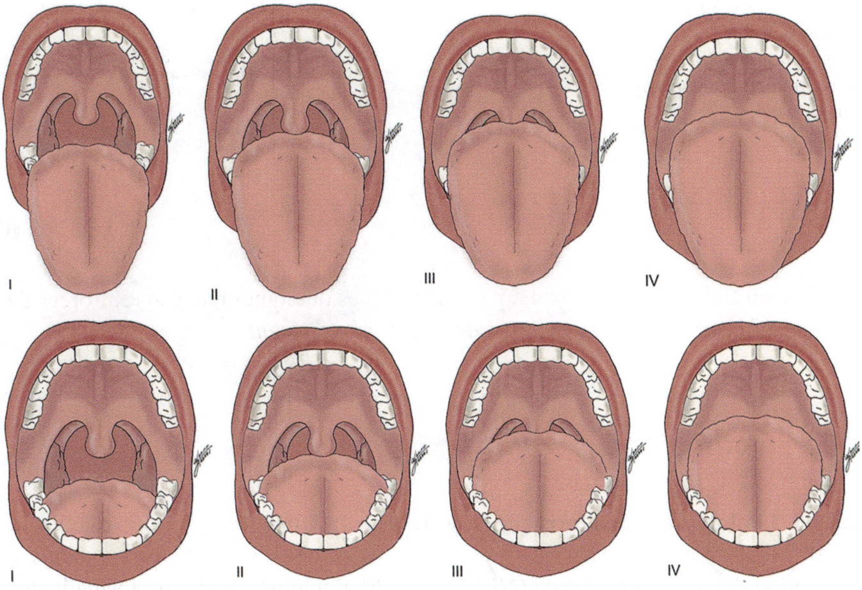

Fig. 1.13 Upper row: modified Mallampati (tongue protruded). Lower row: Friedman tongue position grade (tongue not protruded). (Adapted from Yu and Rosen [81])

thrust responsiveness. Interrater reliability is *fair to moderate* across modern scoring systems (VOTE; PTLTbE), emphasizing the value of standardized protocols and video review [51, 82]. Earlier work reported moderate–substantial agreement for global site attribution, but lower agreement for fine-grained configuration and degree, a pattern echoed in contemporary studies.

Imaging Dynamic (cine) MRI complements DISE by quantifying level-specific narrowing and visualizing soft-tissue motion (palate, tongue, lateral walls), often confirming universal retropalatal involvement and delineating multilevel patterns that guide procedure selection [60].

1.5.4 Therapeutic Framework

General Principles Positive airway pressure (PAP) is first-line for moderate–severe OSA. The 2021 AASM clinical practice guideline recommends discussing surgical referral for adults intolerant of PAP (BMI <40 kg/m^2) and in selected scenarios to facilitate PAP use—framing surgery as a patient-centered option within a multidisciplinary pathway [83].

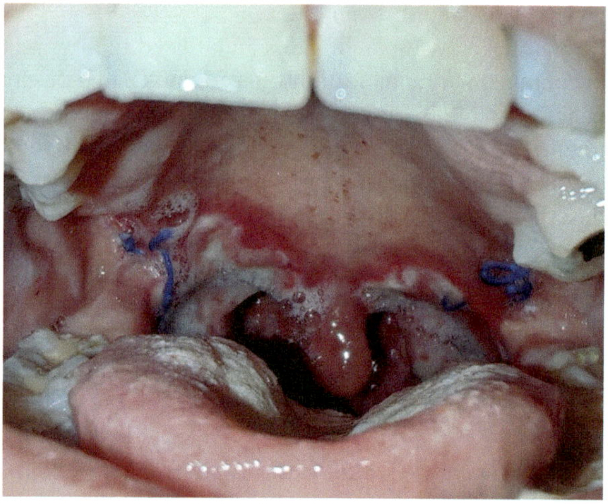

Fig. 1.14 Post-surgical findings after a tonsillectomy and relocation pharyngoplasty after 1 week

1.5.4.1 Palate-Directed Surgery (Fig. 1.14)

- *Uvulopalatopharyngoplasty (UPPP).* UPPP remains widely performed; outcomes vary with anatomy. A meta-analysis shows Friedman Stage I predicts favorable response, while Stage III and low hyoid position predict poorer outcomes—highlighting the need for staging-guided selection and often multilevel planning [84].
- *Expansion sphincter pharyngoplasty (ESP).* By reorienting palatopharyngeus to lateralize and stiffen the velopharyngeal inlet, ESP addresses AP and lateral elements. A randomized controlled trial showed larger AHI reduction and higher success vs. classic UPPP in appropriately selected patients with lateral wall collapse [24]. Subsequent series document durable symptom and PSG improvements with low morbidity and multiyear durability.
- *Barbed techniques (BRP/BP variants).* Barbed reposition pharyngoplasty and related barbed palatopharyngoplasty methods provide efficient lateral wall tensioning and palatal shortening without extensive tissue resection. Meta-analyses report substantial AHI and symptom reduction in uni- and multilevel settings, with operative-time advantages relative to ESP and generally mild, manageable complications. A dedicated safety review catalogs mainly minor short- and long-term effects (e.g., thread extrusion, transient dysphagia, foreign-body sensation).
- *Palatal advancement/transpalatal advancement pharyngoplasty.* In patients with high palatal redundancy or adverse Friedman stage, palatal advancement can outperform classic UPPP for AHI reduction, particularly when lateral wall support is incorporated.

Tonsillectomy (Adults) In adults with large tonsils, isolated tonsillectomy can be highly effective for selected mild–moderate OSA phenotypes, with meta-analytic AHI reductions around 65% and strong responses in lower baseline AHI; however, long-term data suggest that relapse is possible without addressing coexisting levels. These data support integrating tonsillectomy into tailored, often multilevel, palatopharyngeal strategies rather than viewing it as universally definitive in adults.

1.5.4.2 Phenotype-Driven Surgery and Special Considerations

- *Oropharyngeal lateral-wall disease.* Because lateral-wall collapse predicts poorer outcomes if untreated, techniques that tension/reposition the walls (ESP, BRP) should be prioritized when DISE or imaging implicate this segment.
- *Complete concentric palatal collapse (CCC).* CCC at the velum is a strong negative predictor for hypoglossal nerve stimulation candidacy and response, making DISE screening essential when HNS is contemplated. In CCC-dominant phenotypes electing surgery, palatal techniques that robustly address circumferential collapse (e.g., ESP/BRP with lateral-wall emphasis, palatal advancement) are preferred, often within a multilevel plan.

1.5.4.3 Practical, Stepwise Approach

1. *Characterize anatomy and phenotype.* Use standardized oral exam (Mallampati/FTP; tonsil grade) and awake endoscopy to triage patients to DISE and, where available, dynamic MRI.
2. *Map collapse pattern to therapy.* For *AP-dominant* palatal collapse with favorable Friedman stage, UPPP variants may suffice; add tonsillectomy when enlarged tonsils contribute. For *lateral-wall* or *concentric* collapse, favor ESP/BRP or palatal advancement and plan multilevel surgery when the tongue base or other segments contribute.
3. *Set expectations and sequence care.* Align with AASM guidance on surgical referral after PAP intolerance; consider staged approaches with objective reevaluation when outcomes are suboptimal.
4. *Monitor outcomes and morbidity.* Counsel regarding typical palatopharyngeal adverse effects (e.g., transient dysphagia, suture-related symptoms) and the importance of follow-up PSG to verify efficacy.

1.6 Hypopharyngeal and Laryngeal Obstruction in Obstructive Sleep Apnea

Lee Keng Wong, Ahmad Syahir Md Ismail, and Liang Chye Goh

1.6.1 Overview and Anatomical–Physiologic Context (Fig. 1.15)

The *hypopharynx* and *supraglottic larynx* play pivotal roles in maintaining upper airway patency during sleep. Obstruction at these levels is often decisive in determining OSA severity, yet their contribution has historically been underestimated compared with palatal collapse. Their collapsibility reflects a *multifactorial interplay* between static anatomy, neuromuscular tone, and sleep stage-dependent control mechanisms.

From an *anatomical standpoint*, several structures converge to influence hypopharyngeal stability:

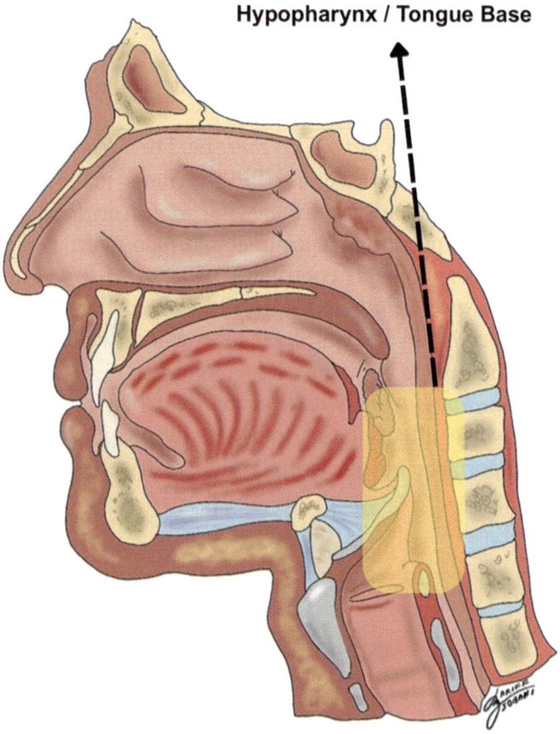

Fig. 1.15 Sagittal cross-section of the upper airway. Shaded area representing the hypopharynx and tongue base

- *Tongue volume*, particularly the posterior third, determines the retroglossal airway caliber. Enlarged tongues—whether due to skeletal crowding, obesity-related lingual fat, or lymphoid hypertrophy—push against the posterior pharyngeal wall, narrowing the airway lumen.
- *Epiglottic morphology*, including its length, curvature, and tissue compliance, dictates whether it resists or succumbs to inspiratory forces. A floppier or elongated epiglottis is more prone to prolapse.
- *Lateral pharyngeal wall (LPW) thickness*, strongly influenced by parapharyngeal fat in obese individuals, contributes significantly to concentric or lateral narrowing.

Overlaying this anatomy is the contribution of *neuromuscular tone*. The *genioglossus muscle* is the primary upper airway dilator, counteracting posterior tongue displacement. During wakefulness, tonic and reflex activation of this muscle maintains retroglossal patency. With sleep onset, however, this tone diminishes, reducing compensatory stiffening. Reflex control of the airway dilator muscles, which varies by sleep stage, further modulates the degree of collapse.

Physiologic studies and imaging have consistently shown how these elements interact. Dynamic imaging demonstrates that posterior displacement of the tongue base, often in combination with medialization of the lateral pharyngeal walls, markedly reduces retroglossal cross-sectional area. Such narrowing may not only increase collapsibility but also prolong respiratory events by limiting airflow recovery. Moreover, *epiglottic prolapse* can cause high-grade obstruction even in the absence of significant palatal disease [40, 85]. This highlights an important clinical principle: severe OSA can arise from predominantly hypopharyngeal and supraglottic collapse, meaning that an apparently "normal palate" does not exclude significant pathology lower in the airway.

t The hypopharynx and supraglottic larynx represent a *dynamic anatomical–physiologic unit*, where structural load, neuromuscular drive, and reflex control intersect. For the surgeon and clinician, understanding this context is essential. It explains why hypopharyngeal obstruction often leads to surgical failures if overlooked, why obesity disproportionately amplifies retroglossal narrowing, and why tailored therapies (tongue-base reduction, lateral wall stiffening, epiglottopexy) are required in selected patients.

1.6.2 Mechanisms and Phenotypes of Collapse

1.6.2.1 Tongue-Base and Lateral Wall Collapse

The *tongue base* is one of the most common and clinically significant sites of obstruction in OSA. During wakefulness, tonic activity of the *genioglossus muscle* maintains anterior tongue position. With the onset of sleep, this neuromuscular tone diminishes. In the *supine position*, gravitational pull accentuates posterior displacement, allowing the tongue base to occlude the airway against the posterior pharyngeal wall [85].

Several anatomic and physiological risk factors amplify this vulnerability:

- *Craniofacial structure* such as micrognathia or retrognathia restricts mandibular space, predisposing the tongue base to posterior crowding.
- *Obesity* contributes via lingual fat infiltration, which both enlarges the tongue and reduces its muscular efficiency.
- *Age-related changes* in muscle tone and connective tissue stiffness further impair compensatory mechanisms.

The *lateral pharyngeal walls (LPWs)* play an equally critical role. Their involvement is frequent, particularly in obese patients where parapharyngeal fat pads exert inward pressure. Collapse here is often concentric or a combined anteroposterior–lateral pattern. This is more than an anatomical curiosity: *LPW collapse is prognostically important*, as it correlates with more severe OSA and predicts surgical failure when unaddressed [86].

Clinically, predictive markers can guide suspicion of retroglossal involvement. The *Friedman tongue position*—a simple, office-based oropharyngeal grading system—correlates with retroglossal crowding and OSA severity. High Friedman grades should prompt further evaluation with imaging or DISE to confirm the degree and pattern of collapse [87].

1.6.2.2 Epiglottic and Aryepiglottic Collapse

The *epiglottis* represents a distinct and underappreciated site of obstruction. Collapse may occur in several forms:

- *Primary anteroposterior prolapse*, where the epiglottis flops backward like a valve.
- *Lateral folding*, where the epiglottic margins collapse medially.
- *Secondary or "downstream" collapse*, in which tongue-base pressure drives the epiglottis posteriorly.

Earlier reports underestimated epiglottic obstruction because *awake exams* rarely reveal it; the epiglottis often appears structurally normal during wakefulness [88]. With the advent of DISE, however, its true prevalence has become clearer. Contemporary series suggest that *epiglottic involvement accounts for roughly 15–20% of OSA cases*, with distinct phenotypes increasingly recognized [64].

This is not a trivial observation. For some patients, epiglottic collapse contributes disproportionately to symptoms. They may present with *positional vulnerability* (worse in supine REM sleep) or *CPAP intolerance*, as the valve-like prolapse of the epiglottis can worsen airflow turbulence when pressurized air is delivered [89]. Such patients may have a relatively modest overall AHI yet experience striking functional impairment.

Recent cohorts have also highlighted *lateral epiglottic collapse* as a recognizable and reproducible phenotype [90]. This has therapeutic implications, as it may not respond predictably to conventional palatal or tongue-base surgery and instead requires tailored strategies such as epiglottopexy, partial epiglottectomy, or barbed repositioning techniques.

1.6.3 Diagnostic Evaluation

1.6.3.1 Awake Endoscopy and Imaging

Baseline flexible nasoendoscopy remains useful to exclude fixed lesions and assess relative tongue-palate space. Structural imaging (CT/MRI) characterizes airway caliber and soft tissues and informs surgical planning [40]. Dynamic or cine-MRI provides frame-by-frame visualization of obstruction during sleep or sedated states, clarifying multilevel collapse [60] (retropalatal nearly universal; retroglossal common; hypopharyngeal variable) and is increasingly leveraged to match phenotype to therapy.

1.6.3.2 Drug-Induced Sleep Endoscopy (DISE)

DISE is the workhorse for dynamic phenotyping of retropalatal, retroglossal/hypopharyngeal, and laryngeal obstruction and for testing mandibular advancement or jaw-thrust responses [88]. While DISE reliably guides site-directed therapy, recent reliability studies show fair–moderate interrater agreement [51, 91] across scoring systems (VOTE and alternatives), underscoring the value of structured protocols, video review, and adjunctive objective metrics where available. Emerging work on automated/assisted DISE scoring suggests feasibility for more consistent grading of collapse severity and configuration [91].

1.6.3.3 Functional Testing During DISE

A positive response to jaw-thrust or simulated mandibular advancement supports candidacy for MADs or maxillomandibular surgery (MMA), while persistent epiglottic prolapse despite jaw-thrust points toward epiglottic surgery or hypoglossal nerve stimulation (HGNS) [28]. DISE can also help predict who will respond to MMA and who may need epiglottic adjuncts.

1.6.3.4 Therapeutic Strategies

First-line Therapy CPAP remains the first-line therapy for moderate–severe OSA; however, adherence challenges—often exacerbated by epiglottic "valving" sensations—necessitate phenotype-specific alternatives [89].

Oral Appliance Therapy and Positional Therapy For retroglossal/hypopharyngeal collapse that improves with jaw-thrust on DISE, mandibular advancement devices are rational and often effective, particularly in nonobese or retrognathic patients [86].

Hypoglossal Nerve Stimulation (HNS) HNS addresses tongue-base collapse by synchronizing hypoglossal activation with inspiration. Contemporary registry and trial follow-up data show durable reductions in AHI and symptom burden at multi-year horizons; efficacy appears consistent across a range of baseline severities when patients are appropriately selected (notably avoiding complete concentric palatal collapse). Importantly, recent analyses suggest that independent epiglottic collapse is not a contraindication and may respond comparably to tongue-base-dependent epiglottic collapse, broadening applicability in laryngeal phenotypes [91].

1.6.4 Surgery for Tongue Base and Hypopharynx

- *Genioglossus advancement (± genioplasty)* and *hyoid suspension* remain foundational procedures for retroglossal collapse, often as part of multilevel plans [28].
- *Tongue-base reduction* techniques include radiofrequency or coblation channeling, midline glossectomy, lingual tonsil reduction, and *transoral robotic surgery (TORS)*. Systematic reviews demonstrate TORS can effectively address tongue-base and/or epiglottic obstruction within multilevel strategies, with acceptable morbidity profiles [92] when performed in experienced centers. Ongoing work is refining patient selection and assessing single-port platforms and hemorrhage-mitigation protocols.
- *Epiglottic surgery.* For primary epiglottic prolapse (anteroposterior or lateral), procedures such as partial epiglottectomy, epiglottopexy, or supraglottoplasty can relieve obstruction while preserving protective function. Contemporary series report meaningful reductions in residual AHI and symptomatic improvement in carefully selected adults—particularly CPAP-intolerant patients with DISE-confirmed epiglottic collapse [64, 89]. When epiglottic obstruction coexists with retroglossal and/or LPW collapse, epiglottic surgery should be integrated into a multilevel plan.

1.7 Role of Surgery in OSA Management

Rajendran Laavanya, Emelda Rose Sebastin, Nor Anis Elini Ismail, and Liang Chye Goh

1.7.1 Introduction and Indications for Surgery

Surgery occupies a well-defined but complementary role in the *multidisciplinary management of obstructive sleep apnea (OSA)*. Continuous positive airway pressure (CPAP) remains the *first-line therapy* for most adults, owing to its robust efficacy across a wide spectrum of phenotypes. However, real-world practice demonstrates that CPAP is far from universally successful. Many patients encounter *intolerance*, *adherence challenges*, or specific *anatomic patterns of collapse* that make PAP delivery ineffective or poorly tolerated. In such cases, surgery serves not as a replacement but as a *strategic adjunct or alternative* in the broader continuum of care.

Contemporary management emphasizes that surgery is *not a one-size-fits-all intervention*, but instead requires:

1. *Careful patient selection*, including assessment of comorbidities, BMI, and airway anatomy.
2. *Endoscopic phenotyping*, particularly with drug-induced sleep endoscopy (DISE), to map the collapse pattern and localize obstruction.
3. *Tailoring procedures* to the identified sites of collapse—whether palatal, tongue base, lateral pharyngeal walls, or epiglottis—often within a *staged or multilevel surgical framework* rather than isolated single-site correction.

Authoritative guidelines from the *American Academy of Sleep Medicine (AASM)* underscore this selective role. They recommend that clinicians *discuss referral to a sleep surgeon* in adults with OSA and body mass index (BMI) <40 kg/m^2 who are *intolerant or unaccepting of PAP therapy*. For patients with *class II or III obesity (BMI ≥ 35 kg/m^2)*, referral to a *bariatric surgeon* is advised as part of the treatment pathway [83]. These recommendations highlight that the type of surgery—upper airway vs. metabolic—should align with the dominant contributor to OSA pathophysiology.

The AASM also recognizes the role of surgery in patients who remain *partially adherent to PAP* but experience *pressure-related side effects*, such as aerophagia, discomfort, or mask intolerance. In these cases, targeted airway surgery may reduce required pressures, improving PAP tolerance rather than replacing it altogether. Conversely, when patients present with a *major anatomic abnormality*—for instance, severe tonsillar hypertrophy or a grossly deviated nasal septum—guidelines still emphasize PAP as the *initial therapy* in most cases, while acknowledging that *individualized exceptions* are appropriate. For example, immediate surgical correction may be reasonable when the abnormality is both a clear driver of obstruction and a barrier to PAP initiation.

In practice, then, the *indications for sleep surgery* are not limited to CPAP failure, but extend to:

- *CPAP intolerance* (complete refusal or inability to tolerate therapy).
- *PAP-related side effects* requiring adjunctive surgical facilitation.
- *Anatomic abnormalities* that strongly suggest surgical benefit.
- *Multilevel disease* in which surgery forms part of a staged treatment plan alongside weight loss, positional therapy, or hypoglossal nerve stimulation.

Taken together, these principles reflect a *modern, patient-centered model* of OSA management. Rather than serving as a "last resort," surgery is best understood as part of a *multimodal therapeutic strategy*, integrated with medical, behavioral, and device-based therapies to optimize outcomes.

1.7.2 Preoperative Evaluation and Patient Selection

Outcomes depend heavily on preoperative phenotyping. Drug-induced sleep endoscopy (DISE) provides [15, 51] a dynamic assessment of the upper airway under sedated conditions that simulate natural sleep and enables grading by the VOTE system (Velum, Oropharyngeal lateral wall, Tongue base, Epiglottis). DISE demonstrates reasonable interrater reliability and helps link specific collapse patterns to targeted therapies—for example, palatal procedures for retropalatal collapse, lateral wall—addressing techniques for lateral pharyngeal collapse, and tongue-directed procedures or neurostimulation for hypopharyngeal collapse. Complete concentric collapse (CCC) [15] of the velum on DISE is particularly relevant: it predicts poor response to certain therapies (e.g., hypoglossal nerve stimulation, see below) and often necessitates palatal lateralization or expansion techniques before or in lieu of neurostimulation.

Shared decision-making incorporates OSA severity, symptom burden, cardiometabolic risk, anatomic phenotype, BMI, comorbidities, and the patient's preferences regarding devices versus operations. Surgical success is typically defined using Sher criteria—a $\geq$ 50% reduction in Apnea–Hypopnea Index (AHI) and a postoperative AHI <20 events/h—recognizing that more stringent targets (e.g., AHI <5–10) may be appropriate in selected patients.

1.7.2.1 Palatal and Lateral Pharyngeal Wall Surgery

Traditional uvulopalatopharyngoplasty (UPPP) has variable efficacy in unselected patients; outcomes improve substantially when procedures specifically address the lateral pharyngeal wall and retropalatal obstruction. Expansion sphincter pharyngoplasty (ESP) repositions [24] the palatopharyngeus to widen and lateralize the velopharyngeal airway. In a randomized trial of carefully selected patients (Friedman stage II–III, lateral wall collapse), ESP produced larger AHI reductions and higher success than UPPP.

Barbed palatopharyngoplasty techniques [93–95] (e.g., barbed reposition pharyngoplasty, BRP) achieve lateral wall stabilization with knotless barbed sutures and have been associated with favorable outcomes and short operative times. Meta-analyses report substantial reductions in AHI (often ~60–70%) with success rates in the 65–90% range in appropriately selected patients; BRP and ESP show broadly comparable efficacy, with BRP frequently faster to perform. Complication profiles are generally acceptable [96], with transient dysphagia, thread extrusion, and velopharyngeal symptoms the most common events.

Key technical principles include preserving palatal function, avoiding excessive tissue resection that predisposes to velopharyngeal insufficiency, and lateralizing rather than simply shortening the palate. Lateral pharyngeal wall collapse—often underrecognized by awake exam—should be directly addressed to avoid residual obstruction after palatal surgery. DISE is instrumental in identifying candidates most likely to benefit.

1.7.2.2 Tongue-Directed Surgery and Hypoglossal Nerve Stimulation

Procedures at the tongue base (e.g., midline glossectomy, lingual tonsillectomy, genioglossus advancement, or hyoid suspension as part of multilevel surgery) can be effective when hypopharyngeal collapse predominates. Evidence quality varies: isolated hyoid surgery yields modest AHI reductions on meta-analysis (~38% overall), while hyoid suspension combined with UPPP [97] within multilevel strategies demonstrates higher success rates in selected series.

Hypoglossal nerve stimulation (HNS) [34, 98, 99] is a nonanatomic, implantable therapy that advances and stiffens the tongue during inspiration. Pivotal (STAR) and subsequent longitudinal cohorts show durable improvements in AHI, sleepiness, and quality of life over 3–5 years with responder rates around 63–75% by Sher-style definitions, and low rates of serious device-related adverse events. Real-world registry data support strong adherence (>90% of patients meeting nightly-use thresholds) and symptom benefits across subgroups. Patient selection typically includes moderate–severe OSA, CPAP intolerance, BMI below payer-specified thresholds, and exclusion of CCC at the velum on DISE.

Regulatory and coverage criteria continue to evolve. Recent updates expanded indications (including higher BMI limits) for some HNS systems, though payer policies may lag and still impose stricter BMI or AHI windows. Selection remains anatomy- and physiology-driven; careful DISE assessment and counseling regarding expectations are essential.

1.7.2.3 Skeletal Surgery (Maxillomandibular Advancement)

Maxillomandibular advancement (MMA) [100, 101] enlarges the entire retropalatal and retrolingual airway by advancing both jaws (often 8–10 mm combined), increasing tension on the soft tissues and tongue base. MMA consistently produces among the largest and most durable AHI reductions of any surgery for adult OSA, including in severe disease and in patients who failed prior soft-tissue procedures. Cohort studies and meta-analyses report mean AHI reductions of ~70–80%, with many patients reaching AHI <5–15 long-term; benefits in sleepiness and oxygenation are sustained over years, though some attenuation in very long-term follow-up has been observed.

MMA is typically reserved for patients with craniofacial deficiency or as definitive therapy for multilevel collapse when other procedures are unlikely to suffice. It requires orthodontic planning, entails longer recovery, and demands thorough counseling—but it remains a high-efficacy option with robust quality-of-life gains in properly selected candidates.

1.7.2.4 Transoral Robotic Surgery (TORS) and Multilevel Strategies

TORS facilitates precise resection of tongue-base soft tissues and lingual tonsils with enhanced visualization. Systematic reviews show meaningful AHI reductions [102], particularly when TORS is combined with palatal and/or nasal procedures in multilevel approaches guided by DISE. Ideal candidates have bulky tongue base or lingual tonsillar hypertrophy contributing to retrolingual collapse.

In practice, many adults benefit from staged or single-session multilevel surgery tailored to their collapse patterns. Contemporary series of multilevel surgery report success rates in the 60–80% range using Sher criteria in severe OSA populations, with meaningful improvements in oxygenation and symptoms.

1.7.2.5 Nasal Surgery: Adjunctive Value and PAP Facilitation

Isolated nasal surgery seldom "cures" OSA, but it improves nasal airflow, can reduce required PAP pressures, and—critically—can transform PAP intolerance into acceptance in patients with prominent nasal obstruction. Systematic reviews/meta-analyses show average reductions [103] of ~2–3 cm H_2O in therapeutic PAP pressures and significant gains in objective or self-reported usage after septoplasty and turbinate reduction; symptom scales (ESS) improve even when AHI changes are modest. Professional society statements reflect these data and endorse nasal surgery as a facilitator of PAP and oral appliance therapy when indicated.

1.7.3 *Perioperative Safety, Complications, and Long-Term Considerations*

When performed in experienced centers with appropriate selection, serious complications are uncommon. Palatal procedures most often cause transient dysphagia or globus; persistent velopharyngeal insufficiency and significant hemorrhage are infrequent. Barbed techniques show low rates of thread-related issues and generally self-limited symptoms. Hyoid and tongue-base procedures carry risks of dysphagia, dental or nerve injury (rare), or wound issues; device-based HNS has a small risk of lead revision, infection, or discomfort. MMA entails osteotomy-related risks (sensory changes, malocclusion, infection) but has a favorable safety profile in specialized hands. Across procedures, meticulous technique, postoperative airway vigilance, and standardized pain and swallow pathways reduce adverse events.

Long-term follow-up is essential. Weight gain, aging-related changes in neuromuscular control, and new comorbidities can erode initial gains; periodic outcomes assessment (symptoms, device downloads for HNS, or repeat sleep testing when indicated) ensures timely rescue measures (adjunctive therapy, weight management, or revisional procedures).

1.7.3.1 Postoperative (General) Management After Surgery for Obstructive Sleep Apnea

Setting and Monitoring

- Admit to an area with continuous pulse oximetry for at least the first postoperative night in patients with moderate–severe OSA, significant comorbidities, or when opioids are required. Consider step-up care (HDU/ICU) for very severe OSA, difficult airway, or major multilevel surgery.

Airway, Breathing, and PAP

- Head-up/lateral positioning, humidified oxygen to maintain baseline saturation, and early incentive spirometry.
- Resume the patient's usual CPAP/BiPAP as soon as it is safe and feasible; if concerned about fresh palatal/nasal wounds, restart at lower pressures with close observation and the surgeon's input.

Analgesia and Antiemesis

- Use multimodal, opioid-sparing analgesia (acetaminophen ± NSAIDs if not contraindicated; local/regional techniques). Avoid long-acting opioids and sedatives; if opioids are necessary, use the lowest effective dose with enhanced monitoring. Pair analgesia with prophylactic antiemetics to reduce retching-related bleeding.

Edema/Bleeding Control

- Short course of steroids may be considered to reduce edema and nausea per institutional practice; maintain blood pressure control; provide clear instructions for delayed hemorrhage (particularly after palatal or tonsillar procedures).

Nasal/Oral Care and Diet

- Saline sprays/irrigations for nasal procedures; gentle oral rinses after transoral surgery. Advance from cool liquids/soft diet as tolerated; emphasize hydration. (Institutional protocols may vary.)

Comorbidity Optimization

- Resume home antihypertensives and antidiabetics when appropriate; employ DVT prophylaxis per risk profile. Coordinate with cardiology for heart-failure patients (PAP adherence reduces postoperative cardiac complications).

Discharge and Follow-up

- Provide written airway-bleeding warnings, driving/operating-machinery cautions if residual sleepiness, and a clear pain plan.
- Reassess sleep-disordered breathing and therapy needs (PAP/oral appliance) after healing; schedule objective outcome testing (e.g., HSAT/PSG) typically 8–12 weeks post-op to guide further management.

1.7.4 Practical Clinical Pathway

1. *Confirm diagnosis and optimize medical therapy* (weight reduction, positional therapy where appropriate) and trial PAP with interface, humidification, and pressure-relief optimization.
2. *Evaluate anatomy dynamically* with DISE (and imaging when indicated) to map collapse.
3. *Match procedure(s) to phenotype*:
    - Retropalatal/lateral wall collapse → ESP or barbed palatopharyngoplasty (often with tonsillectomy).
    - Tongue-base/lingual tonsil hypertrophy → tongue-base reduction, lingual tonsillectomy, or TORS as part of multilevel surgery.
    - Hypoglossal dysfunction without CCC and appropriate BMI → consider HNS.
    - Global multilevel collapse or craniofacial deficiency → consider MMA.
    - Prominent nasal obstruction → septoplasty/inferior turbinate reduction to facilitate PAP or oral appliances.
4. *Set expectations using standardized success definitions* and discuss staged approaches when indicated.
5. *Plan follow-up* with symptom scales, PAP/HNS data, and, when appropriate, polysomnography.

1.8 Outcomes, Success Rates, and Patient Selection for OSA Surgery

Rajendran LaavanyaEmelda Rose Sebastin, Nor Anis Elini Ismail, and Liang Chye Goh

1.8.1 Why Outcomes Matter and How to Define Them

The ultimate goal of surgical intervention for obstructive sleep apnea (OSA) is not merely to modify numbers on a sleep study but to achieve *clinically meaningful improvements*: reducing pathologic respiratory events, restoring restorative sleep, improving daytime function, and mitigating long-term cardiometabolic risk. Surgery is judged not just by whether an airway is anatomically altered, but by whether those changes translate into tangible benefits for the patient and their health trajectory.

1.8.1.1 Traditional Metrics

Historically, outcome reporting has centered almost exclusively on *polysomnographic indices*, with the *Apnea–Hypopnea Index (AHI)* and oxygen desaturation parameters serving as the primary benchmarks. These endpoints are attractive because they are *quantifiable, standardized, and reproducible across institutions.* The most widely adopted composite benchmark remains *Sher's definition of surgical success*: a ≥ 50% reduction in AHI from baseline together with a postoperative AHI <20 events/h [104].

Sher's criteria provided an essential early framework and remain useful for comparing across trials. However, its limitations are increasingly recognized. First, this threshold does not equate to *physiologic "cure,"* as patients may still harbor residual disease at levels sufficient to perpetuate symptoms or risk. Second, it risks *underestimating symptom burden*, especially in phenotypes where sleep fragmentation or REM-specific obstruction persists despite an overall reduction in AHI.

1.8.1.2 Beyond AHI: Contemporary Endpoints

Modern evaluations of surgical outcomes now extend beyond AHI, reflecting the multifaceted impact of OSA. Commonly incorporated measures include:

- *Oxygenation metrics*, such as nadir SpO_2 and cumulative time spent with saturation < 90%, which correlate more directly with hypoxemia burden and cardiovascular risk.
- *Sleep architecture*, including the proportions of REM and NREM sleep, the arousal index, and sleep efficiency. These provide insight into whether surgery restores consolidated, restorative sleep.

- *Patient-reported outcomes*, which capture dimensions not visible on polysomnography. Widely used tools include the *Epworth Sleepiness Scale (ESS)* for daytime sleepiness, the *Functional Outcomes of Sleep Questionnaire (FOSQ)* for daily performance, and disease-specific quality-of-life instruments.
- *Bed-partner observations*, such as snoring intensity, witnessed apneas, and nocturnal restlessness, which often serve as sensitive, real-world correlates of physiologic change.

1.8.2 Toward a Holistic Definition of Success

Given these considerations, contemporary consensus increasingly favors *dual reporting* of outcomes:

1. *Physiologic success*—quantified using Sher's definition or stricter thresholds (e.g., postoperative AHI <10 or <5 events/h, often termed "surgical cure").
2. *Symptomatic benefit*—documented through validated questionnaires, functional measures, and patient/bed-partner feedback.

AHI reduction matters only if it improves daytime function and reduces long-term risk. Moreover, transparent reporting of the proportion of patients reaching more stringent AHI targets provides clarity for both clinicians and patients, ensuring realistic expectations of surgical benefit.

1.8.3 How to Measure Outcomes in Routine Practice and Studies

Accurate and reproducible outcome measurement is essential both for guiding *individual patient care* and for building a reliable evidence base in sleep surgery. Unlike device-based therapies, where adherence can be tracked directly, surgical interventions require structured follow-up to determine whether the procedure has achieved its intended physiologic and symptomatic benefits.

1.8.3.1 Objective Measures

The foundation of outcome assessment remains *sleep testing before and after intervention*. This typically involves full-night polysomnography (PSG), which remains the gold standard, or technically adequate home sleep testing performed with *identical scoring rules* pre- and posttreatment to ensure comparability.

While the Apnea–Hypopnea Index (AHI) is most frequently reported, contemporary practice emphasizes a broader panel of physiologic outcomes:

- *Oxygen Desaturation Index (ODI)*, to quantify the burden of intermittent hypoxemia.
- *Arousal Index*, reflecting the degree of sleep fragmentation.
- *Sleep efficiency* and stage distribution, to evaluate whether restorative REM and slow-wave sleep are being preserved or restored.
- *REM-specific AHI*, which is especially important for REM-predominant OSA phenotypes that may respond differently to interventions.

Tracking these measures provides a more nuanced picture of treatment response, particularly in patients whose overall AHI reduction does not fully capture symptomatic or physiologic benefit.

1.8.3.2 Subjective Measures

Objective data, while indispensable, do not always reflect the lived experience of patients. Therefore, validated *patient-reported outcome measures* are equally important:

- The *Epworth Sleepiness Scale (ESS)* offers a simple, widely recognized tool for assessing changes in daytime sleepiness.
- The *Functional Outcomes of Sleep Questionnaire (FOSQ)* provides a more detailed measure of the impact of sleepiness and fatigue on daily function.

These tools help capture *real-world benefits* that physiologic metrics may miss—for example, in patients with modest AHI improvement but dramatic gains in sleep continuity, alertness, or quality of life.

1.8.4 Timing of Assessments

Consistency in timing is crucial for meaningful interpretation. A *standardized battery of objective and subjective measures* should be collected at *reproducible intervals*—commonly at 3–6 months postoperatively, with longer-term follow-up at 12 months and beyond. This approach facilitates both within-patient assessment and comparison across surgical series, procedures, and institutions.

1.8.4.1 Reporting Standards in Surgical Studies

To ensure transparency and reproducibility, surgical outcome studies should report the following key elements:

1. *Prespecified success definitions*, including Sher's criteria and, where possible, stricter thresholds (e.g., AHI <10 or <5).
2. *Intention-to-treat and per-protocol analyses*, to clarify the impact of dropouts or incomplete follow-up.
3. *Changes in ESS and FOSQ*, or equivalent validated patient-reported measures.
4. *Adverse events and complications*, reported systematically rather than anecdotally.
5. *Durability of outcomes over time*, including weight trajectories, recurrence of symptoms, and the use of adjunctive therapies (e.g., CPAP, mandibular devices, or revision surgery).

1.8.4.2 Defining Surgical Success in Sleep Surgery

Surgical success in obstructive sleep apnea (OSA) has traditionally been benchmarked against *Sher's criteria*—a ≥50% reduction in Apnea–Hypopnea Index (AHI) from baseline and a postoperative AHI <20 events/h. This definition is widely adopted because of its simplicity and reproducibility across studies, yet it does not necessarily equate to cure, nor does it always reflect residual symptom burden in certain phenotypes.

Contemporary outcome reporting increasingly integrates both *objective measures* (AHI, oxygen desaturation index, nadir SpO_2, arousal index, REM-specific AHI) and *subjective metrics* (Epworth Sleepiness Scale [ESS], Functional Outcomes of Sleep Questionnaire [FOSQ], quality-of-life tools). These additional domains help capture meaningful improvements in daytime function, patient satisfaction, and bed-partner reports, even when AHI normalization is incomplete.

To set expectations, it is often helpful to distinguish between:

- *Success*: meeting Sher or similar criteria.
- *Response*: symptomatic or physiologic improvement that falls short of "success."
- *Cure*: AHI normalization (e.g., <5) with resolution of symptoms.

Modern recommendations encourage reporting not only Sher-defined success but also the proportion of patients achieving stricter thresholds (AHI <10 or < 5), alongside changes in patient-reported outcomes. This multidimensional definition provides a more holistic view of surgical effectiveness and facilitates clearer counseling for patients.

1.8.4.3 Success Rates by Procedure (Typical Ranges in Selected Candidates)

These ranges reflect pooled data and representative cohorts; true results depend on anatomy, center expertise, and whether surgery is performed as *single-level* or *multilevel*, guided by drug-induced sleep endoscopy (DISE).

Procedure	Average success rate[a]
Uvulopalatopharyngoplasty (UPPP)	~40–50% as stand-alone
Barbed reposition pharyngoplasty (BRP)	~60–80% in selected cases
Pediatric tonsillectomy (with hypertrophy)	~70–90% in pediatric cases
Genioglossus advancement (GA)	~50–60% (often multilevel)
Tongue-base radiofrequency (RFA)	~30–50% (modest effect; symptom aid)
Hypoglossal nerve stimulation (HNS)	~70–85% in indicated patients
Maxillomandibular advancement (MMA)	~85–90% in selected cases

[a]Success generally reported using Sher's criteria; some series also report AHI <10 or <5 as "near-cure" thresholds.

1.8.5 *Interpreting the Table*

- *UPPP* alone performs best in anatomically favorable palatal phenotypes and often underperforms when oropharyngeal lateral wall or retroglossal collapse is unaddressed.
- *BRP* and related lateralizing palatal techniques improve outcomes where lateral wall components contribute, with acceptable morbidity.
- *Tonsillectomy* can be highly effective in adults with true tonsillar hypertrophy, particularly at lower BMI and with minimal multilevel disease [12].
- *GA and tongue-base procedures* are typically integrated into *multilevel* plans when DISE shows tongue-base collapse.
- *HNS* yields durable improvements in appropriately selected CPAP-intolerant patients; exclusion of complete concentric palatal collapse (CCC) and adherence to device-specific criteria are key [105].
- *MMA* offers the most powerful and durable AHI reduction across severities in properly selected patients, with quality-of-life benefits that persist long-term [12].

1.8.5.1 Patient Selection: Who Benefits Most, and Why

The *single strongest determinant* of surgical success is *matching the procedure to the patient's collapse pattern*, which is most reliably identified with *DISE* in combination with careful awake examination. DISE characterizes *site* (palate, oropharyngeal lateral wall/tonsil, tongue base, epiglottis) and *pattern* (anteroposterior, lateral, concentric), and it helps *rule out poor candidates* for specific therapies (e.g., CCC when considering HNS). Beyond anatomy, *BMI*, *age*, *craniofacial morphology*, *comorbidity burden*, *motivation*, and *realistic expectations* shape outcomes.

Predictors of favorable outcome [105–108] consistently include: well-localized obstruction, lower BMI (commonly <35), younger age, favorable Friedman palate/tongue position, positive jaw-thrust (for mandibular or tongue-directed strategies), and adequate occlusion where skeletal surgery is contemplated. Conversely, diffuse multilevel collapse, CCC at the velum, morbid obesity, and poorly controlled cardiometabolic disease can attenuate benefits and raise risk.

1.8.6 Practical Selection Table

Domain	Favors success	Cautions/risks
Collapse mapping (DISE)	Single dominant site; AP palatal collapse; lateral wall component addressed; tongue-base collapse responsive to jaw-thrust	CCC at the velum; diffuse multilevel without plan; epiglottic collapse unrecognized
Body habitus	BMI <35; stable weight; engaged in weight loss [12]	BMI ≥35 with central adiposity; recent significant weight gain [12]
Craniofacial/occlusion	Retrognathia with correctable occlusion (MMA)	Limited advancement envelope; TMJ disease; malocclusion risk
Age/comorbidity	Younger, low cardiometabolic burden	Severe cardiopulmonary disease; poor peri-op reserve
Motivation/ expectations	Adherent to peri-op pathways; realistic targets	Device intolerance without willingness for alternative therapy

1.8.7 Role of DISE in Planning and Prognostication

DISE is now central to *phenotype-guided* OSA surgery. In addition to anatomic mapping, in-procedure *maneuvers*—jaw-thrust to simulate mandibular advancement, positional changes, chin lift—can predict response to oral appliances, palatal lateralization, or tongue-directed procedures. Identifying *CCC* steers clinicians away from HNS and toward palatal techniques that lateralize or expand the velopharyngeal inlet before considering neuromodulation. DISE also clarifies *epiglottic* behaviors (trapdoor vs. lateral “book-type”), which may require targeted solutions to avoid residual obstruction in otherwise well-executed multilevel plans.

1.8.7.1 Long-Term Considerations and Durability

Even well-selected patients can experience *attenuation of benefit* over time due to *weight gain*, *aging-related muscle tone changes*, or *new sites of collapse* that emerge as anatomy and control systems evolve. Follow-up should therefore include *symptoms*, *ESS/FOSQ*, and *objective testing* when indicated, as well as *reinforcement of weight management* and *sleep-health strategies*. Some patients will require *revision* or *combination therapy* (e.g., adding nasal surgery to enable PAP or oral appliance use; adding HNS after palatal lateralization in non-CCC phenotypes).

1.8.7.2 Safety and Reporting of Adverse Events

Safety profiles vary by procedure. UPPP/palatal operations may cause transient dysphagia or velopharyngeal symptoms; major bleeding is uncommon in experienced hands. Barbed pharyngoplasty series report acceptable, typically minor complications with careful technique [28, 104]. Tongue-base and skeletal procedures carry risks of sensory change, dental injury, malocclusion, or infection; these events are mitigated by meticulous planning and standardized perioperative pathways. For HNS, serious device-related adverse events are uncommon [34], with high long-term adherence and satisfaction in pivotal and registry cohorts.

1.8.7.3 Multidisciplinary Model and Composite Care

Best outcomes arise when surgery is delivered within a *multidisciplinary program* that integrates *PAP*, *oral appliances*, *weight management*, *sleep hygiene*, and *behavioral therapy*. Surgery may be (1) the *primary* path to physiologic control (e.g., MMA for severe, multilevel disease with craniofacial deficiency), (2) an *enabler* of first-line therapy (e.g., nasal surgery to transform PAP intolerance into adherence), or (3) a *component* of staged *multilevel* treatment.

1.9 PAP Therapy Primer for the Sleep Surgeon

Liang Chye GohChee Kuan Wong, and Ahmad Izuanuddin Ismail

1.9.1 Introduction

Positive airway pressure (PAP) therapy remains the *cornerstone of management* for obstructive sleep apnea (OSA), providing a noninvasive and highly effective means of preventing upper airway collapse during sleep. Since its introduction in the early 1980s, PAP has revolutionized the care of patients with sleep-disordered breathing by offering a therapy that is consistently effective across a broad range of phenotypes and severities [6]. Yet despite its status as first-line therapy, real-world outcomes reveal that *adherence remains a major limitation*, with reported long-term compliance rates hovering between 50% and 70% [109]. For sleep surgeons, understanding PAP adherence is essential for setting realistic expectations and deciding when surgery is indicated.:

1.9.1.1 Why PAP Matters to the Surgeon

Historically, surgery and PAP were sometimes viewed as competing strategies. However, modern sleep medicine recognizes them as *complementary tools* rather than alternatives. For many patients, surgery does not eliminate the need for PAP but instead *facilitates its use* by reducing therapeutic pressure requirements, improving comfort, and alleviating nasal or oropharyngeal resistance that interferes with mask tolerance. Conversely, PAP can serve as a bridge before surgery, as a safety net after incomplete surgical response, and as a risk-reduction measure in the perioperative period [110].

The surgeon's perspective is therefore critical. Surgical interventions must be placed in the context of PAP efficacy, limitations, and patient goals. A well-informed surgeon is better equipped to identify patients who may benefit most from surgical modification of the airway, while ensuring that PAP remains an accessible and optimized option for those in whom surgery alone may not be sufficient.

1.9.2 Principles of PAP Therapy

Positive airway pressure (PAP) therapy is the *gold-standard treatment* for obstructive sleep apnea (OSA), with decades of evidence demonstrating robust efficacy across a wide spectrum of disease severities [6]. By delivering a column of pressurized air through a mask interface, PAP acts as a *pneumatic splint* that prevents dynamic collapse of the upper airway during sleep [111]. This stabilizes airflow, reduces apneic and hypopneic events, normalizes oxygen saturation, and restores continuity of sleep.

1.9.2.1 Mechanism of Action (Fig. 1.16)

PAP works through a straightforward but powerful mechanism: it delivers a continuous or variable stream of positive pressure to the upper airway, acting as a *pneumatic splint* that prevents pharyngeal collapse. By maintaining airway patency

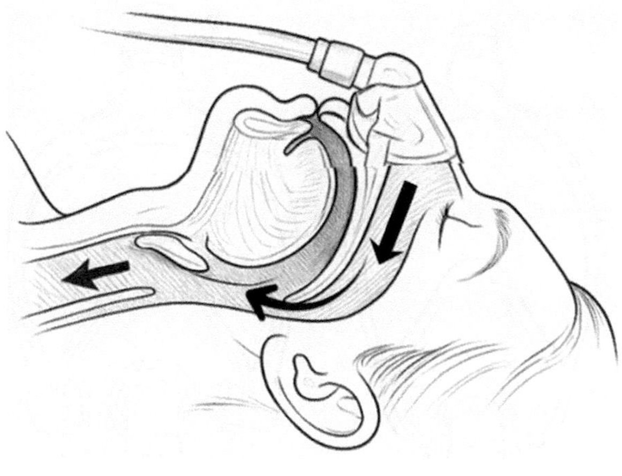

Fig. 1.16 Illustration showing CPAP acting as a pneumatic splint to keep the upper airway patent during sleep

throughout the respiratory cycle, PAP normalizes oxygen saturation, reduces arousals, and restores sleep continuity [111]. These physiologic effects translate into substantial improvements in daytime sleepiness, cognitive function, quality of life, and cardiovascular outcomes [112].

Different modalities exist, including *continuous PAP (CPAP)*, *auto-titrating PAP (APAP)*, and *bilevel PAP (BiPAP/BPAP)*, as well as advanced modes such as *adaptive servo-ventilation (ASV)* for central or complex sleep apnea. Each has specific indications and tolerability considerations, but the overarching principle remains consistent: by splinting the airway open, PAP neutralizes the pathophysiology of OSA at its most fundamental level.

1.9.2.2 Modes of PAP Therapy

Several modalities exist, tailored to patient needs and specific pathophysiologic features:

- *Continuous positive airway pressure (CPAP):* Delivers a fixed, continuous pressure throughout the respiratory cycle. It remains the most studied and widely prescribed modality. The main disadvantages to fixed pressure CPAP is the variability of pressure in different stages of sleep, body position, and other variabilities like nasal congestion.
- *Auto-titrating PAP (APAP):* Adjusts pressure automatically in response to detected events, flow limitation, or snoring. APAP is particularly useful for patients with variable pressure requirements, including positional or REM-predominant OSA [112].
- *Bilevel PAP (BiPAP/BPAP):* Provides a higher pressure during inspiration (IPAP) and lower pressure during expiration (EPAP), improving comfort in patients intolerant of fixed CPAP, those with hypoventilation syndromes, or patients

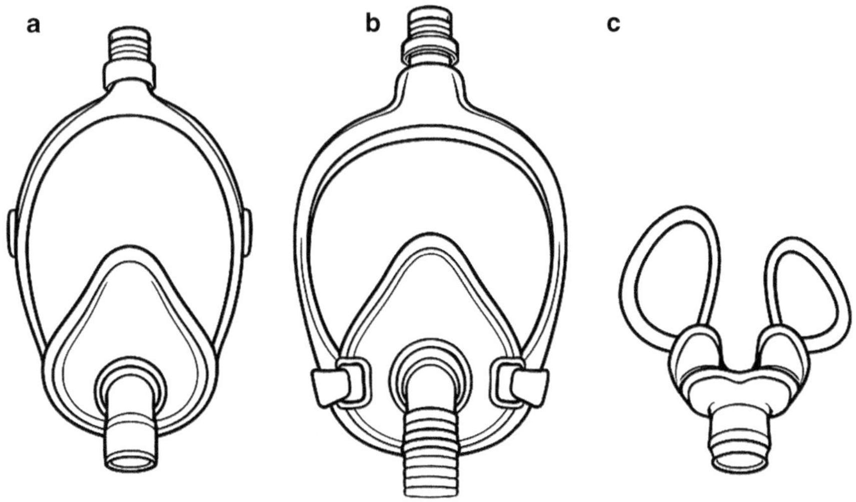

Fig. 1.17 Figure showing tree common mask interface designs used in most CPAPs in the market: (**a**) nasal mask, (**b**) full-face mask, (**c**) nasal pillow

requiring high pressures. Some bilevel PAP also includes backup respiratory rates to ensure minimum respiratory rates are achieved.

- *Adaptive servo-ventilation (ASV):* A more advanced mode designed to treat central sleep apnea and Cheyne–Stokes respiration by dynamically adjusting inspiratory support and backup rate.

1.9.2.3 Interfaces and Delivery Systems (Fig. 1.17)

PAP effectiveness depends not only on the device mode but also on the *mask interface*. Options include:

- *Nasal masks*, which are often most comfortable and associated with better adherence.
- *Nasal pillows*, which are minimally obtrusive and useful in patients with claustrophobia or facial hair.
- *Oronasal (full-face) masks*, required for mouth breathers but often linked to higher leak rates, higher required pressures, and lower adherence [113].

Humidification and heated tubing are additional adjuncts that improve comfort by reducing dryness, congestion, and mucosal irritation, thereby enhancing long-term tolerance.

1.9.3 Indications and Goals of PAP Therapy

1.9.3.1 First-Line Therapy in OSA

PAP therapy remains the *first-line treatment for moderate to severe OSA* across virtually all international guidelines [110]. Its efficacy in eliminating apneas and hypopneas, improving oxygen saturation, and normalizing sleep architecture has been consistently demonstrated in randomized controlled trials. For patients with *mild OSA*, PAP may be indicated if symptoms such as excessive daytime sleepiness, impaired cognition, or cardiovascular comorbidities are present.

The *primary goals* of PAP therapy are to:

1. *Stabilize the upper airway* during sleep by splinting it open with positive pressure.
2. *Restore restorative sleep* by reducing arousals and improving sleep efficiency.
3. *Improve daytime function* by alleviating sleepiness, fatigue, and neurocognitive impairment.
4. *Mitigate long-term health risks*, including cardiovascular disease, metabolic dysfunction, and accident risk [109].

1.9.3.2 PAP in Perioperative and Surgical Contexts

For the sleep surgeon, PAP carries additional significance beyond its role as a primary therapy. It is a *critical adjunct in perioperative management*, particularly in patients undergoing airway or bariatric surgery. Preoperative use of PAP reduces hypoxemia risk, improves blood pressure control, and lowers perioperative complications [114]. Postoperatively, resumption of PAP provides a safety net while surgical edema and healing may transiently exacerbate obstruction.

Furthermore, PAP serves as a *bridge to surgery* in patients with severe OSA who require stabilization before undergoing definitive operative interventions.

1.9.3.3 When PAP Remains Necessary After Surgery

Even after anatomically successful surgical interventions, many patients require ongoing PAP therapy. Factors such as *residual collapse at untreated sites, obesity, positional OSA, or REM-related vulnerability* can limit the durability of surgical results. In these patients, surgery may still confer benefit by reducing the required therapeutic pressure, enabling a switch from an oronasal to nasal mask, or improving comfort—thereby *transforming PAP from intolerable to sustainable*.

1.9.3.4 Expanding Indications Beyond OSA

While OSA remains the primary indication, PAP therapy also plays an important role in other sleep-related breathing disorders:

- *Central sleep apnea (CSA):* treated with adaptive servo-ventilation (ASV) or bilevel PAP with backup rate.
- *Hypoventilation syndromes*: managed with bilevel PAP providing ventilatory support.
- *Overlap syndromes (OSA with COPD or obesity hypoventilation):* where PAP improves both ventilation and oxygenation [115].

1.9.4 Barriers to PAP Success

Despite its proven efficacy, PAP therapy is limited in practice by challenges of *adherence, tolerance, and comfort*. Studies consistently show that up to 30–50% of patients prescribed PAP either abandon therapy within the first year or use it for less than the recommended 4 h/night [109]. For the sleep surgeon, understanding these barriers is essential, because many are *anatomically or surgically modifiable*.

1.9.4.1 Interface-Related Barriers

The *mask interface* is the most immediate determinant of adherence. Poorly fitted masks can cause:

- *Air leaks*, leading to noise, arousals, or inadequate pressure delivery.
- *Discomfort or pressure sores*, especially on the nasal bridge or around the mouth.
- *Claustrophobia or anxiety*, particularly with full-face masks.

Nasal masks and nasal pillow interfaces are generally associated with better comfort and adherence than oronasal masks, but they depend on adequate nasal airflow [116]. Patients with chronic nasal obstruction often default to oronasal masks, which are linked to *higher required pressures, greater leak, and worse compliance* [113].

1.9.4.2 Upper Airway and Nasal Resistance

Nasal obstruction is one of the most common reasons for PAP intolerance. Causes include:

- Structural issues (e.g., deviated septum, turbinate hypertrophy, nasal valve collapse).
- Mucosal disease (e.g., allergic rhinitis, chronic rhinosinusitis).
- Postoperative edema or scarring in multilevel surgery patients.

Elevated *nasal resistance* increases the therapeutic pressures needed to splint the airway and contributes to mouth breathing and oronasal mask dependence. Importantly, several studies demonstrate that reducing nasal resistance surgically (e.g., septoplasty, turbinate reduction) not only improves comfort but also *lowers optimal CPAP pressure requirements* [117].

1.9.4.3 Pressure-Related Intolerance

Even with appropriate interfaces, some patients find PAP intolerable due to:

- *Excessive therapeutic pressures*, especially >15 cm H_2O.
- *Aerophagia* (swallowing of air), leading to bloating and reflux symptoms.
- *Exhalation difficulty*, particularly with fixed-pressure CPAP.

Auto-titrating PAP (APAP) or bilevel PAP (BiPAP) can mitigate some of these issues by tailoring pressure delivery. However, in select patients, surgical reduction of anatomical obstruction can reduce required pressures, transforming PAP from intolerable to sustainable.

1.9.4.4 Behavioral and Psychosocial Factors

Other important barriers include:

- *Lack of symptom perception* (e.g., minimally symptomatic patients prescribed PAP for cardiovascular risk reduction).
- *Psychological factors*, such as anxiety, depression, or perceived stigma associated with PAP use.
- *Poor education or inadequate follow-up*, leading to frustration and discontinuation.

While these are not directly surgical issues, the surgeon's ability to *counsel and reinforce the importance of PAP* plays an important role in long-term success.

1.9.5 How Surgery and PAP Interact

Far from being competing therapies, *surgery and PAP are complementary strategies* in the management of obstructive sleep apnea (OSA). The modern view is that surgery may enhance the effectiveness and tolerability of PAP, while PAP remains an important safety net before, during, and after surgical treatment. Understanding this interplay is crucial for the sleep surgeon to position operative interventions appropriately within the broader care pathway.

1.9.5.1 Surgery as a Facilitator of PAP

One of the most important roles of surgery is to *improve PAP tolerance*. Patients with severe nasal obstruction, tonsillar hypertrophy, or redundant soft tissue often require higher PAP pressures, which can reduce adherence and increase side effects such as aerophagia or mask leak. Surgical correction of these anatomic impediments can:

- *Reduce therapeutic pressures*, sometimes by 2–3 cm H_2O, improving comfort and tolerance [6].
- *Enable use of nasal masks* instead of oronasal interfaces, thereby reducing leak and enhancing adherence [109].
- *Increase nightly adherence*, transforming partial or nonusers into consistent PAP users after nasal or oropharyngeal surgery.

Thus, surgery may not eliminate the need for PAP but can shift patients from "PAP failure" to "PAP success."

1.9.5.2 Adjunctive and Combined Approaches

In patients with severe or multilevel disease, surgery and PAP may function best in *combination*. For example:

- A patient with large tonsils may benefit from tonsillectomy, reducing obstruction and lowering required pressures, yet still require PAP for residual collapse.
- Bariatric surgery may reduce weight and improve airway patency, but PAP is often continued postoperatively to address persistent OSA until weight loss stabilizes.
- In patients with complex anatomy, partial surgical improvement may allow PAP to be delivered at pressures that were previously intolerable.

This *combined approach* reflects a pragmatic, patient-centered strategy that maximizes overall effectiveness.

1.9.5.3 When PAP Remains Necessary Post-surgery

Even after technically successful surgery, many patients continue to demonstrate *residual OSA*. Contributors include obesity, retroglossal collapse, positional vulnerability, or REM-related exacerbation. In such cases, PAP remains an important tool to ensure complete disease control. Importantly, surgery may reduce the *physiologic burden of collapse*, making subsequent PAP use more effective and better tolerated.

1.9.5.4 PAP in the Perioperative Setting

PAP also plays a protective role in the *perioperative period*. Patients with untreated or severe OSA face increased risk of postoperative hypoxemia, arrhythmias, and cardiopulmonary complications. Using PAP preoperatively stabilizes patients and reduces risk during anesthesia and recovery [114]. Postoperatively, PAP can serve as a *bridge therapy*, supporting airway patency while tissues heal and before surgical effects are fully realized.

1.9.6 PAP Titration and Monitoring

For PAP therapy to achieve its full potential, pressures must be appropriately *titrated and monitored* over time. While titration protocols are often the responsibility of sleep physicians and technologists, the sleep surgeon should have a working knowledge of these principles to contextualize surgical decisions, interpret PAP data, and counsel patients effectively.

1.9.6.1 Titration Studies

Polysomnographic PAP titration remains the gold standard for determining the optimal therapeutic pressure. During a dedicated sleep laboratory study, pressure is gradually increased until apneas, hypopneas, snoring, and desaturations are eliminated across all sleep stages and positions [118]. When in-lab titration is not feasible, *auto-titrating PAP (APAP)* devices can provide practical, real-world estimates of required pressures by adjusting dynamically in response to flow limitation, snoring, and events [112].

In patients undergoing surgery, titration studies are especially useful:

- *Preoperatively*, they establish baseline pressure needs and highlight patients with very high requirements who may struggle with tolerance.
- *Postoperatively*, repeat titration can determine whether surgical modification of the airway has reduced pressure requirements or unmasked positional or stage-dependent vulnerabilities.

1.9.6.2 Monitoring Effectiveness

PAP therapy is unique in that it produces large amounts of *objective adherence and efficacy data*. Modern devices track nightly usage, residual events, leak, and pressure profiles, which can be downloaded during clinic visits or transmitted via telemonitoring systems. For the surgeon, familiarity with these metrics is valuable:

- *Usage (hours/night):* The conventional threshold for adherence is ≥4 h/night on ≥70% of nights, though greater usage is associated with more robust symptom and cardiovascular benefit [109].
- *Residual AHI:* Even on PAP, some patients continue to demonstrate elevated AHI due to leak, suboptimal pressure, or central events. Recognizing this helps in differentiating PAP failure from residual anatomic obstruction.
- *Leak:* High leak rates suggest mask/interface problems or untreated nasal obstruction—issues often modifiable by surgical or medical intervention.

1.9.6.3 Longitudinal Monitoring

OSA is a *chronic condition* that can evolve with weight change, aging, or new comorbidities. Accordingly, *ongoing monitoring* is essential. Best practice includes reassessing patients at 3–6 months after PAP initiation, then annually, with interim reviews if symptoms recur. Post-surgical patients should be reevaluated once healing is complete, typically 2–3 months postoperatively, to determine whether PAP pressures or mask interfaces require adjustment. Ongoing monitoring is also required to tackle comorbidities associated with OSA.

1.9.7 The Surgeon's Role in PAP Optimization

Although PAP therapy is usually prescribed and managed by sleep physicians, the *sleep surgeon plays a pivotal role* in optimizing its success. Understanding the barriers to adherence, addressing anatomic impediments, and providing patient-centered counseling are critical contributions that surgeons can make within the multidisciplinary team.

1.9.7.1 Counseling and Patient Education

Many patients approach surgery believing that it will replace PAP entirely. It is therefore essential for surgeons to *set realistic expectations*: while surgery can improve or even resolve OSA in selected patients, it is just as often used to *facilitate ongoing PAP therapy*. Preoperative discussions should emphasize that:

- Surgery may reduce required pressures and improve tolerance, even if PAP remains necessary.
- PAP remains the safest and most reliable therapy for severe OSA, particularly in obese patients.
- Post-surgical reevaluation is important to reassess the role of PAP, rather than assuming discontinuation.

This counseling helps foster *shared decision-making*, ensuring patients understand both the benefits and limitations of surgery within the broader context of OSA care [110].

1.9.7.2 Addressing Nasal and Upper Airway Barriers

Anatomic obstruction is one of the most important contributors to PAP intolerance. The surgeon can directly intervene in cases of:

- *Nasal obstruction:* Septoplasty, turbinate reduction, nasal valve repair, and adenoidectomy in children can significantly reduce nasal resistance, lower PAP pressures, and improve mask tolerance [119].
- *Tonsillar hypertrophy:* Tonsillectomy reduces lateral wall crowding and can improve both airway patency and PAP adherence.
- *Palatal or tongue-base obstruction:* While surgical correction may not eliminate the need for PAP, reducing bulk or collapse at these levels can improve PAP delivery and comfort.

These procedures shift PAP therapy from being intolerable to feasible, effectively transforming nonadherent patients into successful long-term users.

1.9.7.3 Perioperative Considerations

In the perioperative setting, surgeons should integrate PAP into the care plan:

- *Preoperatively*, PAP reduces hypoxemia and cardiopulmonary risk in patients with severe OSA undergoing surgery.
- *Postoperatively*, PAP should be resumed as soon as feasible to stabilize the airway, though timing may vary depending on surgical site and risk of air leak or bleeding. For example, PAP may be delayed or modified after pharyngeal or sinonasal procedures, requiring close collaboration with anesthesiology and sleep medicine [114].
- *Bridging therapy:* In high-risk patients awaiting surgery, PAP provides an essential safety net, reducing perioperative morbidity and mortality.

1.9.7.4 Multidisciplinary Collaboration

Finally, the sleep surgeon's role extends beyond anatomy. By collaborating closely with *sleep physicians, respiratory therapists, and technologists*, surgeons can:

- Interpret PAP download data in the context of surgical anatomy.
- Identify patients who would benefit from re-titration after surgery.
- Provide feedback on how structural interventions have impacted PAP efficacy and tolerance.

This multidisciplinary model not only enhances outcomes but also reinforces the concept of *integrated, phenotype-guided OSA management*.

1.9.8 Future Directions in PAP Therapy

PAP devices are now smaller, more adaptive, and increasingly integrated with remote monitoring. For the sleep surgeon, awareness of these developments is important, as they will increasingly shape how PAP interacts with surgical pathways and patient care in the coming decades.

1.9.8.1 Technological Innovations

Modern PAP devices are smaller, quieter, and more adaptive than earlier generations. Current trends include:

- *Algorithm-driven pressure adjustment:* Next-generation auto-PAP systems employ sophisticated flow and vibration sensors to distinguish obstructive from central events, tailoring therapy in real time with greater accuracy [120].
- *Enhanced comfort features:* Expiratory pressure relief, heated humidification, and advanced leak compensation improve patient tolerance and adherence.
- *Mask technology:* Advances in lightweight, low-profile interfaces and 3D scanning for custom-fitted masks aim to reduce leak and pressure sores, which are common causes of discontinuation.

These innovations reflect a trend toward *making PAP less intrusive and more user-friendly*, potentially expanding its long-term acceptability.

1.9.8.2 Telemonitoring and Remote Care

One of the most transformative changes in recent years is the integration of *telemonitoring platforms*. Many PAP devices now include built-in wireless connectivity, allowing clinicians to track nightly adherence, residual AHI, and leak patterns remotely. Benefits include:

- *Early intervention:* Rapid identification of patients with poor adherence or residual events.
- *Improved engagement:* Patients can review their own usage data through mobile apps, promoting self-management.
- *Population health management:* Clinics can monitor large patient cohorts efficiently, flagging those at risk of dropout [121].

For surgeons, telemonitoring provides an opportunity to evaluate how surgical interventions influence PAP parameters in real time, adding objective feedback to the perioperative process.

1.9.8.3 Personalized Therapy and Endotypes

The future of PAP is also moving toward *precision medicine*. Recognition of distinct OSA endotypes—such as high loop gain, low arousal threshold, or poor dilator muscle responsiveness—suggests that PAP may be optimized differently across subgroups. Emerging approaches include:

- *Targeted pressure profiles* for patients with REM- or supine-predominant OSA.
- *Hybrid therapies* (e.g., combining mandibular advancement with PAP at lower pressures).
- *Surgery + PAP combinations* guided by endotyping, where surgical interventions reduce collapse at specific sites while PAP addresses residual instability [41].

This approach has direct implications for the surgeon: surgical planning will increasingly be informed by how PAP interacts with each patient's phenotype.

1.9.8.4 PAP-NAP as a Strategy to Improve Adherence

An innovative approach to addressing PAP intolerance is the *PAP-NAP*—a daytime, abbreviated sleep laboratory session designed to acclimatize patients to therapy. During a PAP-NAP, patients undergo relaxation training, mask fitting, and brief exposure to PAP under polysomnographic or technologist supervision. This structured environment allows patients to confront anxieties, troubleshoot discomfort, and receive immediate coaching on mask use and breathing techniques. Evidence suggests that PAP-NAP sessions can significantly improve subsequent adherence in patients with initial resistance or anxiety toward PAP initiation, especially those reporting claustrophobia, insomnia, or pressure intolerance [122]. By reframing PAP exposure as a therapeutic trial rather than a burdensome prescription, the PAP-NAP empowers patients, reduces barriers, and fosters long-term engagement with therapy.

1.9.8.5 Integration with Digital Health and AI

Artificial intelligence (AI) and digital health integration hold promise for the *next generation of PAP care*. Machine learning algorithms are being developed to predict adherence risk, identify patients who would benefit from early surgical referral, and personalize PAP titration in real time. Combined with wearable devices that track sleep quality and cardiorespiratory metrics, these tools could create a seamless, data-driven continuum of care [123].

1.10 Sleep Surgery and Obesity Management

Wei Jin Wong and Liang Chye Goh

1.10.1 Introduction

Obstructive sleep apnea (OSA) is a highly prevalent disorder with far-reaching medical, social, and economic implications. Obesity is the most important modifiable risk factor for OSA severity. Excess weight not only increases the likelihood of developing OSA but also amplifies its progression and complicates its management [124].

The relationship between obesity and OSA is multifactorial. Deposition of adipose tissue in the parapharyngeal fat pads and tongue base narrows the upper airway lumen, while central obesity reduces lung volumes and impairs caudal traction, leading to greater pharyngeal collapsibility [125]. Obesity also interacts with ventilatory control mechanisms, promoting instability of breathing during sleep. These pathophysiological changes explain why patients with obesity often demonstrate multilevel collapse on drug-induced sleep endoscopy (DISE), including retropalatal, retrolingual, and lateral pharyngeal wall involvement [126].

From a surgical perspective, obesity presents unique challenges. Patients with a high body mass index (BMI) are known to have lower surgical success rates compared to nonobese counterparts, regardless of whether the intervention targets the palate, tongue base, or hypopharynx. Despite this, obese patients frequently experience the greatest symptomatic burden and are among the most motivated to seek alternatives when conservative therapies, such as continuous positive airway pressure (CPAP), are not tolerated or effective.

Weight loss is therefore central to the long-term care of obese OSA patients. Even modest reductions in body weight have been shown to improve Apnea–Hypopnea Index (AHI), oxygenation, and symptoms of daytime sleepiness. Lifestyle modification and pharmacological therapy, including the use of glucagon-like peptide-1 (GIP/GLP-1) receptor agonists, offer pathways to weight reduction and metabolic improvement. For those with severe obesity, bariatric surgery remains the most effective strategy, consistently producing substantial and sustained improvements in both body weight and OSA severity [127]. However, residual OSA is common after bariatric procedures, reinforcing the need for a combined and multidisciplinary approach to care.

1.10.2 Epidemiology and Clinical Burden

Obstructive sleep apnea (OSA) is a global health problem with significant implications for public health and clinical practice. Among its many risk factors, obesity stands out as the most consistent and modifiable determinant of disease prevalence and severity. Large epidemiological studies estimate that OSA affects up to one billion individuals worldwide, with higher rates in populations experiencing rising trends in overweight and obesity [128]. The prevalence of OSA in the general adult population is reported to range from 9% to 38%, but this figure increases dramatically in individuals with obesity, reaching over 70% in those with morbid obesity [129].

The relationship between body weight and OSA is dose dependent. A 10% increase in weight has been shown to increase the Apnea–Hypopnea Index (AHI) by more than 30%, while a similar degree of weight loss can reduce the severity of OSA by a comparable margin [130]. This association reflects the direct impact of adiposity on upper airway structure and function. Obese individuals are more likely to demonstrate multilevel airway obstruction, tongue-base enlargement, and compromised pharyngeal patency. These anatomical factors are compounded by obesity-related reductions in lung volumes, altered ventilatory control, and systemic inflammation, which collectively amplify the risk of sleep-disordered breathing.

The clinical burden of OSA in obese patients extends beyond disturbed sleep. Recurrent nocturnal hypoxemia and sleep fragmentation contribute to excessive daytime sleepiness, impaired neurocognitive function, mood disturbances, and reduced quality of life. More importantly, untreated OSA is strongly associated with cardiovascular and metabolic comorbidities that disproportionately affect obese individuals. Hypertension, atrial fibrillation, coronary artery disease, stroke, type 2 diabetes, and nonalcoholic fatty liver disease are all more prevalent in this group [131]. The combination of obesity, OSA, and metabolic dysfunction creates a vicious cycle that accelerates morbidity and increases mortality risk.

The economic costs are also substantial. Patients with untreated OSA have higher rates of workplace absenteeism, reduced productivity, and a two- to seven-fold increased risk of motor vehicle accidents. Health-care costs in OSA patients are estimated to be nearly double compared to those without the condition, largely due to the management of associated cardiovascular and metabolic complications. In countries where obesity prevalence is rising rapidly, OSA is expected to become an even greater driver of health-care expenditure.

From a surgical standpoint, these epidemiological realities highlight the importance of careful patient selection and comprehensive management strategies. While surgical interventions can alleviate airway obstruction, addressing the underlying burden of obesity remains essential to long-term outcomes. For the sleep surgeon, understanding the magnitude of OSA in obese populations underscores the need for multidisciplinary collaboration with physicians in sleep medicine, endocrinology, and bariatric surgery to provide effective, durable solutions for this complex patient group.

1.10.3 Impact of Obesity on Sleep Surgery (Fig. 1.18)

Obesity has a profound influence on the outcomes of sleep surgery, shaping not only the anatomical landscape encountered by the surgeon but also the likelihood of achieving long-term therapeutic success. In general, surgical interventions for

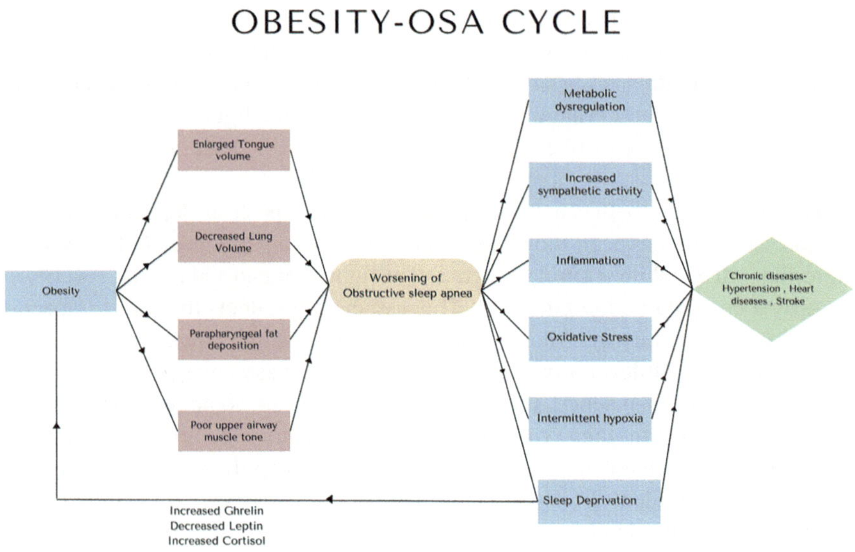

Fig. 1.18 Flow chart demonstrating the vicious cycle of obesity and obstructive sleep apnea

obstructive sleep apnea (OSA) demonstrate lower efficacy in patients with obesity compared to their nonobese counterparts. This observation has been consistent across procedures such as uvulopalatopharyngoplasty (UPPP), tongue-base reduction, and even more advanced multilevel or robotic-assisted surgeries [104].

One of the most important reasons for diminished outcomes lies in the *multilevel nature of obstruction* in obese patients. Drug-induced sleep endoscopy (DISE) frequently reveals collapse occurring at multiple sites, particularly at the retropalatal and retrolingual levels, and often involving lateral pharyngeal wall collapse [12]. This complexity makes single-level surgery less effective, necessitating staged or combined multilevel procedures. Even so, the magnitude of AHI reduction tends to be less dramatic in patients with higher body mass index (BMI).

Several studies have established BMI as an independent predictor of surgical success. Patients with BMI below 30 kg/m^2 typically achieve higher rates of surgical response, while those with BMI above 35 kg/m^2 experience significantly lower success and cure rates. For example, classic UPPP studies have demonstrated success rates exceeding 50% in nonobese patients, but this figure can drop below 30% in obese populations [85, 104]. Similarly, tongue base and hypopharyngeal procedures face greater technical difficulty in obese patients due to enlarged soft-tissue volume, reduced surgical exposure, and higher rates of persistent obstruction.

Beyond efficacy, obesity also contributes to *increased perioperative risks*. Anesthetic management is often more challenging due to a difficult airway, reduced pulmonary reserve, and increased risk of desaturation during induction and emergence. Wound healing complications, including infection and poor tissue recovery, are more frequent in obese patients, particularly in those with metabolic syndrome or diabetes. Additionally, these patients may require prolonged postoperative monitoring, with some necessitating admission to high-dependency or intensive care units to ensure airway safety.

Despite these challenges, surgery remains a reasonable option for selected obese patients, particularly those who are unable or unwilling to tolerate CPAP therapy. Importantly, outcomes in this group should be framed in terms of *symptom improvement and comorbidity reduction* rather than absolute cure. For instance, even modest reductions in AHI may translate into meaningful improvements in daytime sleepiness, blood pressure control, and overall quality of life [133]. This reframing allows for realistic expectations and shared decision-making between patient and surgeon.

A growing body of evidence also suggests that *combining weight management strategies with surgery* yields better long-term outcomes. Patients who undergo bariatric surgery or achieve significant weight loss after airway procedures demonstrate improved surgical durability and lower recurrence of OSA. In this context, sleep surgery should not be viewed as a stand-alone solution but as one component of a multidisciplinary strategy that addresses both airway anatomy and systemic metabolic risk.

Ultimately, obesity does not preclude sleep surgery but rather demands a nuanced and individualized approach. Careful patient selection, multidisciplinary collaboration, and clear counseling on expectations are critical to optimizing outcomes in this challenging but highly prevalent patient population.

1.10.4 Weight Loss as a Therapeutic Strategy

Weight loss represents one of the most effective nonsurgical approaches to improving obstructive sleep apnea (OSA), particularly in individuals where obesity is a primary contributing factor. Because excess body weight contributes to upper airway narrowing, reduced lung volumes, and heightened collapsibility of the pharyngeal walls, weight reduction directly addresses the underlying pathophysiology. Unlike other treatment modalities, weight loss offers broad systemic benefits, improving not only sleep-disordered breathing but also cardiovascular and metabolic health [125].

Several studies have demonstrated a clear and dose-dependent relationship between weight change and Apnea–Hypopnea Index (AHI). A 10% reduction in body weight can decrease AHI by up to 25–30%, while more substantial weight loss has the potential to normalize breathing in some individuals with mild to moderate OSA [130]. The magnitude of improvement is often greatest in patients with higher baseline BMI, reflecting the central role of adiposity in disease severity. Importantly, even in cases where OSA is not fully resolved, weight reduction generally leads to meaningful improvements in daytime sleepiness, blood pressure, and overall quality of life.

1. *Lifestyle and behavioral interventions*

   (a) Lifestyle modification remains the cornerstone of weight management. Structured programs that combine dietary counseling, caloric restriction, and regular exercise have been shown to reduce both weight and OSA severity. However, sustaining long-term weight loss through lifestyle changes alone is notoriously difficult, with high rates of weight regain. Individuals who undergo periods of weight loss and regain, followed by weight loss again ("weight cycling") are more prone to develop metabolic syndrome. Hence, an experienced and dedicated dietitian, physiotherapist, psychologist, and sports medicine specialist are crucial to weight-loss success where lifestyle changes are the therapy of choice. Despite this limitation, lifestyle interventions are strongly recommended as a first-line therapy due to their safety, accessibility, and additional health benefits.

2. *Pharmacological therapy*

   (a) The growing availability of anti-obesity medications has expanded therapeutic options for OSA patients who struggle with weight reduction. Glucagon-like peptide-1 (GLP-1) receptor agonists such as liraglutide and semaglutide have demonstrated significant weight loss in randomized clinical trials, with associated reductions in AHI [133] These agents act by delaying gastric emptying, enhancing satiety, and improving insulin sensitivity. Other agents, such as bupropion–naltrexone or phentermine–topiramate, may also play a role in selected patients. While pharmacotherapy is not a cure for OSA, it can be an important adjunct to improve surgical candidacy or augment the effects of lifestyle modification.

3. *Endoscopic procedures*

   (a) The intragastric balloon has added a new dimension in the armamentarium of treatment for the obesity specialist. Endoscopic ballons offer a safe, simple, and reversible adjunct to weight loss therapies.
   (b) Deployed via either oro-gastroscopy or as a swallowable device, intragastric balloons are then filled with 450–750 cc of saline, occupying the fundus of the stomach and creating a sensation of early satiety. Individuals who have intragastric balloons deployed eat less due to the volume-occupying balloon, and therefore lose weight by entering a calorie-deficit stage.
   (c) More recently, endoscopic sleeve gastroplasty (ESG) has gained popularity. An endoscopic technique, not requiring surgery, with a specialized endoscopic suturing device, ESG reduces gastric volume in a similar manner to traditional sleeve gastrectomy, thus individuals who have the procedure done experience satiety earlier in a manner similar to the intragastric balloon or sleeve gastrectomy. However, as there is no volume-occupying implant, the side effects of ESG are significantly less than the intragastric balloon.
   (d) Long term results on the efficacy of ESG compared to traditional bariatric surgery are pending; however, initial data shows a total weight loss of approximately 15% after ESG, for at least 2 years.

4. *Bariatric surgery as a weight loss strategy*

   (a) For patients with severe obesity, bariatric surgery remains the most effective method of achieving sustained weight reduction. Procedures such as the sleeve gastrectomy, Roux-en-Y gastric bypass, one-anastomosis gastric bypass, and more recently, the so-called sleeve-plus procedures, have been shown to reduce AHI and improve oxygen saturation, often with long-term durability [110].
   (b) The effects of bariatric surgery go far beyond weight loss, individuals who have surgery often experience resolution of metabolic syndrome (diabetes, hypertension, and dyslipidemia), as well as improvement in musculoskeletal-related issues such as osteoarthritis of the joints. In fact, many individuals who were previously indicated for knee or hip replacements do not have their respective orthopedic procedure done after bariatric surgery as the symptom resolution can be dramatic. Bariatric surgery has also been recognized as a bridge to transplant surgery, in particular renal transplant, as the reduction in weight reduces not only the technical complexity of implanting a kidney but also the metabolic burden of the newly implanted kidney.
   (c) The same applies to the donor, who will have to survive with just one kidney. Thus, reducing the metabolic burden on the single kidney in a living-related donor is a paramount importance. With regards to sleep apnea, symptom resolution is directly related to the reduction of soft tissue around the neck, reducing airway collapse in the supine position.
   (d) However, residual OSA is common, and many patients continue to require CPAP or airway-directed procedures postoperatively. This highlights the complementary rather than substitutive role of bariatric surgery in OSA management. The role of combined airway–bariatric surgery remains an area of research importance.

5. *Clinical integration*

   (a) For the sleep surgeon, encouraging weight loss should be an integral part of perioperative planning. Patients who achieve weight reduction prior to airway surgery often experience improved outcomes and lower recurrence rates. Similarly, postoperative weight management is critical to maintaining surgical success. Framing weight loss as a lifelong strategy rather than a short-term preoperative requirement helps align patient expectations and promotes sustainable health benefits.

1.10.4.1 Bariatric Surgery and Sleep Apnea (Figs. 1.19 and 1.20)

Bariatric surgery is the most effective intervention for the management of morbid obesity, producing significant and sustained weight reduction in patients who are unable to achieve meaningful results through lifestyle modification, pharmacotherapy, or endoscopic therapy. Given the strong link between obesity and obstructive sleep apnea (OSA), it is not surprising that bariatric surgery also exerts a marked

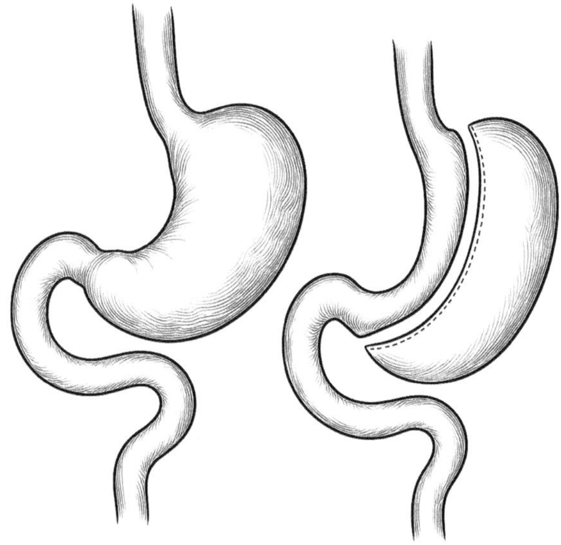

Fig. 1.19 Figure demonstrating a sleeve gastrectomy, an option for bariatric surgery

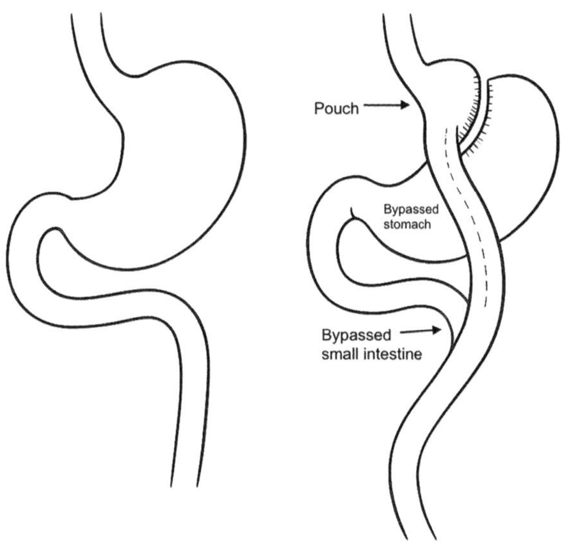

Fig. 1.20 Figure demonstrating a gastric bypass surgery, an option for bariatric surgery

effect on sleep-disordered breathing. For many patients with severe obesity, weight loss through surgical means represents the single most powerful tool to reduce the severity of OSA and its associated health risks.

- *Mechanisms of improvement*

  The benefits of bariatric surgery on OSA are multifactorial. Substantial weight reduction decreases adipose deposition in the parapharyngeal fat pads and tongue base, leading to improved airway caliber. Central obesity is reduced, which improves lung volumes and caudal traction, thereby lowering upper airway collapsibility. Beyond these mechanical effects, improvements in insulin sensitivity, systemic inflammation, and cardiovascular risk factors also contribute to better sleep quality and fewer apneic events [125].

- *Evidence of efficacy*
  - Multiple studies and meta-analyses have confirmed the positive impact of bariatric surgery on OSA. Average reductions in Apnea–Hypopnea Index (AHI) range from 50% to 70% following procedures such as Roux-en-Y gastric bypass and sleeve gastrectomy [127]. Many patients report dramatic improvements in symptoms such as snoring, daytime sleepiness, and fatigue within months of surgery. Importantly, weight loss achieved through surgery is generally more durable compared to lifestyle interventions alone, with long-term improvements in OSA severity observed up to 5 years postoperatively.
  - However, residual OSA is common even after significant weight loss. Studies suggest that while up to 75% of patients demonstrate improvement, only a minority achieve complete remission [127, 134]. Older age, severe baseline OSA, male sex, and craniofacial crowding are predictors of persistent disease despite surgery. This enforces the importance of follow-up sleep studies and ongoing management, as patients may still require CPAP therapy or targeted upper airway procedures.
- *Limitations and considerations*
  - Although bariatric surgery provides substantial benefits, it is not a stand-alone cure for OSA. Patients should be counseled preoperatively that while weight loss will likely improve their condition, many will continue to have residual sleep-disordered breathing. In addition, bariatric surgery carries inherent risks, including nutritional deficiencies, surgical complications, and long-term adherence to dietary modifications. These must be weighed carefully against expected benefits. Weight recidivism, typically 5 years after index bariatric surgery, remains a clinically relevant challenge.
- *Role in comprehensive care*
  - For the sleep surgeon, bariatric surgery should be viewed as a complementary therapy rather than a competing one. In patients with morbid obesity, referral to a bariatric team may significantly enhance long-term OSA outcomes. Eligibility thresholds vary by region and guideline framework: Western guidelines (ASMBS/IFSO 2022) recommend surgery for BMI $\geq$35 kg/m^2 regardless of comorbidities, or $\geq$30 kg/m^2 in the presence of metabolic disease; Asian and Malaysian MOH guidelines apply lower thresholds of $\geq$37.5 kg/m^2, or $\geq$32.5 kg/m^2 with comorbidities such as OSA or type 2 diabetes, reflecting the higher cardiometabolic risk observed at lower BMI in Asian populations. Clinicians should apply the criteria appropriate to their local guidelines and patient population. Referral to a bariatric team may significantly enhance long-term OSA outcomes. Combining bariatric surgery with

airway procedures—either staged or sequentially—can optimize results, especially in those with multilevel obstruction demonstrated on drug-induced sleep endoscopy. Ultimately, integrating bariatric surgery into the management plan highlights the importance of a multidisciplinary approach that addresses both the airway and the metabolic drivers of OSA.

- *Combined and staged surgical approaches*
  - Management of obstructive sleep apnea (OSA) in obese patients often requires more than one intervention. Because obesity contributes to multilevel airway collapse as well as systemic metabolic dysfunction, no single therapy is universally effective. For this reason, combined and staged surgical approaches have gained prominence as a way to maximize outcomes by addressing both the upper airway obstruction and the underlying obesity.
  - Obese patients frequently present with multilevel obstruction, including collapse at the soft palate, tongue base, and lateral pharyngeal walls. In such cases, single-level surgery—such as uvulopalatopharyngoplasty (UPPP)—is unlikely to provide sufficient improvement. Multilevel surgery performed in a single setting, or staged procedures tailored to findings on drug-induced sleep endoscopy (DISE), can yield superior results by addressing multiple points of collapse simultaneously [126].
  - At the same time, weight reduction remains essential for long-term disease control. Bariatric surgery has proven efficacy in reducing Apnea–Hypopnea Index (AHI), but complete remission of OSA is uncommon, particularly in those with severe baseline disease or craniofacial narrowing [135]. This creates an opportunity to combine bariatric surgery with targeted airway interventions. By treating both systemic and local contributors to OSA, combination strategies can provide durable improvements that exceed those achieved with either approach alone.

- *Sequential vs. simultaneous strategies*
  - Staged approaches are often favored, beginning with bariatric surgery to induce weight loss, followed by reassessment of residual OSA. In many cases, weight loss leads to partial improvement, after which airway surgery can be more effective due to reduced tissue volume and better surgical exposure. Alternatively, in patients with severe symptomatic OSA and high surgical risk, initial airway procedures may be necessary to stabilize breathing and facilitate safe bariatric surgery. Careful discussions with the patient, the anesthetic and intensive care teams, and the relevant surgical teams would be of upmost importance to achieve good, sustainable long-term outcomes.
  - Simultaneous approaches—performing bariatric surgery and airway surgery in a single operative session—are less common but may be considered in select patients. These require careful coordination between surgical teams and are generally reserved for highly motivated patients in specialized centers.

1.10.5 *Multidisciplinary Care and Perioperative Considerations*

Obese patients with obstructive sleep apnea (OSA) represent one of the most complex populations for surgical management. Their care requires a coordinated, multidisciplinary approach involving sleep physicians, surgeons, anesthesiologists, dietitians, and in many cases bariatric specialists. The success of surgical therapy in this group depends not only on the technical execution of airway procedures but also on comprehensive perioperative planning and long-term support.

- *Preoperative optimization*
  - Thorough preoperative evaluation is critical. Beyond standard assessment, patients should undergo drug-induced sleep endoscopy (DISE) to identify levels of obstruction, as obese individuals frequently exhibit multilevel collapse. Optimization of comorbid conditions—such as diabetes, hypertension, and dyslipidemia—is essential to reduce perioperative risk. In high-risk patients, initiating or reinforcing adherence to CPAP therapy prior to surgery can stabilize sleep-disordered breathing, reduce perioperative desaturation, and improve recovery [114].
  - Nutritional counseling and weight management strategies should also be initiated preoperatively. Even modest presurgical weight loss can improve anesthetic safety and postoperative outcomes. For patients with severe obesity, referral to bariatric specialists should be considered early in the treatment pathway.
- *Anesthetic challenges*
  - Obesity and OSA pose significant challenges to anesthetic management. Airway intubation can be difficult due to limited neck mobility, macroglossia, and excess soft tissue. Preoxygenation is particularly important, as reduced pulmonary reserve predisposes these patients to rapid desaturation. Intraoperatively, careful titration of sedatives and opioids is required, as these agents exacerbate upper airway collapsibility and depress ventilatory drive [136].
  - Regional anesthesia techniques may be preferable where applicable, but for airway procedures, general anesthesia is typically unavoidable. Anticipating potential complications—such as difficult mask ventilation or reintubation—is crucial, and appropriate equipment (e.g., fiberoptic intubation, video laryngoscopes) should be readily available.
- *Postoperative monitoring and care*
  - The immediate postoperative period is a vulnerable time for obese OSA patients. Residual anesthetics, opioids, and sedatives can worsen airway obstruction and hypoventilation. Extended monitoring in a high-dependency or intensive care setting is often recommended, especially for those with

severe OSA, morbid obesity, or multiple comorbidities. Early mobilization, head-of-bed elevation, and supplemental oxygen may reduce complications. Resuming CPAP therapy as soon as tolerated is strongly advised to prevent desaturation and promote airway stability [137].

- *Long-term multidisciplinary support*
  - Surgery alone rarely resolves OSA in obese patients. Long-term follow-up with sleep physicians, dietitians, and bariatric teams is necessary to monitor weight trends, assess for recurrence of symptoms, and reinforce adherence to CPAP or adjunctive therapies. The surgeon plays a vital role in this continuum, not only by performing targeted interventions but also by integrating surgical care into a broader framework of lifestyle and medical management.
- *Clinical perspective*
  - Perioperative planning for obese OSA patients should be proactive, not reactive. By working collaboratively across specialties, clinicians can reduce perioperative risk, improve surgical outcomes, and address the systemic drivers of disease. This team-based approach is the cornerstone of safe and effective surgical care in this challenging population.

1.10.6 Future Directions and Conclusion

Management of obesity-related OSA is changing, and future directions in management reflect both technological innovation and a broader, system-level approach to care. While traditional therapies such as CPAP, bariatric surgery, and airway surgery remain central, new strategies aim to personalize treatment, improve outcomes, and reduce the global burden of disease.

One promising area lies in *precision medicine*. Increasing evidence suggests that OSA is not a uniform disorder but a heterogeneous condition influenced by distinct anatomical, physiological, and metabolic phenotypes. For obese patients, this means moving beyond a "one-size-fits-all" strategy toward individualized treatment plans. Drug-induced sleep endoscopy (DISE) combined with imaging modalities such as dynamic MRI and computational modeling can help identify dominant sites of obstruction, guiding tailored surgical and medical therapies [126].

Another emerging frontier is the use of *pharmacological weight-loss agents*. Glucagon-like peptide-1 (GLP-1) receptor agonists and dual incretin mimetics are demonstrating dramatic and sustained weight reduction in obesity trials. Their role in OSA is under active investigation, with early results suggesting meaningful improvements in AHI and cardiometabolic outcomes [133]. As access to these agents expands, they may serve as a bridge or adjunct to surgery, improving both candidacy and long-term success.

Advances in bariatric and metabolic surgery are also reshaping the field. Less invasive procedures, including endoscopic sleeve gastroplasty and duodenal mucosal resurfacing, are being studied for their ability to achieve weight reduction with lower complication rates. These may offer alternatives for high-risk OSA patients who are not candidates for traditional bariatric surgery [136].

Technology will also play an increasing role in perioperative care. *Artificial intelligence (AI) and machine learning* are being applied to automate DISE video analysis, predict surgical outcomes, and stratify perioperative risk. Remote monitoring through wearable devices and telemedicine platforms is expected to become routine, enabling continuous assessment of treatment adherence and recurrence of symptoms [137].

Finally, there is growing recognition of the need for *integrated, multidisciplinary care models*. Obesity-related OSA is not solely a surgical or respiratory problem; it is a systemic disease requiring long-term engagement from sleep physicians, bariatric surgeons, endocrinologists, anesthesiologists, and dietitians. Future practice will likely center around multidisciplinary "sleep-obesity clinics" that combine surgical expertise with structured weight management, lifestyle coaching, and cardiometabolic monitoring.

1.10.7 Conclusion

Obesity exerts a profound impact on both the development of OSA and the outcomes of its surgical management. While sleep surgery remains a critical option for patients intolerant of CPAP or with significant anatomical obstruction, its success in obese populations is often limited by multilevel collapse, higher perioperative risks, and systemic metabolic drivers of disease. Weight loss, achieved through lifestyle, pharmacotherapy, or bariatric surgery, is therefore central to long-term disease control.

The future of managing OSA in obese patients lies in *combining airway surgery with weight management strategies*, supported by technological advances and multidisciplinary care. Surgeons must counsel patients that success should be measured not only by reductions in AHI but also by improvements in symptoms, quality of life, and comorbidity burden. By integrating surgical expertise with evolving metabolic and pharmacological therapies, clinicians can provide more durable and comprehensive outcomes.

1.11 Powered Instruments in Sleep Surgery

Ng Boon Han Kevin and Liang Chye Goh

1.11.1 Introduction

Modern sleep surgery has evolved in lockstep with advances in powered instruments—devices that transform energy (radiofrequency, plasma/coblation, laser light, ultrasonic vibration, or high-speed rotary power) into controlled tissue effects. Compared with cold steel alone, powered tools enable precise, hemostatic dissection in a highly vascular, compact airway; they can reduce thermal spread, shorten operative time for selected steps, and support DISE-directed, multilevel strategies while preserving function [22, 138–140].

Early temperature-controlled *radiofrequency ablation (RFA)* studies established that submucosal energy delivery can stiffen or volumetrically reduce palate/tongue tissue with low pain and minimal speech/swallow effects, enabling office-based therapy for snoring and mild OSA. Foundational work by Powell et al. on palatal RFA and tongue-base reduction demonstrated symptom improvement, tissue shrinkage on imaging, and favorable safety that catalyzed broader adoption and parameter standardization [22, 141]. Subsequent multilevel RFA series showed durable AHI reductions in appropriately selected patients, reinforcing its role as a minimally invasive option or adjunct within staged care pathways [139, 140, 142].

Coblation (radiofrequency plasma in saline) extends this paradigm by operating at lower tissue temperatures (~40–70 °C), allowing submucosal channeling of the tongue or targeted palatal debulking with fine hemostasis and often less postoperative pain. In a multicenter trial combining modified UPPP with coblation tongue-channeling, median AHI fell from 23.1 to 5.6 with low morbidity—illustrating how powered technology can amplify outcomes when integrated with reconstructive pharyngoplasty [143]. Contemporary reviews and pediatric applications confirm coblation's precision and favorable morbidity profile [144, 145].

For bulk tissue removal, the *microdebrider* couples suction with a rotating blade to resect lymphoid tissue efficiently while maintaining a clean field—useful in lingual tonsillectomy and adenoidectomy. Contemporary evidence (pediatric and adult) shows significant AHI improvements when lingual tonsillectomy is deployed as part of DISE-guided multilevel surgery, with acceptable bleeding/readmission rates—benefits facilitated by powered resection tools such as the microdebrider [19, 146–149]. Intracapsular tonsillectomy series also validate microdebrider efficacy for sleep-disordered breathing, supporting faster recovery in many centers [146].

Lasers (e.g., CO_2, diode, KTP) offer micrometer-level precision with strong coagulative capability, enabling procedures such as LAUP, partial epiglottectomy, or lingual tonsil work where bloodless visualization is critical. Early LAUP cohorts documented objective snoring reduction [150, 151], while long-term results and modern refinements continue to support selective use in mild OSA and anatomic niches [152–154].

Traditional *monopolar electrocautery/diathermy* remains indispensable for rapid cutting and coagulation, though at the cost of greater thermal spread. Recent comparative data suggest no significant difference in post-tonsillectomy hemorrhage versus plasma blade or thermal welding systems [155–158], while pain and operative time nuances vary—highlighting that tool choice should balance cost, thermal profile, and case goals rather than defaulting to any single technology.

At the bony level, *high-speed drills/burrs* and increasingly *piezoelectric (ultrasonic) osteotomes* underpin skeletal airway surgery (e.g., genioglossus advancement, MMA). Piezosurgery selectively cuts mineralized tissue while sparing soft tissue, enhancing safety near neurovascular structures but with slower cutting speed and higher cost—trade-offs relevant in delicate maxillofacial maneuvers [159–162]. These technologies support MMA, which consistently delivers the largest AHI reductions across sleep surgeries with favorable safety profiles [29, 163]—making powered bone instrumentation central to best-in-class outcomes.

Powered tools are not mere conveniences; they are enablers of precision medicine in sleep surgery. By tailoring energy modality and instrument mechanics to tissue targets (mucosa, lymphoid tissue, muscle, bone), surgeons can: (1) optimize hemostasis and visualization, (2) minimize collateral injury and pain, (3) execute complex, multilevel reconstructions efficiently, and (4) expand candidacy for patients who cannot tolerate CPAP—ultimately improving quality-of-life and physiologic endpoints [22, 29, 138–140].

1.11.2 Coblation (Controlled Ablation)

1.11.2.1 Technology Overview

Coblation represents a distinct advancement in surgical energy delivery systems. It uses bipolar radiofrequency energy within a conductive saline medium to generate a plasma field that is capable of breaking molecular bonds, resulting in precise tissue disintegration rather than bulk thermal destruction. Unlike traditional electrocautery, which operates at significantly higher temperatures, coblation functions at a lower thermal range of approximately 40–70 °C [143–145, 164]. This reduction in heat not only minimizes collateral damage to surrounding tissues but also preserves mucosal integrity and reduces the risk of scarring.

From a surgical perspective, these features translate into several practical advantages. Coblation allows for controlled resection with improved hemostasis, a cleaner operative field, and the potential for more accurate sculpting of delicate upper airway structures. Clinically, patients benefit through reduced postoperative discomfort, faster recovery, and lower incidence of complications such as excessive bleeding or prolonged edema. For sleep surgeons, these properties make coblation particularly attractive in procedures targeting the tonsils, turbinates, tongue base, and other airway sites where precision and preservation of adjacent tissue are paramount.

1.11.2.2 Common Systems

- ArthroCare ENT Coblation (e.g., Reflex Ultra, EVac 70, EVac Xtra)
- Celon ProSleep Plus (Olympus)—a bipolar RF-induced thermal lesioning platform

1.11.2.3 Clinical Applications

Coblation has been applied successfully in:

- Tongue-base reduction (coblation channeling technique)
- Inferior turbinate reduction
- Soft-palate debulking

- Adenoid and lingual tonsil ablation [143–145]

In a multicenter Australian trial, modified uvulopalatopharyngoplasty (UPPP) combined with coblation tongue-channeling reduced median AHI from 23.1 to 5.6, with low morbidity and excellent patient tolerance [143]. Subsequent reviews and pediatric studies further support coblation as a safe and versatile instrument for airway surgery [144, 145].

1.11.2.4 Surgical Considerations

- Preoperative mapping of channeling points is essential, particularly near the foramen cecum and lingual frenulum, to avoid vascular or neurogenic injury.
- The wand should be dipped in saline before activation to reduce resistance.
- Energy delivery is optimized by activating before tissue contact and using a gentle swirling motion within the tissue.
- Standard settings: Coblate 5, Coagulation 3, ~15 s per channel [144, 164].

1.11.2.5 Advantages

- Minimal postoperative pain
- Excellent intraoperative hemostasis
- Submucosal ablation with mucosal preservation [144, 164]

1.11.2.6 Limitations

- High cost of disposable wands
- Risk of incomplete results if channeling depth is insufficient
- Limited ability to coagulate larger vessel bleeds [144, 164]

1.11.3 Microdebrider

1.11.3.1 Technology Overview

The microdebrider is a powered surgical instrument that integrates precise mechanical resection with continuous suction. It consists of a hollow outer sheath encasing a rapidly rotating or oscillating inner blade, which shaves targeted tissue while aspirating debris and blood simultaneously [143, 146, 155]. This dual function provides the surgeon with a consistently clear operative field, minimizing intraoperative interruptions and enhancing visualization of delicate anatomical structures.

Because of its efficiency and precision, the microdebrider is particularly well suited for resecting soft, friable, or hypertrophic lymphoid tissue, such as enlarged adenoids, turbinates, or residual tonsillar tissue. Compared with conventional cold steel or cautery techniques, the microdebrider reduces operative time, offers greater control over the volume of tissue removed, and allows for sculpting rather than en bloc excision. Clinically, these features can translate into decreased blood loss, reduced postoperative pain, and faster recovery, making it a versatile and valuable tool in modern airway and sinonasal surgery [143, 146, 155].

1.11.3.2 Common Systems

- Medtronic Straightshot M4
- Karl Storz Unidrive ENT System
- Olympus DIEGO Elite

1.11.3.3 Clinical Applications

Microdebriders are widely used in:

- *Lingual tonsillectomy*—often as part of DISE-guided multilevel sleep surgery
- *Adenoidectomy*—especially when performed endoscopically
- *Intranasal surgery*—including turbinoplasty and as an adjunct in septoplasty
- *Palatal tissue debulking* [19, 146–149]

Clinical series confirm that *lingual tonsillectomy* with the microdebrider leads to significant improvements in AHI and symptom burden in both adults and children, with acceptable bleeding and readmission rates [147, 149]. Intracapsular tonsillectomy performed with a microdebrider also demonstrates favorable recovery profiles, reduced pain, and faster return to normal diet and activity [146].

1.11.3.4 Surgical Considerations

- Optimal rotational speed: 1000–5000 RPM, depending on tissue consistency.
- Continuous suction maintains visibility, reduces blood pooling, and improves safety.
- Surgeons must remain cautious to avoid *deep muscular trauma*, especially in the posterior tongue base where access is limited [19, 146].

1.11.3.5 Advantages

- Clear operative field due to simultaneous suction
- Reduced operative time
- Precise resection with less collateral trauma [146, 147, 149]

1.11.3.6 Limitations

- Bulky handpiece may limit access to posterior oral cavity
- Less effective in fibrotic tissue, which may clog the blade
- Requires careful handling to avoid deep-tissue injury [19, 146]

1.11.4 Radiofrequency Ablation (RFA)

1.11.4.1 Technology Overview

Radiofrequency ablation (RFA) is a minimally invasive technique that employs high-frequency alternating current, typically in the range of 350–500 kHz, to generate controlled thermal injury within targeted tissues [22, 138–142, 146, 149, 156]. The alternating current produces rapid ionic agitation, which in turn creates localized heating and induces submucosal coagulative necrosis. Unlike surface-based cautery, RFA is designed to confine its effect to the submucosal layer, thereby preserving the integrity of the overlying mucosa.

Following treatment, a cascade of wound-healing responses leads to progressive fibrosis and scarring, resulting in tissue contraction and volumetric reduction over several weeks. This delayed remodeling effect is particularly advantageous in managing conditions such as turbinate hypertrophy, tongue-base enlargement, and other obstructive sites where bulk reduction is desired without extensive resection. Clinically, RFA is valued for its precision, relatively low perioperative morbidity, and ability to be performed in outpatient or office-based settings, offering patients a less invasive alternative to conventional surgical excision [22, 138–142, 146, 149, 156].

1.11.4.2 Common Systems

- Celon ProSleep Plus (Olympus)
- Somnus RFA System
- Ellman Surgitron

1.11.4.3 Clinical Applications

- *Soft palate stiffening* (palatal RFA, pillar implants)
- *Tongue-base reduction*
- *Nasal turbinate reduction* [22, 138–142, 151]

RFA has been shown to significantly improve *snoring* and *mild-to-moderate OSA* with low complication rates. Powell and colleagues pioneered RFA of the palate and tongue base, reporting symptom improvement, tissue shrinkage, and favorable safety [22, 141]. Later studies confirmed durable reductions in AHI when used in multilevel approaches [139, 140, 142].

1.11.4.4 Surgical Considerations

- Can be performed under local anesthesia in the office or under sedation.
- Therapeutic effect is delayed, with maximal benefit appearing *4–6 weeks post-procedure*.
- Multiple treatment sessions may be required for optimal outcomes [142, 146, 149, 156].

1.11.4.5 Advantages

- Minimally invasive, with short downtime
- Low complication rate and minimal pain
- Suitable for office-based settings [22, 138–142]

1.11.4.6 Limitations

- Requires multiple sessions in many cases
- Limited efficacy in severe anatomical collapse
- Delayed therapeutic effect [146, 149, 156]

1.11.5 Lasers

1.11.5.1 Technology Overview

Lasers harness concentrated, coherent light energy to vaporize, incise, or coagulate soft tissue with exceptional precision. Their clinical utility in upper airway and otolaryngologic surgery arises from the ability to selectively target tissues while simultaneously achieving hemostasis. The effect of a laser is largely determined by its wavelength, which dictates depth of penetration, absorption characteristics, and coagulative potential [150–154].

For example, the *CO_2 laser* (10.6 μm) is highly absorbed by water, enabling extremely precise and superficial ablation with minimal thermal spread, making it ideal for delicate mucosal procedures. The *diode laser* (810–980 nm), in contrast, penetrates deeper into tissue and generates stronger coagulative effects, which are useful for volume reduction or treating hypertrophic tissue. The *KTP laser* (532 nm), with its affinity for oxyhemoglobin, provides excellent hemostasis in vascular tissues and is especially valuable for tonsillar surgery or epiglottic procedures. Collectively, lasers offer versatility, excellent visualization, and reduced intraoperative bleeding, though their use requires careful training and adherence to safety protocols [150–154].

1.11.5.2 Common Lasers

- CO_2 laser with micromanipulator
- Diode laser
- KTP laser

1.11.5.3 Clinical Applications

- *Laser-assisted uvulopalatoplasty (LAUP)* for snoring and mild OSA
- *Partial epiglottectomy* for supraglottic collapse
- *Lingual tonsil reduction*
- *Nasopharyngeal stenosis management* [150–154]

Early studies demonstrated measurable reductions in snoring intensity following LAUP [150, 151]. Long-term series further supported its role in selected patients with mild OSA [152], while refinements, including dual-laser techniques (Nd:YAG and Er:YAG), continue to expand its applications [154].

1.11.5.4 Surgical Considerations

- Strict laser safety protocols: protective eyewear, smoke evacuation, and fire precautions.
- CO_2 lasers are often used with micromanipulators under an operating microscope or robotic arm.
- Risk of airway fire mandates careful use with supplemental oxygen.

1.11.5.5 Advantages

- Micrometer-level precision
- Excellent hemostasis
- Minimal postoperative swelling [150–154]

1.11.5.6 Limitations

- High equipment cost
- Steep learning curve and safety requirements
- Potential risk of airway fire if misused [150, 154]

1.11.6 Electrocautery and Monopolar Diathermy

1.11.6.1 Technology Overview

Monopolar electrocautery, also referred to as monopolar diathermy, is one of the most traditional and widely used energy-based surgical modalities in otolaryngology and sleep surgery. It delivers high-frequency alternating current through a single active electrode, usually a fine metal tip, with the return current passing through a grounding pad on the patient. This circuit enables the surgeon to perform both cutting and coagulation functions by varying the waveform and power settings [155–158].

The technique is valued for its *accessibility, versatility, and cost-effectiveness*, making it a mainstay in both high-resource and resource-limited settings. However, because it operates at higher thermal ranges compared with newer technologies such as coblation or thermal welding, it produces greater *collateral heat spread*. This can result in more extensive tissue injury, postoperative pain, and delayed healing. Despite these drawbacks, electrocautery remains indispensable due to its reliability, rapid hemostatic ability, and adaptability across a wide range of procedures in sleep and airway surgery [155–158].

1.11.6.2 Common Systems

- Valleylab Force FX
- ERBE VIO
- Integrated cautery units in operating tables

1.11.6.3 Clinical Applications

- Palatal incisions during pharyngoplasty
- Tonsillectomy
- Epiglottectomy
- Coagulation of muscle flaps [155, 156]

1.11.6.4 Surgical Considerations

- Provides rapid cutting and coagulation but produces a wider thermal zone of injury.
- Risk of delayed healing and postoperative pain due to eschar formation.
- Hemostasis is effective, but recurrence of bleeding may occur with larger vessels.

1.11.6.5 Advantages

- Widely available and inexpensive
- Efficient for both cutting and coagulation
- Reliable for routine tonsil and palate work [155, 156]

1.11.6.6 Limitations

- Greater postoperative pain
- Increased risk of delayed healing
- More collateral tissue injury compared with coblation [155–157]

1.11.7 High-Speed Drills and Burrs

1.11.7.1 Technology Overview

High-speed drills are precision instruments that employ rapidly rotating burrs to cut, contour, or remove bone with efficiency and control. In sleep surgery, they are indispensable for *skeletal-level interventions*, where airway expansion requires modification of bony structures rather than soft tissue alone. Their role is particularly critical in *maxillomandibular advancement (MMA)* and *genioglossus advancement*, procedures that enlarge the pharyngeal airway by repositioning skeletal landmarks [29, 163].

The high rotational speeds of these drills enable smooth bone removal with minimal chatter, which is essential when working near vital structures. Continuous irrigation is required during use to dissipate frictional heat and avoid thermal osteonecrosis, underscoring the need for meticulous surgical technique. While they demand a skilled operator and carry risks of nerve or tooth root injury, their efficiency, precision, and adaptability make them a cornerstone of skeletal sleep surgery. [29, 163].

1.11.7.2 Common Systems

- Stryker CORE Drill
- Medtronic Midas Rex
- Aesculap ELAN 4

1.11.7.3 Clinical Applications

- Piriform aperture drilling for nasal valve stabilization
- Maxillomandibular advancement (MMA)
- Genioglossus advancement (anchor site preparation) [29, 163]

1.11.7.4 Surgical Considerations

- Burr selection is critical to prevent chatter and ensure precise osteotomy.
- Copious irrigation is required to dissipate heat.
- Guarded burrs improve safety in tight anatomic spaces.

1.11.7.5 Advantages

- Precise bony removal
- Versatile burr types for different applications
- Effective in dense skeletal tissue [29]

1.11.7.6 Limitations

- Generates significant heat
- Requires advanced surgical skill
- Risk of nerve or vessel injury if misapplied [29]

1.11.8 Piezoelectric Surgery (Piezosurgery)

1.11.8.1 Technology Overview

Piezoelectric surgery, also known as piezosurgery, employs ultrasonic microvibrations in the range of 25–30 kHz to achieve selective cutting of mineralized tissue while sparing adjacent soft tissue [159–162]. The vibrating tip generates cavitation effects in the surrounding irrigation fluid, which contributes to both cooling and microdissection. This mechanism allows surgeons to perform *atraumatic osteotomies* with reduced risk of collateral injury and minimal thermal damage compared with conventional rotary drills.

The selectivity of piezoelectric systems is especially advantageous when operating close to delicate structures such as neurovascular bundles, tooth roots, or sinus membranes. As a result, it enhances procedural safety in craniofacial and maxillomandibular advancement surgery, where precision is paramount. However, the trade-off is a *slower cutting speed* relative to high-speed drills, which can prolong operative time in dense bone. Despite this limitation, piezosurgery is increasingly valued for its precision, safety profile, and ability to facilitate fine skeletal modifications in sleep surgery [159–162].

1.11.8.2 Common Systems

- Mectron Piezosurgery®
- Acteon Piezotome®
- EMS Piezon®

1.11.8.3 Clinical Applications in Sleep Surgery

- *Maxillomandibular advancement (MMA):* precise osteotomies near neurovascular bundles
- *Genioglossus advancement:* controlled mandibular window osteotomy
- *Nasal valve/nasofacial augmentation:* precise bone modification for nasal airway improvement [159–162]

1.11.8.4 Surgical Considerations

- Requires copious irrigation to avoid overheating.
- Specialized tips (bone saw, scalpel, chisel) must be selected for the site.
- Cutting speed is slower than drills, demanding patience and tactile familiarity.

1.11.8.5 Advantages

- Preserves soft-tissue integrity
- Minimal bleeding
- Improved postoperative bone healing (osteoconduction)
- Reduced mechanical trauma [159, 160]

1.11.8.6 Limitations

- Slower than conventional drills
- More expensive and less widely available
- Requires specific training [159, 162] (Table 1.1)

Table 1.1 Comparison of powered instruments in sleep surgery

Instrument	Mechanism of action	Common applications	Advantages	Limitations	Typical use setting
Coblation [143–145, 164]	Bipolar RF plasma field in saline	Tongue-base channeling, palate reduction, turbinates	Low heat, precise ablation, mucosal preservation	Disposable wand cost, limited coagulation of large vessels	OR (GA)
Microdebrider [19, 146–149]	Rotary blade + Continuous suction	Lingual tonsillectomy, adenoidectomy, palate trimming	Clear field, efficient, precise	Bulky handpiece, clogging in fibrotic tissue	OR (GA)
Radiofrequency [22, 138–142]	High-frequency palate current → submucosal necrosis	Minimally stiffening, tongue-base ablation, turbinates	Minimally invasive, office-friendly, low pain	Repeat sessions, delayed effect	Clinic/ day surgery/ OR
Lasers [150–154]	Focused light LAUP, energy	Partial epiglottectomy, lingual tonsil reduction, LAUP	Precision, excellent hemostasis, minimal swelling	Safety concerns, learning curve	OR (GA/ LA)
Electrocautery [155–158]	Heat from electric current	Tonsillectomy, pharyngoplasty	Widely available, inexpensive, efficient	Greater pain, thermal spread	
High-speed drill [29, 163]	Mechanical burr	MMA, genioglossus advancement	Precise bony removal	Heat generation, neurovascular risk	OR (skeletal-level)
Piezoelectric [159–162]	Ultrasonic vibrations	MMA, genioglossus advancement	Soft tissue sparing, minimal bleeding	Slower, expensive, limited access	OR (skeletal-level)

1.12 Surgical Management of Pediatric Obstructive Sleep Apnea

Nurul Asma Che Ab Rahim and Jeyasakthy Saniasiaya

1.12.1 Introduction

Pediatric obstructive sleep apnea (OSA) is the most prevalent sleep-related breathing disorder, which afflicts approximately 2–4% of the pediatric population. Yet, the actual prevalence is estimated to be much higher due to subclinical diagnoses.

Pediatric OSA is a part of sleep-disordered breathing characterized by intermittent or prolonged partial or complete upper airway obstruction, resulting in disruption of normal sleep ventilation and sleep fragmentation. Adenotonsillar hypertrophy has been considered to be a significant contributing factor to pediatric OSA. Nonetheless, the prevalence of OSA is much higher in children with comorbidities such as obesity, Down syndrome, craniofacial anomaly, neurological condition, musculoskeletal impairment, and high loop gain—exaggerated ventilatory response to respiratory perturbations. In these children, sleep-disordered breathing often arises from multifactorial causes, including multilevel upper airway obstruction, leading to persistent OSA following adenotonsillectomy.

Traditionally, parents or caretakers of children with OSA present nighttime symptoms with complaints of snoring, apnea, gasping/choking, frequent change of body positions, mouth opening, neck hyperextension, enuresis, and sweating during sleeping. Daytime symptoms in these children include hyperactive behavior, daytime somnolence in older children, morning headache, and inability to concentrate in school. Long-standing, untreated pediatrics OSA can lead to behavioral problems, poor school performance, neurocognitive deficit, systemic complications such as pulmonary hypertension.

Management of pediatric obstructive sleep apnea remains a challenge as no consensus exists to date pertaining to the best treatment option for each child. It is pertinent to note that the "one-size-fits-all" rule cannot be implemented in managing OSA in children as treatment needs to be tailored individually.

The choice of treatment depends on factors such as age, underlying comorbidities, night and daytime symptoms, risk factors, and findings from physical examinations and investigations, including overnight pulse oximetry (OPO) or polysomnography (PSG). Treatment of pediatric OSA encompasses surgical and nonsurgical modalities. Notable nonsurgical treatment options include behavioral modifications such as weight loss, orthodontic appliances, noninvasive mask ventilation (e.g., continuous positive airway pressure, CPAP), myofunctional therapy, and anti-inflammatory medications. Among the myriad surgical treatment choices, adenotonsillectomy is the most favored and has been regarded as the first-line surgical option. This is then followed by other surgical options depending on the age and location of the obstruction. The advent of instrumentation has revealed several prominent modes of investigation, such as sleep magnetic resonance imaging (MRI) and drug-induced sleep endoscopy (DISE), which aid in detecting the exact site of collapse during sleep. Surgical treatment modalities of pediatrics OSA have been discussed in this chapter.

1.12.2 Surgical Management

1.12.2.1 Adenotonsillectomy

Adenotonsillectomy is a relatively standard surgical procedure among pediatric patients, which encompasses the surgical removal of palatine tonsils and adenoids. Adenotonsillectomy has been traditionally regarded as the gold standard or first-line treatment for pediatric OSA [165], as adenotonsillar hypertrophy is considered a notable risk factor of pediatric OSA [166].

Adenotonsillectomy procedure requires general anesthesia and is performed in the operating theatre either as a day-care procedure or requiring an overnight stay. The palatine tonsils are surgically removed by numerous techniques, including cold-instrument technique using blunt dissection, bipolar cautery, harmonic scalpel, radiofrequency ablation, coblation, laser, microdebrider as well as the guillotine knife technique [167].

Adenoidectomy, on the other hand, involves the surgical removal of the adenoids or pharyngeal tonsil from the nasopharynx. Several techniques, such as blind curettage, suction curettage, endoscopic microdebrider, and the coblation technique, have been widely used.

Surgical removal of the adenoid and the tonsils increases the upper airway dimensions, resulting in a decrease in upper airway collapsibility during sleep. A randomized controlled trial by the Childhood Adenotonsillectomy Trial (CHAT) demonstrated improvement in symptoms and reduced apnea in 79% of participants post-adenotonsillectomy, compared to patients who underwent watchful waiting, where only 46% showed improvement in apnea [168]. Albeit the striking improvement among children with sleep-disordered breathing, the success rate in pediatric OSA has been highly variable [169]. Hence, postoperative or follow-up polysomnography (PSG) following adenotonsillectomy is recommended, especially in children with preoperative moderate to severe OSA, syndromic children, children with underlying comorbidities such as chronic lung disease, neurological impairment, and cardiovascular disease.

Adenotonsillectomy in children has several complications, including respiratory distress following surgery, [170]. Negative pressure pulmonary edema is among the causes of respiratory compromise following adenotonsillectomy requiring oxygen supplementation, post-surgery intensive care unit (ICU) care, and, in some cases, reintubation. Post-adenotonsillectomy bleeding, either primary or secondary bleeding, is another notable complication that requires attention. Besides that, throat pain and dehydration from refusal of oral intake are among other known complications.

It is noteworthy that parents are informed that the success rate of adenotonsillectomy in treating OSA in pediatric patients is not 100%.

1.12.2.2 Intracapsular Tonsillectomy (ICT) Versus Extracapsular Tonsillectomy (ECT)

Intracapsular tonsillectomy (ICT) has recently gained popularity due to its faster recovery rate, which has been widely reported. ICT encompasses partial removal of tonsillar tissue while prese [171]. During a conventional extracapsular tonsillectomy (ECT), the lateral muscular wall of the pharynx can be damaged, leading to an inflammatory response and superinfection by oral bacterial flora, which may contribute to significant post-tonsillectomy pain. In ICT, the capsule of the tonsil can act as a barrier to inflammation and infection of the pharyngeal musculature, which

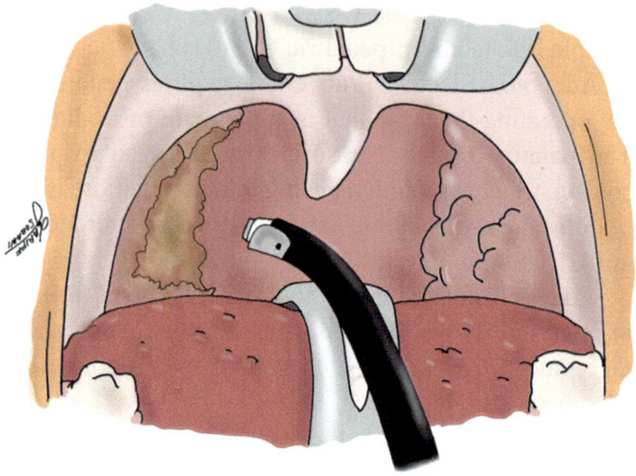

Fig. 1.21 Coblator-assisted intracapsular tonsillectomy

is also termed as a "biological dressing." Therefore, reduced postoperative pain and bleeding, as well as an earlier return to daily activities and oral intake, have been reported with ICT [170]. However, the drawback of ICT is the possibility of recurrence, and repeated surgery is higher due to tonsil regrowth as compared to the ECT [171]. In a recent cross-sectional survey study among pediatric otolaryngologists, ECT remains the most commonly performed technique. Most respondents primarily used ECT (44.5%), followed by those who performed both techniques equally (34.8%), and those who favored intracapsular tonsillectomy (20.5%) [172]. ECT was considered ideal for patients with recurrent tonsillitis, recurrent peritonsillar abscesses, and OSA, whereas ICT was preferred for OSA and patients with bleeding disorders. The ICT technique is expected to become more widespread as long-term data and cost-effective studies emerge (Fig. 1.21).

1.12.3 Tongue-Base Surgery

Among the various obstructive sites identified in cases of residual OSA following adenotonsillectomy (AT), the tongue base is one of the most frequently encountered. Three main types of abnormalities have been described at this level: lingual tonsillar hypertrophy, glossoptosis, and macroglossia. This site of obstruction is particularly common in children with comorbidities such as obesity, Down syndrome, and Pierre Robin Sequence. To address tongue-base obstruction, several surgical techniques have been described in the literature, including lingual tonsillectomy, glossectomy, tongue-base reduction, genioglossus advancement, and tongue lip adhesions. Regardless of the specific approach used, the primary objective of tongue-base surgery is to adequately clear the vallecular space to improve airway patency.

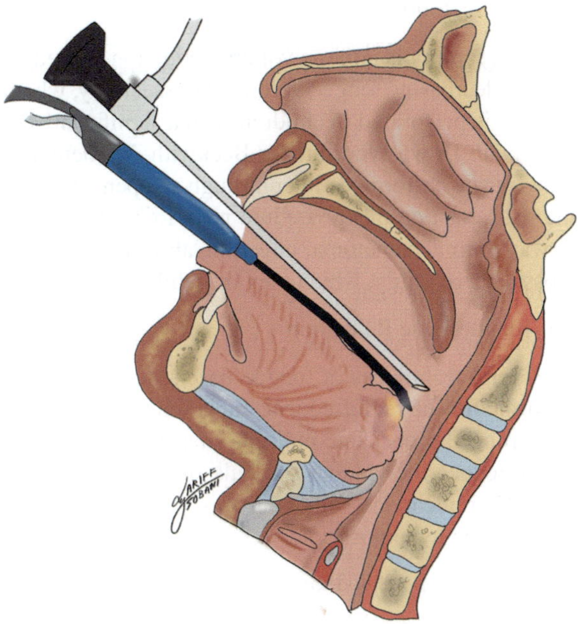

Fig. 1.22 Coblator assisted lingual tonsillectomy

(a) Lingual Tonsillectomy

The lingual tonsil is found at the tongue base and is a part of the Waldeyer ring of lymphoid tissue [165]. Enlarged lingual tonsil causes airway narrowing prominently during sleep, causing OSA in children. Lingual tonsillar hypertrophy can be visualized in the clinic during flexible nasopharyngolaryngoscopy. However, it can be prominently seen during a drug-induced sleep endoscopy (DISE). Besides that, MRI or CT can also be used to evaluate the size of the lingual tonsil [173]. Meta-analysis by Kang et al. revealed promising results ensuing lingual tonsillectomy, as AHI reduction of 8.9 events/h was demonstrated with a minimum rise of oxygen saturation of 6.0% [173]. It is worth noting that in children with prior adenotonsillectomy, reactive lymphoid hyperplasia leads to OSA. Apart from that, lingual hypertrophy may occur secondary to obesity, laryngopharyngeal reflux, and allergic rhinitis. Lingual tonsillar hypertrophy has been regarded as the most prominent cause of residual OSA in children following adenotonsillectomy [173].

Lingual tonsillectomy is performed through a transoral approach using mouth gags or laryngoscopes to expose the vallecular area. Several techniques may be used, including coblation, microdebrider-assisted excision, and laser modalities, such as CO_2 or KTP lasers, each allowing for the controlled removal of hypertrophic lingual tonsil tissue. Coblation provides low-temperature ablation with good hemostasis. The microdebrider enables precise mechanical debulking, and laser techniques allow tissue vaporization with excellent visualization, all aiming to safely reduce tissue bulk and restore a clear vallecular space. Complications of lingual tonsillectomy include postoperative pain, airway edema, bleeding and transient dysphagia, with rare risks of airway compromise (Fig. 1.22).

(b) Glossectomy

Glossectomy is a tissue volume reduction procedure aimed at increasing airway size by decreasing tongue volume. Glossectomy, which includes a wedge of tongue muscle, is performed in children with a significantly hypertrophied tongue, such as those with Down syndrome or Beckwith–Wiedemann syndrome. Midline glossectomy can be performed either through an open approach or submucosally [174]. Yet, the risks ensuing this procedure need to be discussed with parents, such as upper airway edema, hematoma, infection, abscess, and injury to the nerve, such as hypoglossal nerve injury, which may be debilitating [175].

(c) Tongue-Base Reduction

Several techniques of tongue-base reduction have been described. Powell et al. advocate for the radiofrequency ablation technique, which involves the insertion of two-pronged probes into multiple sites of the tongue base, generating thermal damage to reduce the volume and bulk of the tongue-base tissue through fibrosis [22, 176]. Complications following this procedure include ulceration, infection, and injury to the hypoglossal nerve.

(d) Tongue Lip Adhesion

Tongue lip adhesion (TLA) is a surgical procedure used primarily in infants with Pierre Robin Sequence to temporarily advance the tongue by suturing its anterior surface to the lower lip, thereby preventing posterior tongue collapse and relieving upper airway obstruction. The aim is to stabilize the airway while the mandible grows, thereby improving feeding and breathing until definitive correction, such as mandibular distraction osteogenesis, is possible. TLA is most effective in cases of isolated tongue-base airway obstruction and is a less invasive alternative to tracheostomy or mandibular distraction osteogenesis [177, 178].

1.12.4 Oropharyngeal Surgery

Besides tonsillectomy, other adjunct oropharyngeal surgeries that can be carried out include lateral pharyngoplasty, expansion sphincter pharyngoplasty, and uvulopalatopharyngoplasty. Lateral pharyngoplasty involves suturing the two tonsillar pillars together after the removal of the tonsils, in order to minimize pharyngeal collapse. [23] Expansion sphincter pharyngoplasty involves rotation and suspension of the palatopharyngeal muscle onto the soft palate, sparing the uvula in order to widen the diameter of the oral airway while stiffening the soft palate to prevent further collapse. Uvulopalatopharyngoplasty, on the other hand, is a more technical procedure that involves the removal of the soft palate and uvula while widening the oral airway. Interestingly, uvulopalatopharyngoplasty has been reported to have a good outcome in children with neurological impairment such as cerebral palsy [180].

Notable complications following this surgery include nasopharyngeal stenosis, palatal incompetence, and speech difficulties.

1.12.5 Nasal Surgery

The nose is the main gate for inspired air to enter the lungs. Hence, it is paramount to address and correct the nasal deformity, especially when a multilevel surgery is planned. Additionally, the adequate patency of the nose is crucial in children who require nasal CPAP to maintain and open the airway during sleep [181].

Surgical correction of the nose encompasses septoplasty, submucous resection, turbinoplasty, endoscopic sinus surgery, and even balloon sinuplasty, depending on the site of deformity or obstruction [181].

Septoplasty, which involves the surgical correction of a deformed septum, is performed with caution in younger children, as it is believed to disrupt normal craniofacial growth. Limited septoplasty is traditionally favored in children and has shown promising results. Complications include bleeding, septal hematoma, and septal perforation [182].

Turbinate reduction surgery in children can be performed via coblation-assisted inferior turbinoplasty, microdebrider-assisted reduction, and radiofrequency ablation [182].

Coblation techniques utilize a narrow electrode or wand that generates a low-temperature plasma field of approximately 40–70 °C, allowing effective tissue dissolution followed by fibrosis. The procedure is performed by inserting the coblation wand in ablation mode into the submucosal tissue of the turbinate, advancing it longitudinally along the lower anterior portion, whereas microdebrider-assisted inferior turbinoplasty is performed by making an anterior–inferior turbinate incision, introducing the microdebrider into the submucosal plane, and debriding the hypertrophied tissue to reduce turbinate volume. Cheng et al. incorporated inferior turbinate reduction using microdebrider along with adenotonsillectomy in pediatric patients with OSA and allergic rhinitis and found that the concurrent turbinoplasty and adenotonsillectomy group of children had significant improvement in terms of objective and subjective outcomes as compared to the group of children who underwent only adenotonsillectomy [183].

On comparing all the above techniques, coblation and microdebrider-assisted turbinoplasty are similarly effective overall. Coblation offers advantages in terms of reduced intraoperative bleeding, shorter operative time, and less postoperative pain, whereas the microdebrider provides superior endoscopic outcomes, greater symptomatic improvement, and reduced postoperative crusting [184] (Fig. 1.23)

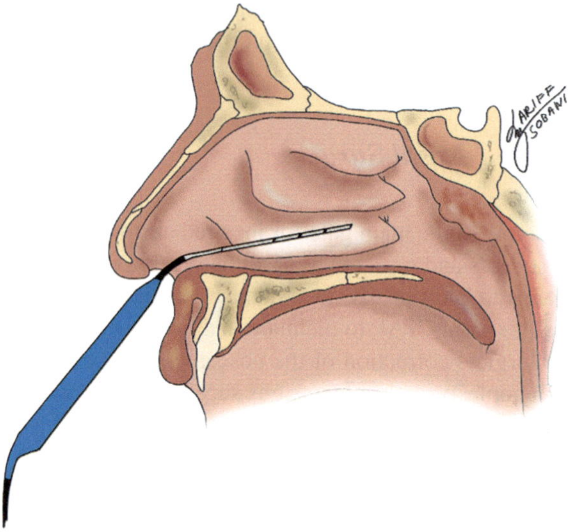

Fig. 1.23 Coblator-assisted turbinoplasty

1.12.6 Supraglottoplasty

Laryngomalacia is the most common congenital cause of upper airway obstruction in children, characterized by the presence of redundant supraglottic tissue that collapses and obstructs the airway. Laryngomalacia is recognized as a significant contributor to pediatric obstructive sleep apnea [185, 186]. Laryngomalacia during sleep is known as sleep-exclusive laryngomalacia [187], occult laryngomalacia [188], late-onset laryngomalacia [189], state-dependent laryngomalacia [190], and sleep-dependent laryngomalacia. Traditionally, laryngomalacia affects infants; however, sleep-related laryngomalacia may also affect older children between 2 and 18 years of age, with an approximate prevalence of 3.9% [191]. Drug-induced sleep endoscopy has demonstrated sleep-induced laryngomalacia in 77% of children [187].

The spontaneous nature of this entity allows for a watch-and-wait period. Yet, in cases where the infants exhibit respiratory distress, failure to thrive, or persistent symptoms, surgical intervention is deemed necessary. Supraglottoplasty has been the gold standard treatment for laryngomalacia, a condition resulting from redundant upper airway tissue that collapses. Nonetheless, promising results post-surgery, especially improvement in AHI, have been reported supporting supraglottoplasty as a choice of surgery in pediatric OSA [188, 189].

Supraglottoplasty is a surgical procedure that entails epiglottoplasty and aryepiglottoplasty, and can be performed via several techniques, including cold instruments, microdebrider, and laser, with a comparable success rate [192, 193]. (Fig. 1.24)

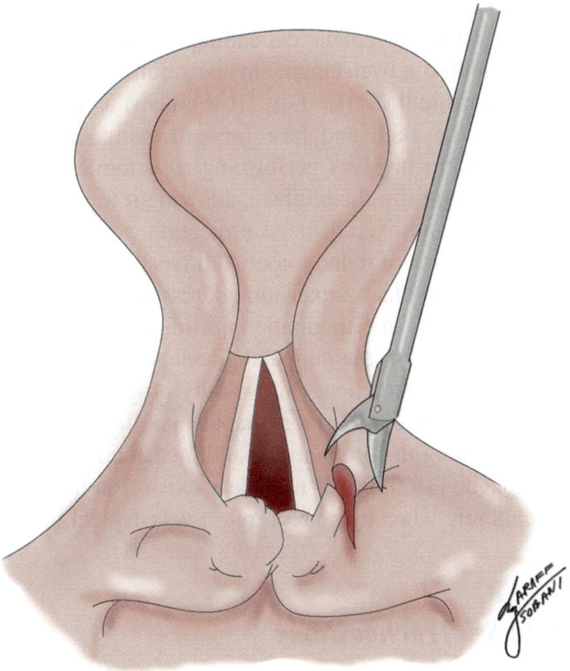

Fig. 1.24 Supraglottoplasty

1.12.7 Craniofacial Surgery

The shape and dimensions of the upper airway, among others, are determined by craniofacial morphology. Children with craniofacial anomalies, e.g., Pierre Robin Sequence (PRS) with micrognathia, retrognathia, glossoptosis with or without cleft lip/palate, have an increased risk of OSA due to upper airway obstruction as the tongue is relatively large compared to the mandibular structures and tends to prolapse backwards.

Children with midface and mandibular hypoplasia, e.g., Syndromic Craniosynostosis and Treacher Collins syndrome, exhibit variable severity of OSA, which correlates with the degree of hypoplasia. Maxillomandibular hypoplasia, combined with a retro-positioned mandible, is associated with epipharynx and mesopharynx stenosis, leading to upper airway obstruction. Airway obstruction in these groups can be severe and results in intermittent hypoxia that may impair long-term cognitive and intellectual development.

Surgery to address mandibular anomalies includes mandibular advancement and mandibular distraction osteogenesis, which involves fracturing and advancing the jaw into a new position to widen the airway dimension. Mandibular advancement, also known as orthognathic surgery, involves repositioning the jaw in a new position immediately. Mandibular distraction osteogenesis, on the other hand, involves dividing and advancing the mandible in stages to induce histogenesis, leading to mandible elongation [194].

Management of maxillary hypoplasia includes Monobloc advancement and Le Fort II/ III advancement, depending on the severity and level of midface deficiency. A Monobloc advancement involves cutting and mobilizing the forehead (frontal bone) and midface (Le Fort III segment) as one piece, then advancing the entire front of the skull and face forward using distraction devices. A Le Fort II/III advancement involves performing osteotomies at the respective Le Fort II or III levels to mobilize the midface, allowing it to be advanced to enhance airway space, occlusion, and overall facial projection. Success rate following advancement surgeries in terms of reduction of AHI has been lauded in recent publications [195].

Rapid maxillary expansion addresses upper jaw constriction [196] by applying forces through an orthodontic mini-implant across the midpalatal suture. This separates and realigns the midpalatal zone, allowing collagen fibers to reorganize in the direction of distraction, followed by progressive ossification that results in maxillary widening. Furthermore, rapid maxillary expansion has contributed indirectly by increasing the oropharyngeal dimension through altering the resting position of the tongue [197]. Rapid maxillary expansion has reported a long-term success rate in children, whereby no recurrence was evident upon 12-year follow-up [198].

1.12.8 Tracheostomy

Tracheostomy is a surgical procedure in which a tube is inserted through an opening into the trachea. As tracheostomy bypasses the upper airway, it has been considered a definitive treatment in patients with severe OSA with hypoxaemia [199]. In children, tracheostomy has been the treatment option, especially for those with severe and refractory OSA, craniofacial anomalies, and neuromuscular disease, whereby other modalities have failed [199].

It is worth noting that, although significant improvement is reported post-tracheostomy, it is linked to significant long-term complications such as tracheostomy dependence, frequent infections, decannulation, death, and even reduces the child's quality of life. Furthermore, having a child with a tracheostomy requires great effort by caretakers, as constant care is required. Hence, the decision for tracheostomy is reserved only when all other options have failed or are deemed impossible.

1.12.9 Hypoglossal Nerve Stimulation

Hypoglossal nerve stimulation (HGNS) is a surgically implanted upper airway stimulation that has recently gained popularity among adult patients with OSA, due to its promising success rate. It is currently FDA-approved for the treatment of OSA in adults [34] and for children with Down syndrome over the age of 13. HGNS addresses upper airway obstruction by stabilizing the posterior tongue and palate, which are the structures most prone to collapse during inspiration. The fundamental principle of this device is based on the a priori assumption that upper airway patency is primarily maintained by genioglossus muscle activation [200]. During apnea, when upper airway muscle drive decreases [201], the device counteracts this by delivering unilateral hypoglossal nerve stimulation to restore airway patency [34]. The procedure involves surgically implanting a small generator in the upper chest and placing a stimulation lead around the hypoglossal nerve to activate tongue-protruding branches during inspiration. The latest version features a built-in accelerator that directly senses inspiration, allowing the system to synchronize stimulation with each breath. A recent publication revealed an average reduction of 85% of AHI in children with Down syndrome with persistent severe OSA who previously underwent adenotonsillectomy and failed CPAP [202].

References

1. Burwell CS, Robin ED, Whaley RD, Bickelmann AG. Extreme obesity associated with alveolar hypoventilation: a Pickwickian syndrome. Am J Med. 1956;21(5):811–8. https://doi.org/10.1016/0002-9343(56)90094-8.
2. Heinberg CJ. A surgical procedure for the relief of snoring. Eye Ear Nose Throat Mon. 1955;34(6):389. passim.
3. Motta J, Guilleminault C, Schroeder JS, Dement WC. Tracheostomy and hemodynamic changes in sleep-inducing apnea. Ann Intern Med. 1978;89(4):454–8. https://doi.org/10.7326/0003-4819-89-4-454.
4. Gastaut H, Tassinari CA, Duron B. Polygraphic study of the episodic diurnal and nocturnal (hypnic and respiratory) manifestations of the Pickwick syndrome. Brain Res. 1966;1(2):167–86. https://doi.org/10.1016/0006-8993(66)90117-X.
5. Kuhlo W, Doll E, Franck MC. Erfolgreiche Behandlung eines Pickwick-Syndroms durch eine Dauertrachealkanüle. Dtsch Med Wochenschr. 1969;94(24):1286–90. https://doi.org/10.1055/s-0028-1110279.
6. Sullivan CE, Issa FG, Berthon-Jones M, Eves L. Reversal of obstructive sleep apnoea by continuous positive airway pressure applied through the nares. Lancet. 1981;1(8225):862–5.
7. Yaremchuk K, Garcia-Rodriguez L. A history of sleep surgery. Adv Otorhinolaryngol. 2017;80:17–21.
8. Fujita S, Conway W, Zorick F, Roth T. Surgical correction of anatomic abnormalities in obstructive sleep apnea syndrome: uvulopalatopharyngoplasty. Otolaryngol Head Neck Surg. 1981;89(6):923–34.
9. Simmons FB, Guilleminault C, Silvestri R. Snoring and some obstructive sleep apnea can be cured by oropharyngeal surgery. Arch Otolaryngol. 1983;109(8):503–7.
10. Li HY. Palatal surgery: from ablation to reconstruction. Sleep Med Clin. 2019;14(1):51–8.
11. Gottlieb DJ, Punjabi NM. Diagnosis and management of obstructive sleep apnea: a review. JAMA. 2020;323(14):1389–400. https://doi.org/10.1001/jama.2020.3514.
12. Sher AE, Schechtman KB, Piccirillo JF. The efficacy of surgical modifications of the upper airway in adults with obstructive sleep apnea syndrome. Sleep. 1996;19(2):156–77.
13. Caples SM, Rowley JA, Prinsell JR, et al. Surgical modifications of the upper airway for obstructive sleep apnea in adults: a systematic review and meta-analysis. Sleep. 2010;33(10):1396–407. https://doi.org/10.1093/sleep/33.10.1396.
14. Croft CB, Pringle M. Sleep nasendoscopy: a technique of assessment in snoring and obstructive sleep apnoea. Clin Otolaryngol Allied Sci. 1991;16(5):504–9.

15. Kezirian EJ, Hohenhorst W, de Vries N. Drug-induced sleep endoscopy: the VOTE classification. Eur Arch Otorrinolaringol. 2011;268(8):1233–6. https://doi.org/10.1007/s00405-011-1633-8.
16. Riley RW, Powell NB, Guilleminault C. Obstructive sleep apnea syndrome: a review of 306 consecutively treated surgical patients. Otolaryngol Head Neck Surg. 1993;108(2):117–25. https://doi.org/10.1177/019459989310800203.
17. Kamami YV. Laser CO2 for treatment of snoring. Acta Otorhinolaryngol Belg. 1990;44(4):451–6.
18. Littner M, Kushida CA, Hartse K, Anderson WM, Davila D, Johnson SF, Wise MS, Hirshkowitz M, Woodson BT. Practice parameters for the use of laser-assisted uvulopalatoplasty: an update for 2000. Sleep. 2001;24(5):603–19.
19. Powell NB, Riley RW, Troell RJ, Li KK, Blumen MB, Guilleminault C. Radiofrequency volumetric tissue reduction of the palate in subjects with sleep-disordered breathing. Chest. 1998;113(5):1163–74.
20. Li KK, Powell NB, Riley RW, Troell RJ, Guilleminault C. Radiofrequency volumetric reduction of the palate: an extended follow-up study. Otolaryngol Head Neck Surg. 2000;122(3):410–4. https://doi.org/10.1016/S0194-5998(00)70057-X.
21. Maturo SC, Mair EA. Submucosal minimally invasive lingual tonsillectomy: a new approach to lingual tonsil hypertrophy. Otolaryngol Head Neck Surg. 2006;135(3):487–8.
22. Powell NB, Riley RW, Troell RJ, Guilleminault C. Radiofrequency tongue base reduction in sleep-disordered breathing: a pilot study. Otolaryngol Head Neck Surg. 1999;120(5):656–64.
23. Cahali MB. Lateral pharyngoplasty: a new treatment for obstructive sleep apnea hypopnea syndrome. Laryngoscope. 2003;113(11):1961–8.
24. Pang KP, Woodson BT. Expansion sphincter pharyngoplasty: a new technique for the treatment of obstructive sleep apnea. Otolaryngol Head Neck Surg. 2007;137(1):110–4.
25. Li HY, Lee LA. Relocation pharyngoplasty for obstructive sleep apnea. Laryngoscope. 2009;119(12):2472–7. https://doi.org/10.1002/lary.20634.
26. Friedman M, Ibrahim HZ, Vidyasagar R, et al. Z-palatoplasty (ZPP): a technique for patients without tonsils. Otolaryngol Head Neck Surg. 2004;131(1):89–100. https://doi.org/10.1016/j.otohns.2004.02.051.
27. Mantovani M, Minetti A, Torretta S, Pincherle A, Pignataro L. The velo-uvula-pharyngeal lift: a step forward for the treatment of snoring and obstructive sleep apnea. Acta Otorhinolaryngol Ital. 2012;32(2):48–53.
28. Vicini C, Hendawy E, Campanini A, Eesa M, Bahgat A, AlGhamdi S, et al. Barbed reposition pharyngoplasty (BRP) for OSAHS: a feasibility, safety, efficacy and teachability pilot study. Eur Arch Otorrinolaringol. 2015;272(10):3065–70. https://doi.org/10.1007/s00405-015-3628-3.
29. Holty JEC, Guilleminault C. Maxillomandibular advancement for the treatment of obstructive sleep apnea: a systematic review and meta-analysis. Sleep Med Rev. 2010;14(5):287–97. https://doi.org/10.1016/j.smrv.2009.11.003.
30. Li KK, Powell NB, Riley RW, Zonato AI, Troell RJ, Guilleminault C. Postoperative airway findings after maxillomandibular advancement for obstructive sleep apnea syndrome. Laryngoscope. 2000;110(2 Pt 1):325–7.
31. Vicini C, Dallan I, Canzi P, Frassineti S, La Pietra MG, Montevecchi F. Transoral robotic tongue base resection in obstructive sleep apnoea-hypopnoea syndrome: a preliminary report. ORL J Otorhinolaryngol Relat Spec. 2010;72(1):22–7. https://doi.org/10.1159/000284352.
32. Schwartz AR, Bennett ML, Smith PL, De Backer W, Hedner J, Boudewyns A, Van de Heyning P, Ejnell H, Hochban W, Knaack L, Podszus T, Penzel T, Peter JH, Goding GS Jr, Erickson DJ, Testerman R, Ottenhoff FA, Eisele DW. Therapeutic electrical stimulation of the hypoglossal nerve in obstructive sleep apnea. Arch Otolaryngol Head Neck Surg. 2001;127(10):1216–23. https://doi.org/10.1001/archotol.127.10.1216.
33. Eastwood PR, Barnes M, Walsh JH, et al. Treating obstructive sleep apnea with hypoglossal nerve stimulation. Sleep. 2011;34(11):1479–86.

34. Strollo PJ Jr, Soose RJ, Maurer JT, et al. Upper-airway stimulation for obstructive sleep apnea. N Engl J Med. 2014;370(2):139–49. https://doi.org/10.1056/NEJMoa1308659.
35. U.S. Food and Drug Administration. Premarket approval (PMA) P130008: inspire II upper airway stimulator. Decision date: April 30, 2014. Accessed January 20, 2026. https://www.accessdata.fda.gov/scripts/cdrh/cfdocs/cfpma/pma.cfm?id=P130008.
36. Woodson BT, Strohl KP, Soose RJ, et al. Upper airway stimulation for obstructive sleep apnea: 5-year outcomes. Otolaryngol Head Neck Surg. 2018;159(1):194–202. https://doi.org/10.1177/0194599818762383.
37. Malhotra A, Grunstein RR, Engleman HM, et al. Tirzepatide for the treatment of obstructive sleep apnea and obesity. N Engl J Med. 2024;391(13):1193–1205. https://doi.org/10.1056/NEJMoa2404881.
38. Eckert DJ, White DP, Jordan AS, Malhotra A, Wellman A. Defining phenotypic causes of obstructive sleep apnea: identification of novel therapeutic targets. Am J Respir Crit Care Med. 2013;188(8):996–1004. https://doi.org/10.1164/rccm.201303-0448OC.
39. Jordan AS, McSharry DG, Malhotra A. Adult obstructive sleep apnoea. Lancet. 2014;383(9918):736–47.
40. Schwab RJ. Upper airway imaging. Clin Chest Med. 1998;19(1):33–54.
41. Eckert DJ, Malhotra A. Pathophysiology of adult obstructive sleep apnea. Proc Am Thorac Soc. 2008;5(2):144–53.
42. Remmers JE, deGroot WJ, Sauerland EK, Anch AM. Pathogenesis of upper airway occlusion during sleep. J Appl Physiol Respir Environ Exerc Physiol. 1978;44(6):931–8.
43. McKeown P, O'Connor-Reina C, Plaza G. Breathing re-education and phenotypes of sleep apnea: a review. J Clin Med. 2021;10(3):471.
44. Younes M. Contributions of upper airway mechanics and control mechanisms to severity of obstructive apnea. Am J Respir Crit Care Med. 2003;168(6):645–58.
45. Malhotra RK, Kirsch DB, Kristo DA, Olson EJ. American Academy of Sleep Medicine Board of Directors. Polysomnography for obstructive sleep apnea should include arousal-based scoring: an American Academy of Sleep Medicine position statement. J Clin Sleep Med. 2018;14(7):1245–7.
46. Hillman DR, Platt PR, Eastwood PR. The upper airway during anaesthesia. Br J Anaesth. 2003;91(1):31–9.
47. Smith PL, Wise RA, Gold AR, Schwartz AR, Permutt S. Upper airway pressure-flow relationships in obstructive sleep apnea. J Appl Physiol. 1988;64(2):789–95.
48. Kazemeini E, Van de Perck E, Dieltjens M, Willemen M, Verbraecken J, Op de Beeck S, et al. Critical to know Pcrit: a review on pharyngeal critical closing pressure in obstructive sleep apnea. Front Neurol. 2022;13:775709.
49. Landry SA, Joosten SA, Eckert DJ, Jordan AS, Sands SA, White DP, et al. Therapeutic CPAP level predicts upper-airway collapsibility in OSA. Sleep. 2017;40(6):zsx056.
50. Verbraecken J, Dieltjens M, Op de Beeck S, Vroegop A, Braem M, Vanderveken O, Randerath W. Non-CPAP therapy for obstructive sleep apnoea. Breathe (Sheff). 2022;18(3):220164.
51. Kezirian EJ, White DP, Malhotra A, Ma W, McCulloch CE, Goldberg AN. Interrater reliability of drug-induced sleep endoscopy. Arch Otolaryngol Head Neck Surg. 2010;136(4):393–7.
52. Carberry JC, Jordan AS, White DP, Wellman A, Eckert DJ. Upper airway collapsibility (Pcrit) and pharyngeal dilator muscle activity are sleep stage dependent. Sleep. 2016;39(3):511–21.
53. Isono S, Tanaka A, Nishino T. Lateral position decreases collapsibility of the passive pharynx in patients with obstructive sleep apnea. Anesthesiology. 2002;97(4):780–5.
54. Srijithesh PR, Aghoram R, Goel A, Dhanya J. Positional therapy for obstructive sleep apnoea. Cochrane Database Syst Rev. 2019;5:CD010990.
55. Mo JH, Lee CH, Rhee CS, Yoon IY, Kim JW. Positional dependency in Asian patients with obstructive sleep apnea and its implication for hypertension. Arch Otolaryngol Head Neck Surg. 2011;137(8):786–90.
56. De Vito A, Carrasco Llatas M, Ravesloot MJ, Kotecha B, De Vries N, Hamans E, Maurer J, Bosi M, Blumen M, Heiser C, Herzog M, Montevecchi F, Corso RM, Braghiroli A, Gobbi R,

Vroegop A, Vonk PE, Hohenhorst W, Piccin O, Sorrenti G, et al. European position paper on drug-induced sleep endoscopy: 2017 update. Clin Otolaryngol. 2018;43(6):1541–52.
57. Zhou N, Ho JTF, de Vries N, Bosschieter PFN, Ravesloot MJL, de Lange J. Evaluation of drug-induced sleep endoscopy as a tool for selecting patients with obstructive sleep apnea for maxillomandibular advancement. J Clin Sleep Med. 2022;18(4):1073–81.
58. Wray CM, Thaler ER. Hypoglossal nerve stimulation for obstructive sleep apnea: a review of the literature. World J Otorhinolaryngol Head Neck Surg. 2016;2(4):230–3.
59. Chao TN, Chang MW, Hake MM, Mirza N. Predictors of success in hypoglossal nerve stimulator implantation for obstructive sleep apnea. World J Otorhinolaryngol Head Neck Surg. 2020;7(1):40–4.
60. Volner K, Chao S, Camacho M. Dynamic sleep MRI in obstructive sleep apnea: a systematic review and meta-analysis. Eur Arch Otorrinolaringol. 2022;279(2):595–607.
61. Schwab RJ, Pasirstein M, Pierson R, et al. Identification of upper airway anatomic risk factors in obstructive sleep apnea with volumetric MRI. Am J Respir Crit Care Med. 2003;168(5):522–30.
62. Francia-Lugo J, Godoy-Febres R, Luna-Anguiano M, et al. Classification of epiglottic collapse patterns in obstructive sleep apnea using drug-induced sleep endoscopy. Healthcare (Basel). 2023;11(21):2874.
63. Vallianou K, Chaidas K. Surgical options for epiglottic collapse in adult obstructive sleep apnea: a systematic review. Life (Basel). 2022;12(11):1845.
64. Francia C, Lugo R, Moffa A, Casale M, Giorgi L, Iafrati F, et al. Defining epiglottic collapse patterns in obstructive sleep apnea: the Francia–Lugo classification. Healthcare (Basel). 2023;11(21):2874.
65. Chen LY, Chen YH, Hu SW, Lin MT, Lee PL, Chiang AA, Tu YK. In search of a better CPAP interface: a network meta-analysis comparing nasal masks, nasal pillows and oronasal masks. J Sleep Res. 2022;31(6):e13686.
66. Zonato AI, Rosa CFA, Oliveira L, Bittencourt L. Comparing CPAP masks during initial titration for obstructive sleep apnea syndrome: one-year experience. Braz J Otorhinolaryngol. 2022;88(Suppl 5):S100–7.
67. Schoustra E, van Maanen P, den Haan C, Ravesloot MJL, de Vries N. The role of isolated nasal surgery in obstructive sleep apnea therapy: a systematic review. Brain Sci. 2022;12(11):1446.
68. Correa EJ, Conti DM, Moreno-Luna R, Sánchez-Gómez S, O'Connor RC. Role of nasal surgery in adult obstructive sleep apnea: a systematic review. Sleep Sci. 2024;17(3):e310–21.
69. Trosman I. Childhood obstructive sleep apnea syndrome: a review of the 2012 American Academy of Pediatrics guidelines. Pediatr Ann. 2013;42(10):195–9.
70. Redline S, Amin R, Beebe D, Chervin RD, Garetz SL, Giordani B, et al. The Childhood Adenotonsillectomy Trial (CHAT): rationale, design, and challenges of a randomized controlled trial evaluating a standard surgical procedure in a pediatric population. Sleep. 2011;34(11):1509–17.
71. Rhee JS, Weaver EM, Park SS, Baker SR, Hilger PA, Kriet JD, et al. Clinical consensus statement: diagnosis and management of nasal valve compromise. Otolaryngol Head Neck Surg. 2010;143(1):48–59.
72. Hsu YB, Liu SY, Lan MY, Huang YC, Tzeng IS, Lan MC. Role of rhinomanometry in the prediction of therapeutic positive airway pressure for obstructive sleep apnea. Respir Res. 2020;21(1):115.
73. Hoel HC, Kvinnesland K, Berg S. Outcome of nasal measurements in patients with OSA: mounting evidence of a nasal endotype. Sleep Med. 2023;103:131–7.
74. Ishman SL, Maturo S, Schwartz S, McKenna M, Baldassari C, Boss EF, et al. Expert consensus statement: management of pediatric persistent obstructive sleep apnea after adenotonsillectomy. Otolaryngol Head Neck Surg. 2023;168(2):115–30.
75. Modica DM, Marchese D, Lorusso F, Speciale R, Saraniti C, Gallina S. Functional nasal surgery and use of CPAP in OSAS patients: our experience. Indian J Otolaryngol Head Neck Surg. 2018;70(4):559–65.

76. Kempfle JS, BuSaba NY, Dobrowski JM, Westover MB, Bianchi MT. A cost-effectiveness analysis of nasal surgery to increase continuous positive airway pressure adherence in sleep apnea patients with nasal obstruction. Laryngoscope. 2017;127(4):977–83.
77. Liming BJ, Ryan M, Mack D, Ahmad I, Camacho M. Montelukast and nasal corticosteroids to treat pediatric obstructive sleep apnea: a systematic review and meta-analysis. Otolaryngol Head Neck Surg. 2019;160(4):594–602.
78. Ehsan Z, Ishman SL, Soghier I, Almeida FR, Amin R, et al. Management of persistent, post-adenotonsillectomy obstructive sleep apnea in children: an official American Thoracic Society clinical practice guideline. Am J Respir Crit Care Med. 2024;209(3):248–61.
79. Green KK, Kent DT, D'Agostino MA, Hoff PT, Lin HS, Soose RJ, et al. Drug-induced sleep endoscopy and surgical outcomes: a multicenter cohort study. Laryngoscope. 2019;129(3):761–70.
80. Lv C, Yang L, Ngan P, Xiao W, Zhao T, Tang B, et al. Role of the tonsil–oropharynx ratio on lateral cephalograms in assessing tonsillar hypertrophy in children seeking orthodontic treatment. BMC Oral Health. 2023;23(1):836.
81. Yu JL, Rosen I. Utility of the modified Mallampati grade and Friedman tongue position in the assessment of obstructive sleep apnea. J Clin Sleep Med. 2020;16(2):303–8.
82. Mitsikas D, Jakob B, Janjic V, Hasler C, Tschopp S. Interrater reliability of different scoring systems for drug-induced sleep endoscopy. Sleep Breath. 2024;29(1):27.
83. Kent DT, Stanley JJ, Aurora RN, Levine C, Gottlieb DJ, Spann MD, et al. Referral of adults with obstructive sleep apnea for surgical consultation: an American Academy of Sleep Medicine clinical practice guideline. J Clin Sleep Med. 2021;17(12):2499–505.
84. Choi JH, Cho SH, Kim SN, Suh JD, Cho JH. Predicting outcomes after uvulopalatopharyngoplasty for adult obstructive sleep apnea: a meta-analysis. Otolaryngol Head Neck Surg. 2016;155(6):904–13.
85. Sériès F. Upper airway muscles awake and asleep. Sleep Med Rev. 2002;6(3):229–42.
86. Sung CM, Tan SN, Shin MH, Lee J, Kim HC, Lim SC, et al. The site of airway collapse in sleep apnea, its associations with disease severity and obesity, and implications for mechanical interventions. Am J Respir Crit Care Med. 2021;204(1):103–6.
87. Friedman M, Hamilton C, Samuelson CG, Lundgren ME, Pott T. Diagnostic value of the Friedman tongue position and Mallampati classification for obstructive sleep apnea: a meta-analysis. Otolaryngol Head Neck Surg. 2013;148(4):540–7.
88. Ravesloot MLJ, de Vries N. One hundred consecutive patients undergoing drug-induced sleep endoscopy: results and evaluation. Laryngoscope. 2011;121(12):2710–6.
89. Jeong SH, Sung CM, Lim SC, Yang HC. Partial epiglottectomy improves residual apnea-hypopnea index in patients with epiglottis collapse. J Clin Sleep Med. 2020;16(9):1607–10.
90. Wang TY, Huyett P, Yang H, Sumner J, Sands SA, Calianese D, et al. Lateral epiglottic collapse in obstructive sleep apnea is associated with laterally directed pharyngeal collapse. J Clin Sleep Med. 2025;21(4):649–54.
91. Mitsikas D, Jakob B, Janjic V, Hasler C, Tschopp S. Inter-rater reliability of different scoring systems for drug-induced sleep endoscopy in patients with obstructive sleep apnea. Sleep Breath. 2024;29(1):27.
92. Mouratidou S, Chaidas K. Transoral robotic surgery for obstructive sleep apnoea: a systematic literature review of current practices. Life (Basel). 2024;14(12):1700.
93. Neruntarat C, Khuancharee K, Saengthong P. Barbed reposition pharyngoplasty versus expansion sphincter pharyngoplasty: a meta-analysis. Laryngoscope. 2021;131(6):1420–8.
94. Iannella G, Lechien JR, Perrone T, Meccariello G, Cannavicci A, Cammaroto G, et al. Barbed reposition pharyngoplasty (BRP) in obstructive sleep apnea treatment: state of the art. Am J Otolaryngol. 2022;43(1):103197.
95. Saenwandee P, Neruntarat C, Saengthong P, Worapairoj P, Vichianan Y. Barbed pharyngoplasty for obstructive sleep apnea: a meta-analysis. Am J Otolaryngol. 2022;43(2):103306.
96. Moffa A, Giorgi L, Cassano M, Lugo R, Baptista P, Casale M. Complications and side effects after barbed pharyngoplasty: a systematic review. Sleep Breath. 2023;27(1):31–8.

97. Van Tassel J, Chio E, Silverman D, Nord RS, Platter D, Abidin MR. Hyoid suspension with uvulopalatopharyngoplasty for the treatment of obstructive sleep apnea. Ear Nose Throat J. 2023;102(5):NP212–9.
98. Woodson BT, Strohl KP, Soose RJ, Gillespie MB, Maurer JT, de Vries N, et al. Upper airway stimulation for obstructive sleep apnea: 5-year outcomes. Otolaryngol Head Neck Surg. 2018;159(1):194–202.
99. Huyett P. Early objective adherence to hypoglossal nerve stimulation therapy. J Clin Sleep Med. 2022;18(2):631–6.
100. Zhou N, Ho JTF, Huang Z, Zou D, Stepan L, Teng Y, et al. Maxillomandibular advancement versus multilevel surgery for treatment of obstructive sleep apnea: a systematic review and meta-analysis. Sleep Med Rev. 2021;57:101471.
101. Camacho M, Noller MW, Del Do M, Wei JM, Gouveia CJ, Zaghi S, et al. Long-term results for maxillomandibular advancement to treat obstructive sleep apnea: a meta-analysis. Otolaryngol Head Neck Surg. 2019;160(4):580–93.
102. Rosero EB, Joshi GP. Outcomes of sleep apnea surgery in outpatient and inpatient settings. Anesth Analg. 2021;132(5):1215–22.
103. Ishii LE, Roxbury CR, Godoy A, Ishman SL, Ishii M. Does nasal surgery improve obstructive sleep apnea in patients with nasal obstruction and OSA? A meta-analysis. Otolaryngol Head Neck Surg. 2015;153(3):326–33.
104. Kezirian EJ, Weaver EM, Yueh B, Khuri SF, Henderson WG, Daley J. Risk factors for serious complication after uvulopalatopharyngoplasty. Arch Otolaryngol Head Neck Surg. 2006;132(10):1091–8.
105. Ramar K, Dort LC, Katz SG, Lettieri CJ, Harrod CG, Thomas SM, et al. Clinical practice guideline for the treatment of obstructive sleep apnea and snoring with oral appliance therapy: an update for 2015. J Clin Sleep Med. 2015;11(7):773–827.
106. Carvalho B, Hsia J, Capasso R. Surgical therapy of obstructive sleep apnea: a review. Neurotherapeutics. 2012;9(4):710–6.
107. Holty JEC, Guilleminault C. Surgical options for the treatment of obstructive sleep apnea. Med Clin North Am. 2010;94(3):479–515.
108. Kent D, Stanley J, Aurora RN, Levine C, Gottlieb DJ, Spann MD, et al. Referral of adults with obstructive sleep apnea for surgical consultation: an American Academy of Sleep Medicine systematic review, meta-analysis, and GRADE assessment. J Clin Sleep Med. 2021;17(12):2507–31.
109. Weaver TE, Grunstein RR. Adherence to continuous positive airway pressure therapy: the challenge to effective treatment. Proc Am Thorac Soc. 2008;5(2):173–8.
110. Epstein LJ, Kristo D, Strollo PJ Jr, et al. Clinical guideline for the evaluation, management and long-term care of obstructive sleep apnea in adults. J Clin Sleep Med. 2009;5(3):263–76.
111. Marín JM, Carrizo SJ, Vicente E, Agustí AG. Long-term cardiovascular outcomes in men with obstructive sleep apnoea–hypopnoea with or without CPAP treatment: an observational study. Lancet. 2005;365(9464):1046–53.
112. Masa JF, Corral J, Pereira R, et al. Therapeutic decision-making for sleep apnea and hypopnea syndrome using home respiratory polygraphy: a large multicenter study. Am J Respir Crit Care Med. 2011;184(8):964–71.
113. Teo M, Amis T, Lee S, Falland K, Lambert S, Wheatley J. Equivalence of nasal and oronasal masks during initial CPAP titration for obstructive sleep apnea syndrome. Sleep. 2011;34(7):951–5.
114. Kaw R, Chung F, Pasupuleti V, Mehta J, Gay PC, Hernandez AV. Meta-analysis of the association between obstructive sleep apnoea and postoperative outcome. Br J Anaesth. 2012;109(6):897–906.
115. Randerath WJ, Verbraecken J, Andreas S, et al. Non-CPAP therapies in obstructive sleep apnoea: ERS Task Force report. Eur Respir J. 2011;37(5):1000–28.
116. Mortimore IL, Kochhar P, Douglas NJ. Effect of posture, route of respiration, and negative pressure on palatal muscle activity in humans. J Appl Physiol (1985). 1995;79(2):448–54.

117. Sugiura T, Noda A, Nakata S, et al. Influence of nasal resistance on initial acceptance of continuous positive airway pressure in obstructive sleep apnea syndrome. Respiration. 2007;74(1):56–60.
118. Kushida CA, Chediak A, Berry RB, et al. Clinical guidelines for the manual titration of positive airway pressure in patients with obstructive sleep apnea. J Clin Sleep Med. 2008;4(2):157–71.
119. Li HY, Wang PC, Chen YP, Lee LA, Fang TJ, Wang CY. Critical appraisal and meta-analysis of nasal surgery for obstructive sleep apnea. Am J Rhinol Allergy. 2011;25(1):45–9.
120. Malhotra A, White DP. Obstructive sleep apnoea. Lancet. 2002;360(9328):237–45.
121. Fox N, Hirsch-Allen AJ, Goodfellow E, et al. Impact of a telemedicine monitoring system on positive airway pressure adherence in obstructive sleep apnea: randomized controlled trial. Sleep. 2012;35(4):477–81.
122. Goh LC, Rajendram N, Lim BWW, Kulasegarah J, Govindaraju R, Soo CI, Wong CK. Comparative study on CPAP compliance: PAP-NAP followed by CPAP trial vs CPAP trial alone. Sleep Sci. 2025;18(3):e301–6.
123. Pépin JL, Bailly S, Rinder P, et al. CPAP therapy termination rates by OSA phenotype: a French nationwide database analysis. J Clin Med. 2021;10(5):936.
124. Young T, Peppard PE, Taheri S. Excess weight and sleep-disordered breathing. J Appl Physiol (1985). 2005;99(4):1592–9.
125. Schwartz AR, Patil SP, Laffan AM, Polotsky V, Schneider H, Smith PL. Obesity and obstructive sleep apnea: pathogenic mechanisms and therapeutic approaches. Proc Am Thorac Soc. 2008;5(2):185–92.
126. Eichler C, Sommer JU, Stuck BA, Hörmann K, Maurer JT. Does drug-induced sleep endoscopy change the treatment concept of obstructive sleep apnea? Sleep Breath. 2013;17(1):63–8.
127. Greenburg DL, Lettieri CJ, Eliasson AH. Effects of surgical weight loss on measures of obstructive sleep apnea: a meta-analysis. Am J Med. 2009;122(6):535–42.
128. Benjafield AV, Ayas NT, Eastwood PR, et al. Estimation of the global prevalence and burden of obstructive sleep apnoea: a literature-based analysis. Lancet Respir Med. 2019;7(8):687–98.
129. Young T, Peppard PE, Gottlieb DJ. Epidemiology of obstructive sleep apnea: a population health perspective. Am J Respir Crit Care Med. 2002;165(9):1217–39.
130. Peppard PE, Young T, Palta M, Dempsey J, Skatrud J. Longitudinal study of moderate weight change and sleep-disordered breathing. JAMA. 2000;284(23):3015–21.
131. Redline S, Yenokyan G, Gottlieb DJ, et al. Obstructive sleep apnea-hypopnea and incident stroke: the sleep heart health study. Am J Respir Crit Care Med. 2010;182(2):269–77.
132. Weaver EM, Kapur VK, Yueh B. Polysomnography vs self-reported measures in patients with sleep apnea. Arch Otolaryngol Head Neck Surg. 2004;130(4):453–8.
133. Blackman A, Foster GD, Zammit G, et al. Effect of liraglutide 3.0 mg in individuals with obesity and moderate or severe obstructive sleep apnea: the SCALE Sleep Apnea randomized clinical trial. Int J Obes. 2016;40(8):1310–9.
134. Sarkhosh K, Switzer NJ, El-Hadi M, et al. The impact of bariatric surgery on obstructive sleep apnea: a systematic review. Obes Surg. 2013;23(3):414–23.
135. Chung F, Liao P, Yegneswaran B, Shapiro CM, Kang W. Postoperative changes in sleep-disordered breathing and sleep architecture in patients with obstructive sleep apnea. Anesthesiology. 2014;120(2):287–98.
136. Lopez-Nava G, Asokkumar R, Rull A, et al. Endoscopic sleeve gastroplasty for the treatment of obesity: a multicenter study of 248 patients with 24 months follow-up. Obes Surg. 2017;27(10):2649–55.
137. Vigil L, Zapata T, Grau A, Bonet M, Montaña M, Piñar M. Innovación en sueño [Sleep Innovation]. Open Respir Arch. 2025;6(Suppl 2):100402.
138. Blumen MB, Dahan S, Fleury B, Hausser-Hauw C, Chabolle F. Radiofrequency ablation for the treatment of mild to moderate obstructive sleep apnea. Laryngoscope. 2002;112(11):2086–92.

139. Steward DL, Weaver EM, Woodson BT. Multilevel temperature-controlled radiofrequency for obstructive sleep apnea: extended follow-up. Otolaryngol Head Neck Surg. 2005;132(4):630–5.
140. Herman H, Stern J, Alessi DM, Swartz KA, Gillespie MB. Office-based multilevel radiofrequency ablation for mild-to-moderate obstructive sleep apnea. OTO Open. 2023;7(1):e19. Published 2023 Feb 17.
141. Steward DL. Effectiveness of multilevel (tongue and palate) radiofrequency tissue ablation for patients with obstructive sleep apnea syndrome. Laryngoscope. 2004;114(12):2073–84.
142. Birkent H, Soken H, Akcam T, Karahatay S, Gerek M. The effect of radiofrequency volumetric tissue reduction of soft palate on voice. Eur Arch Otorrinolaringol. 2008;265(2):195–8.
143. MacKay SG, Carney AS, Woods C, et al. Modified uvulopalatopharyngoplasty and coblation channeling of the tongue for obstructive sleep apnea: a multicentre Australian trial. J Clin Sleep Med. 2013;9(2):117–24.
144. Goyal A, Chavan P, Shinde V, et al. A comparative study between coblation-assisted tonsillectomy and conventional dissection and snare tonsillectomy. Cureus. 2024;16(8):e68281.
145. Inada H, Hirata M, Kimura A, et al. Comparison of classical method and microdebrider technique for adenoidectomy in pediatric patients with obstructive sleep apnea. Fujita Med J. 2024;10(2):49–52.
146. Sorin A, Bent JP, April MM, Ward RF. Complications of microdebrider-assisted powered intracapsular tonsillectomy and adenoidectomy. Laryngoscope. 2004;114(2):297–300.
147. Williamson A, Morrow VR, Carr MM, Coutras SW. Safety and efficacy of lingual tonsillectomy in multilevel airway surgery for pediatric obstructive sleep apnea. J Clin Sleep Med. 2024;20(2):189–99.
148. Kandogan T, Olgun L, Ozüer MZ. Management of lingual tonsillar hypertrophy using microdebrider. Kulak Burun Bogaz Ihtis Derg. 2008;18(5):323–5.
149. DeMarcantonio MA, Senser E, Meinzen-Derr J, Roetting N, Shott S, Ishman SL. The safety and efficacy of pediatric lingual tonsillectomy. Int J Pediatr Otorhinolaryngol. 2016;91:6–10.
150. Ferguson KA, Heighway K, Ruby RR. A randomized trial of laser-assisted uvulopalatoplasty in the treatment of mild obstructive sleep apnea. Am J Respir Crit Care Med. 2003;167(1):15–9.
151. Kamami YV. Outpatient treatment of snoring with CO_2 laser: laser-assisted UPPP. J Otolaryngol. 1994;23(6):391–4.
152. Neruntarat C. Laser-assisted uvulopalatoplasty: short-term and long-term results. Otolaryngol Head Neck Surg. 2001;124(1):90–3.
153. Shiffman HS, Khorsandi J, Cauwels NM. Minimally invasive combined Nd:YAG and Er:YAG laser-assisted uvulopalatoplasty for treatment of obstructive sleep apnea. Photobiomodul Photomed Laser Surg. 2021;39(8):550–7.
154. Fontenot A, Liu SY, Dewan K. CO_2 laser lingual tonsil reduction as a treatment for tongue discomfort during hypoglossal nerve stimulation: a case report. J Clin Sleep Med. 2024;20(11):1857–61.
155. Albazee E, Alshammari B, Alotaibi M, Tripathi KM, Abuawad A. Thermal welding tonsillectomy versus monopolar electrocautery tonsillectomy: a systematic review and meta-analysis of randomized clinical trials. Turk Arch Otorhinolaryngol. 2023;61(2):83–90.
156. Karatzias GT, Lachanas VA, Sandris VG. Thermal welding versus bipolar tonsillectomy: a comparative study. Otolaryngol Head Neck Surg. 2006;134(6):975–8.
157. Lee YC, Hsin LJ, Lin WN, Fang TJ, Tsai YT, Luo CM. Adolescents and adults undergoing temperature-controlled surgical instruments vs electrocautery in tonsillectomy: a systematic review and meta-analysis of randomized clinical trials. JAMA Otolaryngol Head Neck Surg. 2020;146(4):339–46.
158. Chen AW, Chen MK. Comparison of post-tonsillectomy hemorrhage between monopolar and plasma blade techniques. J Clin Med. 2021;10(10):2051.
159. Pavlíková G, Foltán R, Horká M, Hanzelka T, Borunská H, Sedý J. Piezosurgery in oral and maxillofacial surgery. Int J Oral Maxillofac Surg. 2011;40(5):451–7.

160. Rana M, Gellrich NC, Rana M, Piffkó J, Kater W. Evaluation of surgically assisted rapid maxillary expansion with piezosurgery versus oscillating saw and chisel osteotomy - a randomized prospective trial. Trials. 2013;14:49. Published 2013 Feb 17
161. Bettega G, Pépin JL, Veale D, Deschaux C, Raphaël B, Lévy P. Obstructive sleep apnea syndrome: 51 consecutive patients treated by maxillofacial surgery. Am J Respir Crit Care Med. 2000;162(2 Pt 1):641–9.
162. Vercellotti T. Technological characteristics and clinical indications of piezoelectric bone surgery. Minerva Stomatol. 2004;53(5):207–14.
163. Merta M, Heliövaara A, Leikola J, Suojanen J. Early experience of wafer-free Le Fort I osteotomy with patient-specific implants in cleft lip and palate patients. J Plast Reconstr Aesthet Surg. 2023;77:78–86.
164. Svistushkin VM, Starostina SV, Toldanov AV. Possibilities of coblation in otorhinolaryngology: an analytical review. Eur Arch Otorrinolaringol. 2022;279(4):1655–62.
165. Yu JL, Afolabi-Brown O. Updates on management of pediatric obstructive sleep apnea. Pediatr Invest. 2019;3:228–35.
166. Marcus CL, Brooks LJ, Draper KA, et al. Diagnosis and management of childhood obstructive sleep apnea syndrome. Pediatrics. 2012;130:e714–55.
167. Sunkaraneni V, Ismail-Koch H, Salib R, et al. Guillotine tonsillectromy: a neglected technique. J Laryngol Otol. 2009;123(8):907–8.
168. Marcus CL, Moore RH, Rosen CL, Giordani B, Garetz SL, Taylor HG, Mitchell RB, Amin R, Katz ES, Arens R, Paruthi S, Muzumdar H, Gozal D, Thomas NH, Ware J, Beebe D, Snyder K, Elden L, Sprecher RC, Willging P, Jones D, Bent JP, Hoban T, Chervin RD, Ellenberg SS, Redline S; Childhood Adenotonsillectomy Trial (CHAT). A randomized trial of adenotonsillectomy for childhood sleep apnea. N Engl J Med. 2013;368(25):2366–76. https://doi.org/10.1056/NEJMoa1215881. Epub 2013 May 21. PMID: 23692173; PMCID: PMC3756808.
169. Brietzke SE, Gallagher D. The effectiveness of tonsillectomy and adenoidectomy in the treatment of pediatric obstructive sleep apnea/hypopnea syndrome: a meta-analysis. Otolaryngol Head Neck Surg. 2006;134(6):979–84.
170. Benedek P, Balakrishnan K, Cunningham MJ, et al. International Pediatric Otolaryngology group (IPOG) consensus on the diagnosis and management of pediatric obstructive sleep apnea (OSA). Int J Pediatr Otorhinolaryngol. 2020;138:110276.
171. Koltai PJ, Solares CA, Koempel JA, et al. Intracapsular tonsillar reduction (partial tonsillectomy): reviving a historical procedure for obstructive sleep disordered breathing in children. Otolaryngol Head Neck Surg. 2003;129:532–8.
172. Spencer GM, Wilson CA, Davidson J, et al. Global tonsillectomy practice patterns - a survey study of pediatric otolaryngologists. Int J Pediatr Otorhinolaryngol. 2025;191:112276.
173. Kang KT, Koltai PJ, Lee CH, et al. Lingual tonsillectomy for treatment of pediatric obstructive sleep apnea: a meta-analysis. JAMA Otolaryngol Head Neck Surg. 2017;143(6):561–8. https://doi.org/10.1001/jamaoto.2016.4274.
174. Woodson BT, Fujita S. Clinical experience with ligualplasty as part of the treatment of severe obstructive sleep apnea. Otolaryngol Head Neck Surg. 1992;107:40–8.
175. Maturo SC, Mair EA. Submucosal minimally invasive lingual excision: an effective, novel surgery for pediatric tongue base reduction. Ann Otol Rhinol Laryngol. 2006;115:624–30.
176. Wooten CT, Shott SR. Evolving therapies to treat retroglossal and base-of-tongue obstruction in pediatric obstructive sleep apnea. Arch Otolaryngol Head Neck Surg. 2010;136:983–7.
177. Mermans JF, Lissenberg-Witte BI, et al. Tongue lip adhesion in the treatment of Robin sequence. J Craniofac Surg. 2018;29(8):2327–33.
178. Zhang RS, Hoppe IC, Taylor JA, Bartlett SP. Surgical management and outcomes of Pierre Robin sequence: a comparison of mandibular distraction osteogenesis and tongue-lip adhesion. Plast Reconstr Surg. 2018;142(2):480–509.
179. Guilleminault C, Li K, Quo S, et al. A prospective study on the surgical out-comes of children with sleep-disordered breathing. Sleep. 2004;27(1):95–100.

180. Seid AB, Martin PJ, Pransky SM, Kearns DB. Surgical therapy of obstructive sleep apnea in children with severe mental insufficiency. Laryngoscope. 1990;100(5):507–10.
181. Pang KP. The role of nasal surgery in the treatment of OSA. Curr Otorhinolaryngol Rep. 2013;1:20–4.
182. Sulman CG. Pediatric sleep surgery. Front Pediatr. 2014;2:51.
183. Cheng PW, Fang KM, Su HW, Huang TW. Improved objective outcomes and quality of life after adenotonsillectomy with inferior turbinate reduction in pediatric obstructive sleep apnea with inferior turbinate hypertrophy. Laryngoscope. 2012;122:2850–4.
184. Bhagat PR, Bathla M, Doshi H, Solanki K, Gajjar R. A study of comparison of outcomes of submucous diathermy, coblation and micro-debrider assisted inferior turbinoplasty in patients having inferior turbinate hypertrophy. Indian J Otolaryngol Head Neck Surg. 2024;76(3):2548–56.
185. Thorne MC, Garetz SL. Laryngomalacia: review and summary of current clinical practice in 2015. Paediatr Respir Rev. 2016;17:3–8.
186. Bedwell J, Zalzal G. Laryngomalacia. Semin Pediatr Surg. 2016;25:119–22.
187. Camacho M, Dunn B, Torre C, Sasaki J, Gonzales R, Liu SY, et al. Supraglottoplasty for laryngomalacia with obstructive sleep apnea: a systematic review and metaanalysis. Laryngoscope. 2016;126:1246–55.
188. Chan DK, Truong MT, Koltai PJ. Supraglottoplasty for occult laryngomalacia to improve obstructive sleep apnea syndrome. Arch Otolaryngol Head Neck Surg. 2012;138:50–4.
189. Revell SM, Clark WD. Late-onset laryngomalacia: a cause of pediatric obstructive sleep apnea. Int J Pediatr Otorhinolaryngol. 2011;75:231–8.
190. Oomen KP, Modi VK. Occult laryngomalacia resulting in obstructive sleep apnea in an infant. Int J Pediatr Otorhinolaryngol. 2013;77:1617–9.
191. Thevasagayam M, Rodger K, Cave D, et al. Prevalence of laryngomalacia in children presenting with sleep-disordered breathing. Laryngoscope. 2010;120:1662–6.
192. Denoyelle F, Mondain M, Gresillon N, Roger G, Chaudre F, Garabedian EN. Failures and complications of supraglottoplasty in children. Arch Otolaryngol Head Neck Surg. 2003;129(10):1077–80.
193. Rastatter JC, Schroeder JW, Hoff SR, Holinger LD. Aspiration before and after Supraglottoplasty regardless of technique. Int J Otolaryngol. 2010;2010:912814.
194. Natu SS, Ali I, Alam S, Giri KY, Agarwal A, Kulkarni VA. The biology of distraction osteogenesis for correction of mandibular and craniomaxillofacial defects: a review. Dent Res J (Isfahan). 2014;11:16–26.
195. Noller MW, Guilleminault C, Gouveia CJ, Mack D, Neighbors CL, Zaghi S, et al. Mandibular advancement for pediatric obstructive sleep apnea: a systematic review and meta-analysis. J Craniomaxillofac Surg. 2018;46:1296–302.
196. Pirelli P, Saponara M, Guilleminault C. Rapid maxillary expansion in children with obstructive sleep apnea syndrome. Sleep. 2004;27:761–6.
197. Principato JJ. Upper airway obstruction and craniofacial morphology. Otolaryngol Head Neck Surg. 1991;104:881–90.
198. Pirelli P, Saponara M, Guilleminault C. Rapid maxillary expansion (RME) for pediatric obstructive sleep apnea: a 12-year follow-up. Sleep Med. 2015;16:933–5.
199. Rizzi CJ, Amin JD, Isaiah A, Valdez TA, Jeyakumar A, Smart SE, Pereira KD. Tracheostomy for severe pediatric obstructive sleep apnea: indications and outcomes. Otolaryngol Head Neck Surg. 2017 Aug;157(2):309–13.
200. Remmers JE, Issa FG, Suratt PM. Sleep and respiration. J Appl Physiol. 1985;68:1286–9.
201. Schwartz AR, Bennett ML, Smith PL, et al. Therapeutic electrical stimulation of the hypoglossal nerve in obstructive sleep apnea. Arch Otolaryngol Head Neck Surg. 2001;127:1216–23.
202. Caloway CL, Diercks GR, Keamy D, et al. Update on hypoglossal nerve stimulation in children with down syndrome and obstructive sleep apnea. Laryngoscope. 2020;130:E263–7.

Chapter 2
Drug-Induced Sleep Endoscopy (DISE)

Chun Hong Yeap, Siti Nadzrah Yunus, Jeremy Sin Hun Tan, Mohd Ayzam Ahmad, and Maythad Uataya

2.1 Preoperative Assessment Framework for Sleep Apnea Surgery

Chun Hong Yeap and Siti Nadzrah Yunus

2.1.1 Introduction

Sleep apnea is an independent predictor of postoperative pulmonary, cardiovascular, and airway complications, and is associated with increased resource utilization and mortality [1, 3, 13, 16]. It amplifies the depressant effects of anesthetic agents and opioids while diminishing physiological reserve [3, 6, 16]. A structured preoperative assessment (Fig. 2.1), therefore, serves the following three key purposes:

C. H. Yeap · S. N. Yunus (✉) · J. S. H. Tan
Department of Anesthesiology, Faculty of Medicine, Universiti Malaya, Kuala Lumpur, Malaysia
e-mail: chunhong@um.edu.my; siti.nadzrah@ummc.edu.my; jeremy.tansh@um.edu.my

M. A. Ahmad (✉)
Department of Otorhinolaryngology, Hospital Sultanah Bahiyah, Alor Setar, Kedah, Malaysia

M. Uataya
Department of Otorhinolaryngology, Faculty of Medicine, Siriraj Hospital, Mahidol University, Bangkok, Thailand
e-mail: maythad.uat@mahidol.ac.th

L. C. Goh, S. T. Toh (eds.), *Sleep Surgery in a Nutshell*,
https://doi.org/10.1007/978-981-95-9749-9_2

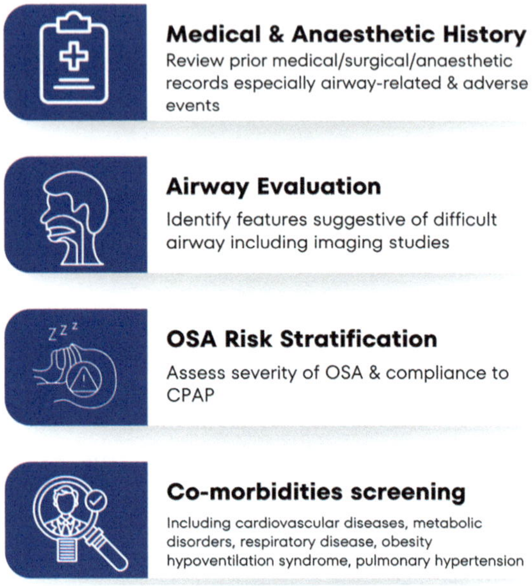

Fig. 2.1 Structured preoperative assessment

1. to quantify disease control,
2. to identify and optimize comorbid conditions, and
3. to align the surgical, anesthetic, and nursing teams on intra- and postoperative management.

2.1.1.1 Sleep Apnea Severity and Stratification

Accurate characterization of current disease burden underpins every downstream decision.

1. Record the Apnea–Hypopnea Index (AHI) and nocturnal nadir SpO_2 from the most recent sleep study [7, 15]. Both AHI and polysomnography or oximetry-derived hypoxemia parameters may help identify patients at higher risk of postoperative respiratory and cardiovascular events [1, 7, 15].
2. Confirm continuous positive airway pressure (CPAP) adherence by inspecting the 30-day usage download; ≥4 h of nightly use is associated with a ~50% reduction in postoperative desaturation and unplanned ICU admission [32]. This criteria satisfies national criteria for day-surgery eligibility [2, 6, 33].

When to update testing

Repeat home sleep apnea testing (HSAT) or schedule drug-induced sleep endoscopy (DISE) if the sleep study is >12 months ago **or** body weight has increased by >10 kg or worsening of OSA symptoms [8, 34].

HSAT may be used as an alternative diagnostic modality when formal polysomnography is unavailable or impractical and would delay surgery [8].

2.1.1.2 Comprehensive Medical Evaluation (3C Worksheet)

Sleep apnea-related morbidity is amplified by cardiovascular, cerebrovascular, and pulmonary disease [1, 11, 13, 16]. A structured one-page worksheet ensures nothing is overlooked:

Domain	Component of assessment	Escalation criteria[a]
Cardiovascular	Blood pressure (BP) control History of myocardial infarction (MI) Class of heart failure	Get a cardiology consultation if: BP >180/110 mmHg New York heart association (NYHA) class III–IV or features of heart failure MI <3 months
Cerebrovascular	History of stroke/transient ischemic attack (TIA) Antithrombotic therapy	Seek neurology consultation when: Stroke/TIA <3 months Suitability to withhold antithrombotic therapy
Respiratory	Chronic obstructive pulmonary disease (COPD)/asthma Require domiciliary O_2 Record the lowest SpO_2 from the sleep study	Get a respiratory review and request for echocardiogram to rule out pulmonary hypertension if [7, 11, 15, 35]: Nadir SpO_2 <70% Daytime SpO_2 <90%

[a]Baseline complete blood count (to look for polycythemia), serum bicarbonate (acceptable cut off value of < 27mmol/L) and electrocardiogram (for evidence of right ventricular strain pattern) can provide information on disease control; chest X-ray, arterial blood gas, or transthoracic echocardiogram are required only when escalation triggers are present. Cardiopulmonary exercise test (CPET) is reserved for patients with poor effort tolerance or uncontrolled systemic disease

2.1.1.3 Airway and Surgical Specific Assessment

Securing the airway is the single greatest technical challenge in sleep apnea surgery; a detailed structural assessment therefore precedes every operative decision. By systematically documenting morphologic risk factors, the team can anticipate both surgical exposure and the degree of anesthetic difficulty, allocate appropriate equipment, and avert unplanned airway emergencies.

- *Airway morphology*: the presence of neck circumference >40 cm, BMI $\geq$30 kg m^{-2}, modified Mallampati III–IV, micro/retrognathia, macroglossia, tonsillar hypertrophy, high-arched palate may suggest the likelihood of a difficult airway [9, 14].
- *History of difficult mask ventilation/intubation* and prior DISE findings with complex anatomical structures [9].
- *Cephalometric or CT data* (if already available) may guide surgical planning, but are not routinely required.

2.1.1.4 Preoperative Optimization and Patient Engagement

Perioperative risk in sleep apnea is modifiable. A focused 4 to weeks optimization period, emphasizing CPAP adherence, medical stabilization, and behavioral change, has been shown to improve oxygen reserve and cardiovascular resilience markedly [2, 6, 36]. Because success hinges on patient participation, every intervention is paired with clear written guidance and objective targets, transforming the patient from a passive recipient into an active partner in their perioperative safety.

Intervention	Target/action	Rationale
CPAP	Nightly CPAP/NIPPV ≥4 h for 4 to 6 weeks [33]; Address CPAP intolerance (consider mask refit, humidification, nasal decongestant); Patient brings device and usage print-out on admission	Reduces airway oedema, airway hyperreactivity and postoperative events; Nonadherence (<4 h per night or <70% of nights) [32] correlates with adverse outcomes [2, 6]
Medical optimization	BP <160/100; HbA1c <8.5%	Limits cardiovascular decompensation
Lifestyle modification	Complete alcohol/tobacco abstinence minimum of 4 weeks; Encourage any preoperative weight loss; Refer BMI ≥35 kg m^{-2} to metabolic/obesity team	Improves oxygen reserve and wound healing
Education	One-page leaflet detailing perioperative CPAP use and mobilization plan	Written material doubles retention compared to verbal counselling [37]

2.1.1.5 Elective Surgery Delay Criteria

Postpone surgery if any of the following persist despite optimization:

- Systolic BP >180 mmHg or diastolic BP >110 mmHg.
- Recent myocardial infarction or stroke (<3 months).
- Decompensated heart failure or newly detected arrhythmia.
- $PaCO_2$ >45 mmHg in obesity hypoventilation syndrome (OHS) without prior CPAP acclimatization [11].
- Active upper airway infection.

Special Considerations

- *Inpatient vs outpatient surgery*: decide based on sleep apnea severity, comorbid burden, anticipated opioid need, and facility capability (continuous monitoring, trained staff) [3, 4, 16].
- *Uncontrolled systemic disease, severe pulmonary hypertension, or resting hypoxemia* mandates inpatient management and possible critical care admission before surgery [1, 11, 15].

2.1.2 Perioperative Management Plan

Once disease status and comorbidities are defined, an integrated anesthetic–surgical roadmap converts risk stratification into practical bedside actions.

Diagnosed sleep apnea—CPAP adherent
Continue CPAP throughout perioperative period; Extubate head-up onto CPAP
Diagnosed sleep apnea—CPAP non adherent
Initiate supervised PAP trial preoperatively or arrange in hospital titration; Address barriers (mask leak, pressure intolerance).
High clinical suspicion, no confirmed study
Proceed with HSAT/oximetry; If surgery cannot be delayed, manage as high-risk per guideline

2.1.3 Postoperative Disposition

Rigorous postoperative surveillance is the final safeguard against late hypoxemia, opioid-induced ventilatory depression and cardiovascular decompensation in patients with sleep apnea [3, 12, 16]. Bed allocation must therefore be dictated by objective risk metrics rather than theatre logistics or bed availability [3, 4, 12, 16].

Criterion (any single factor)	Required level of care
AHI >30 h^{-1} *or* Epworth sleepiness Scale (ESS) ≥ 11	High-dependency unit (HDU) with CPAP; minimum postanesthetic care unit (PACU) stay ≥3 h after last respiratory event
BMI ≥35 kg m^{-2} *and* long-acting opioid use	HDU or step-down ward with continuous capnography
Cardiopulmonary escalation trigger	HDU or ICU
Low-risk profile	Standard surgical ward; hourly SpO_2 checks for the first 4 h; maintain baseline room-air SpO_2 before transfer

Red-flag symptoms for escalation trigger: persistent desaturation <90%, uncontrolled pain, excessive somnolence

Summary Points

- AHI, nadir SpO_2, and CPAP adherence are the pillars of risk stratification [2, 6, 7, 15].
- Cardiovascular, cerebrovascular, and pulmonary comorbidities must be optimized before anesthesia [1, 11, 13, 16].
- A 4 to 6 weeks optimization bundle (CPAP, lifestyle modification, medical tuning) yields measurable perioperative benefit [2, 6].
- Postoperative disposition should match the patient's therapeutic needs [3, 4, 12, 16] and objective risks to an appropriate monitored environment, rather than be based solely on bed availability.
- Success hinges on coordinated, multidisciplinary care, and clear patient engagement.

2.2 Drug-Induced Sleep Endoscopy (DISE): Anesthesia Preparation and Perioperative Care

Siti Nadzrah Yunus and Jeremy Sin Hun Tan

2.2.1 *Introduction*

Drug-induced sleep endoscopy (DISE) is a diagnostic procedure that employs pharmacologically induced sleep to visualize upper airway obstruction and guide definitive treatment for obstructive sleep apnea (OSA). Anesthetic management plays a central role i the validity and safety of DISE. The objective is not simply to sedate the patient, but to achieve a stable level of sedation that approximates natural sleep closely enough to permit meaningful endoscopic assessment while preserving spontaneous ventilation, maintaining oxygenation and avoiding arefactual airway collapse caused by over-sedation [19–22]. Success hinges on meticulous risk stratification, precise sedative titration and coordination with endoscopy procedure, and structured recovery monitoring [18–20, 22].

2.2.2 *DISE 3-Step Safety Framework*

Perioperative care for DISE can be outlined by the DISE 3-step safety framework that steers the patient from initial assessment to discharge (Fig. 2.2).

2.2.2.1 Step 1: Preoperative Risk Stratification and Optimization

Building on the comprehensive preoperative evaluation detailed in the preceding chapter, safe conduct of DISE begins with a focused, evidence-based appraisal across the five domains below that determines both risk level and day-case eligibility [18–20, 22].

Domain	Red flag	Action/optimization
OSA severity	Apnea–hypopnea Index (AHI) >30 h^{-1} [19, 20, 22] Nadir pulse oximetry <90% [19, 20, 22] Body mass index (BMI) > 35 kg m^{-2} [19, 20, 22]	CPAP initiation and optimization Postoperative high-dependency unit (HDU) monitoring
Continuous positive airway pressure (CPAP) adherence	Therapy interrupted >48 h [18, 19] Residual AHI on device download >15 h^{-1} [18, 19]	Reinstate nightly CPAP up to operative day [18, 19] Patient to bring the mask and device on the day of surgery If noncompliant, upgrade to the inpatient pathway

Domain	Red flag	Action/optimization
Systemic comorbidities	Symptoms of heart failure Recent ischemic event Uncontrolled systemic diseases [18–20, 24] On sedative medication(s) for mood disorder/chronic opioid use	Optimize medical status (speciality referral as needed) [18–20, 24] Consider deferring surgery if symptomatic Perioperative medication management as per institutional protocol Consider HDU monitoring
Anticipated airway difficulty	Macroglossia Mouth opening <3 cm Craniofacial anomalies Limited neck extension Previous difficult airway history	Senior anesthetist and advanced airway equipment present according to the difficult airway society (DAS) guideline [19, 21] Crisis algorithm is mandatory [19, 20] (sudden airway obstruction, hypoxemia, laryngospasm, aspiration, anaphylaxis)
Postoperative pulmonary complication (PPC) risk	STOP-BANG ≥5 Untreated OSA [18–20] Cardiorespiratory comorbidities Concurrent sedative/opioid therapy Active smoker	Smoking cessation >24 h before operation Fasting >6 h of solid and >2 h of clear fluid Aspiration prophylaxis when indicated Consider HDU monitoring [18–20]

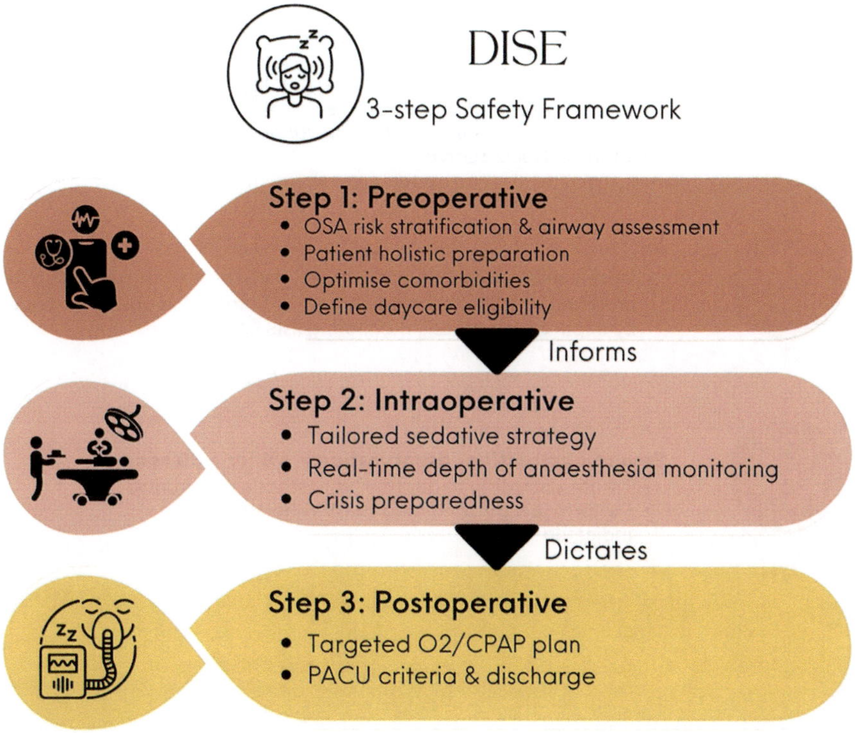

Fig. 2.2 DISE 3-step safety framework

Day-Case DISE Exclusion Criteria [18–20, 22]

AHI >30 h^{-1} | BMI >35 kg m^{-2} | use of sedative/opioid therapy | uncontrolled systemic disease or systemic disease with end-organ damage | features of difficult airway

Morning Checklist

Confirm fasting ≥6 h solids & ≥2 h clear fluid, verify CPAP used overnight and device is in theatre, secure an IV access, and brief the team on airway plan and crisis cart location [19, 20].

2.2.2.2 Step 2: Intraoperative Management

01 PREPARATION

- *Involves deliberate* ***MONITORED AIRWAY OBSTRUCTION*** *with risk of hypoxaemia, potential airway maneuvers or invasive airway rescue*
- **Monitoring**: *ECG, NIBP, SpO2, EtCO2 by nasal cannula, depth of anaesthesia monitoring such as BIS/Sedline*
- Adjuncts:
  - Antisialagogue: IV Glycopyrrolate 200µg
  - Aspiration prophylaxis (BMI > 35kg/m² or gastro-esophageal reflux symptoms): IV Ranitidine 50mg, IV Metoclopramide 10mg
  - Laryngeal oedema prophylaxis: IV Dexamethasone 0.15mg/kg

02 SETTING UP

- **Goal**: to induce Stage N1/N2 Sleep
- *Ensure quiet & dimmed theatre*
- *Patient is lying supine in their usual sleeping* posture
- Start on NpO2 3L/min

03 INDUCTION & TITRATION STRATEGY

- Once personnel and equipments are ready, begin induction using the preferred sedation technique. Titrate until snoring is observed, guided by depth of anaesthesia monitoring (BIS 50–70)

04 DEPTH ADJUSTMENT

Severe obstruction/ desaturation > 4% for > 60 secs

- Titrate according to depth of anaesthesia monitoring
- Perform jaw thrust +/- bag mask ventilation when indicated

The table below provides an at-a-glance comparison of the main anesthetic regimens reported for DISE, summarizing typical dosing, key advantages, and known limitations. The regimen marked with ★ is our center's choice, offering the optimal balance of physiological sleep fidelity and day-case suitability.

#	Technique and delivery	Dosage pattern	Key advantages (sleep fidelity/workflow)	Main pitfalls and cautions
1	Propofol—Manual incremental bolus [19–21, 24]	1 mg kg^{-1} induction → 20 mg bolus q2 min to snore–apnea cycle (SAC)	Fast onset; inexpensive; equipment-light	Abrupt depth changes; higher risk of overshoot apnea
2	Propofol—Target-controlled infusion (TCI) [19, 20, 22, 24]	Start at 1.5μg mL^{-1} (slow) or 2.5μg mL^{-1} (rapid) ↑ 0.2μg mL^{-1} q2 min to SAC	Smooth titration; reproducible multilevel collapse; rapid recovery	Needs TCI pump; dose-dependent respiratory depression
3	Dexmedetomidine infusion [19–21, 24]	Bolus of 1μg kg^{-1} over 10 min→maintain with 0.2–0.7μg kg^{-1} h^{-1}	Minimal ventilatory depression; physiologic sleep stage N1/N2	Slow onset; bradycardia; may need propofol rescue
4	★ Propofol + dexmedetomidine [19, 20, 24]	Slow bolus of dexmedetomedine 0.25μg kg^{-1} of lean body weight → propofol TCI 2.0μg mL^{-1} (titrate ±0.2μg mL^{-1})	Synergistic: Rapid titratability (propofol) + airway stability (dexmedetomidine); shorter discharge times; excellent for daycare DISE [19, 20, 24]	Requires TCI pumps and vigilance for cumulative depth
5	Midazolam [30] induction → propofol maintenance [20, 21, 24]	Midazolam 0.05–0.1 mg kg^{-1} IV bolus → propofol infusion/ bolus as needed	Anxiolysis; inexpensive	Greater tongue-base collapse, respiratory drive suppression; variable recovery [20, 24, 30]; flumazenil sometimes needed

2.2.2.3 Step 3: Postoperative Care and Monitoring

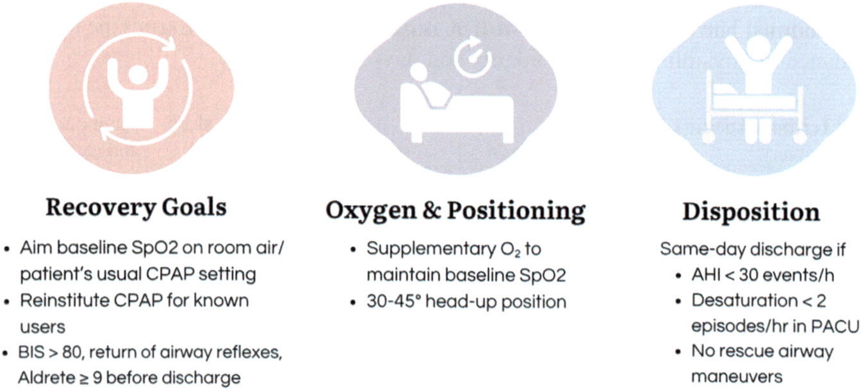

Allow *discharge* to the planned disposition (home for day-case), once SpO_2 >94% on room air, airway patency is confirmed, and Modified Aldrete ≥9 [18, 19].

Escalate to HDU if any exclusion criterion is met, such as: desaturation ≥5% below baseline for more than 30 min, recurrent obstruction requiring airway maneuvers, uncontrolled pain or nausea, or hemodynamic instability [18–20].

Summary Points

- *AHI, nadir SpO_2, BMI, and CPAP adherence* are the primary filters for determining whether DISE can proceed as a day-case or requires inpatient care [5, 18, 19, 20, 22, 24, 31].
- *A five-domain risk screen* comprising OSA severity, CPAP adherence, comorbidities, airway difficulty, PPC risk) guides clinical optimization and escalation [18–20, 22, 24].
- *Dexmedetomidine plus propofol TCI* best balances physiologic sleep fidelity with fast recovery for an outpatient workflow [19, 20, 24].
- *Discharge only when* room-air SpO_2 ≥94% for 15 min and the Aldrete ≥9; otherwise, admit to the HDU [18, 19].
- *Crisis algorithms* for hypoxemia and airway events must be visible and rehearsed before every list.

2.3 Drug-Induced Sleep Endoscopy (DISE)

Mohd Ayzam Ahmad and Maythad Uataya

2.3.1 Introduction

Obstructive sleep apnea (OSA) is characterized by recurrent episodes of partial or complete upper airway obstruction during sleep, resulting in intermittent hypoxemia, sleep fragmentation, and sympathetic activation. Management is individualized and typically spans behavioral measures (weight reduction, positional therapy, alcohol avoidance), continuous positive airway pressure (CPAP), oral appliance therapy (OAT), and surgery. CPAP remains the first-line treatment for most patients with moderate-to-severe OSA because it reliably splints the pharyngeal airway and abolishes apneic and hypopneic events when used consistently. Nevertheless, a substantial minority of patients struggle with tolerance or adherence; for them, alternative or adjunctive options—including customized mandibular advancement devices and site-directed surgery—should be considered within a structured, phenotype-guided pathway.

Accurate identification of the anatomic *level(s)* and *pattern(s)* of collapse is central to selecting and sequencing non-CPAP therapies. Conventional evaluations—physical examination, awake flexible nasopharyngolaryngoscopy (including Müller's maneuver), and imaging—provide valuable anatomic context but are limited in two important ways. First, they are performed during wakefulness, when upper airway dilator muscle tone is higher and reflex compensation is active; second, they capture largely static snapshots rather than the dynamic behavior of the airway under sleep-like conditions. As a result, findings on Müller's maneuver, for example, do not consistently predict the site or severity of collapse during actual sleep. This recognition underpins the shift toward *dynamic*, sleep-state assessments to guide therapy [23]

Drug-induced sleep endoscopy (DISE), first described by Croft and Pringle in 1991, was developed to fill this gap. Using carefully titrated sedation to reproduce the sleep state, DISE provides real-time visualization of the velum, lateral pharyngeal walls/tonsillar pillars, tongue base, and supraglottic structures during snoring and obstructive events. Standardized frameworks—most commonly the VOTE system [23, 24]—allow the examiner to document the *level* of obstruction (Velum, Oropharyngeal lateral wall, Tongue base, Epiglottis), the *configuration* (anteroposterior, lateral, or concentric), and the *degree* (partial vs complete). This information has practical consequences [24]: it helps identify candidates for oral appliance therapy (e.g., jaw-thrust responsive, tongue-predominant collapse), select palatal techniques that lateralize and stiffen the velopharyngeal segment when lateral wall collapse is present, and determine when tongue-base or epiglottic procedures should be added in a multilevel plan. DISE is also used to screen for complete concentric palatal collapse, a pattern that can influence candidacy for hypoglossal nerve stimulation.

Like all tests, DISE has limitations [26–28]. Sedation approximates but does not perfectly replicate natural sleep; interobserver variability exists and improves with training and standardized reporting; and results must be interpreted in the context of body position, nasal patency, and sleep-stage effects. Nonetheless, when performed within a disciplined protocol (including airway safety, appropriate sedative selection, and reproducible scoring), DISE meaningfully enhances diagnostic precision and has been associated with more rational procedure selection and improved surgical outcomes. In contemporary practice, it serves as a bridge between static anatomy and dynamic physiology, enabling clinicians to move beyond a one-size-fits-all approach and to tailor therapy to the patient's specific pattern of collapse [27–29].

2.3.2 *Indications [24, 29]*

1. Patients with OSA or snoring
2. Patients with OSA inadequate CPAP compliance or unwillingness to accept CPAP therapy
3. Surgical planning for multilevel upper airway obstruction
4. Candidate evaluation for hypoglossal nerve stimulation (HGNS)
5. Patients with residual disease after prior upper airway surgery for OSA
6. Pediatric patients with persistent OSA post adenotonsillectomy
7. Patients with complex or positional OSA patterns

2.3.3 *Contraindications*

1. Absolute contraindication
   (a) Severe cardiopulmonary instability
   (b) High-risk sedation patients (e.g., BMI >50 with comorbidities)
   (c) Patients allergic to sedative agents or with a history of anaphylaxis to related foods (e.g., eggs, egg products, soybeans, soy products) should avoid propofol [26]
   (d) Inability to tolerate nasal endoscopy
   (e) Pregnant patients [23]
2. Relative contraindications
   (a) Patients with morbid obesity are generally not good candidates for upper airway surgery or oral appliance therapy.
   (b) Patients with markedly severe OSA

2.3.4 Pre-Procedure Preparation

1. *Informed consent*: Discuss the rationale, risks (airway compromise, desaturation), and benefits of DISE.
2. *Preoperative assessment*: Review comorbidities, previous sleep study results, BMI, and airway anatomy.
3. *Fasting*: Minimum 6 h for solids, 2 h for clear fluids.
4. *Monitoring setup*: Continuous monitoring of:

   - Oxygen saturation (SpO_2)
   - Heart rate
   - Blood pressure
   - BiS monitoring probe [21, 31]

2.3.5 Equipment and Setup

- Flexible nasopharyngoscope (3.5–4.0 mm)
- Endoscope video recording system
- Oxygen delivery device (nasal cannula or face mask)
- Suction apparatus
- Resuscitation equipment
- Sedative agents (commonly propofol, dexmedetomidine, or midazolam)
- Topical decongestant and local anesthetic for nasal cavity
- Bispectral index (BIS) monitor (Figs. 2.3 and 2.4)

2.3.6 Procedure Steps

- Patient preparation: complete history and physical examination including Müller's maneuver should be done in clinic during initial consultation. All patients must be well explained and consented.
- Selected cases will be referred to anesthesia clinic.
- Patient is kept nil by mouth at least 6 h prior to procedure.
- Nasal decongestants, local nasal anesthesia, and antisecretory agents (atropine, glycopyrrolate) have been described as optional preparatory measures. However, these interventions may influence upper airway dynamics and respiratory control, and therefore should be used with caution.
- Patient should lie in a supine position and attempt to mimic the sleeping habits at home.
- Awake flexible nasopharyngolaryngoscopy (FNPLS) performed prior to sedation can be used to confirm adequate topical anesthesia. This examination also allows the anesthesia and surgical team to visualize the airway before sedating a

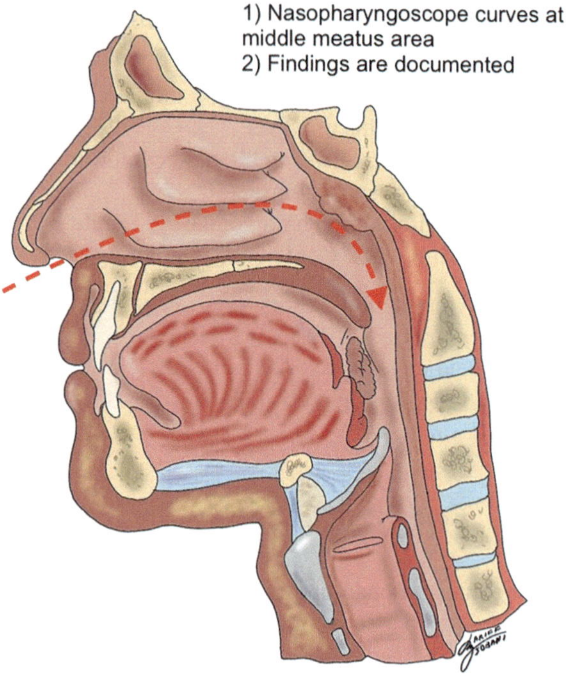

Fig. 2.3 Diagram demonstrating direction (dotted red) of flexible nasopharyngoscope, which goes through the middle meatus and into the nasopharynx

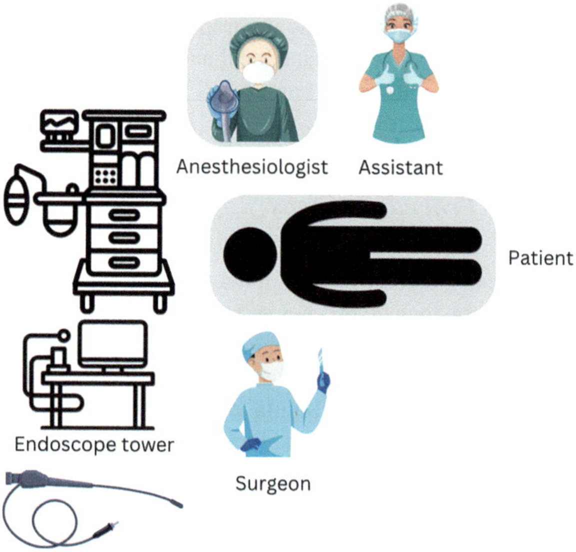

Fig. 2.4 Example of OT set-up during drug-induced sleep endoscopy (DISE)

patient with sleep-disordered breathing, providing an additional measure of reassurance, and can be used to compare the level and severity of obstruction with those observed during sleep.

- The operating room should be dimly lit and quiet, maintained at a comfortable temperature.
- The sedation agent depends on the personnel anesthetist preference [21], but several criteria are suggested, which include short half-life, available in infusion type, minimal impact on respiratory drive, minimal impact on muscle tone/REM, specific and rapid antidote, i.e., propofol, midazolam, or dexmedetomidine [19, 20, 21].
- Sedation given and titrated until patient reached a desired sleep state, defined as loss of consciousness with no response to verbal stimulation at normal conversational volume, corresponding approximately to a modified Ramsay score of 5, or *Bispectral Index (BIS) monitoring of 65–75 (60–80)* [21, 31].
- Observation should be performed during a stable level of sedation with a consistent breathing pattern. Following an observation period of at least two respiratory cycles or 1 min, FNPLS is introduced to initiate the assessment with simultaneous audiovisual recording.
- Special attention is paid to the following levels: *soft palate, lateral pharyngeal wall, palatine tonsil, tongue base/lingual tonsil, and epiglottis.*
- The *VOTE classification* is widely recognized to characterize the DISE finding that focuses on the specific structures that contribute at the following levels: Velum, Oropharyngeal, Tongue base, and Epiglottis.
- Additional procedures during DISE may be performed, such as changing to the lateral position for supine position-related OSA, Esmarch's maneuver [23, 24] (which adds value in assessing the potential effectiveness of mandibular advancement surgery), jaw thrust to zero overjet or mandibular advancement device titration, closing the mouth in patients with open-mouth breathing, using a nasopharyngeal airway bypass to evaluate primary or secondary epiglottic collapse originating from the palate, or PAP-assisted evaluation can uncover causes of persistent residual AHI in therapy-adherent patients [24].
- The finding then recorded and the surgical management then proceeded accordingly.

2.3.7 Documentation and Reporting Template

2.3.7.1 Sample Structured Report

Patient ID:
Date:
Sedative Used:
Lowest Oxygen Saturation during DISE:
Events Observed:

BiS range Achieved:

Position+ Supine, head at natural position

Documentation

Level	Collapse Configuration	Degree	Remarks
Velum	AP/lateral/concentric/none	0/1/2/X	
Oropharynx	Lateral/none	0/1/2/X	
Tongue	AP/none	0/1/2/X	
Epiglottis	AP/lateral/none	0/1/2/X	

Remarks
0 = No obstruction (<50% collapse)
1 = Partial obstruction (50–75% collapse)
2 = Complete obstruction (>75% Collapse)
X = No observation made
AP = Anteroposterior

2.3.7.2 Alternative or Additional Systems

- *NOHL*: Nose, Oropharynx, Hypopharynx, Larynx
- *Palate-Tongue-Epiglottis (PTE)* score
- *European Position Paper Scoring* (includes pattern, configuration, level, and behavior)

2.3.8 Risk and Potential Complications

- Nasal trauma
- Local pain on intravenous infusion
- Allergic reaction to medications
- Laryngospasm
- Pulmonary aspiration
- Hypercapnia, desaturation and loss of airway
- Cardiac dysrhythmias
- Systemic hypertension

Images Demonstrating Various Airway Configuration of the Velum (Figs. 2.5, 2.6, 2.7, 2.8, 2.9, 2.10, 2.11, and 2.12)

2.3.9 Post-Procedural Care

Following drug-induced sleep endoscopy (DISE), careful post-procedural management is essential to ensure patient safety and optimize diagnostic yield. Although DISE is generally regarded as a low-risk procedure, the use of sedatives and airway manipulation necessitates structured monitoring and standardized discharge criteria.

- *Recovery and monitoring*

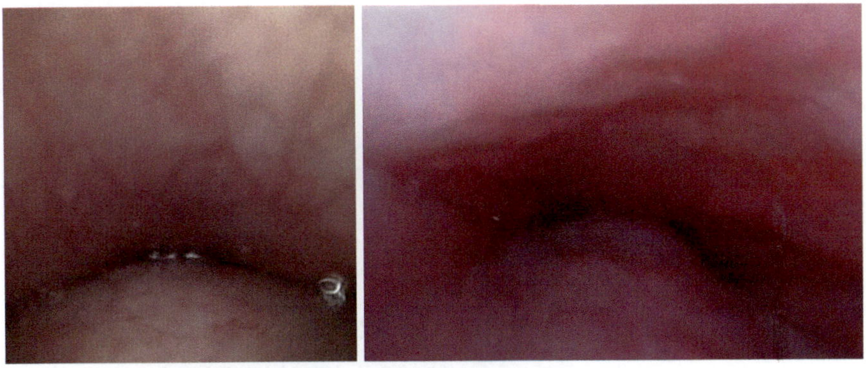

Fig. 2.5 Velum: complete AP obstruction

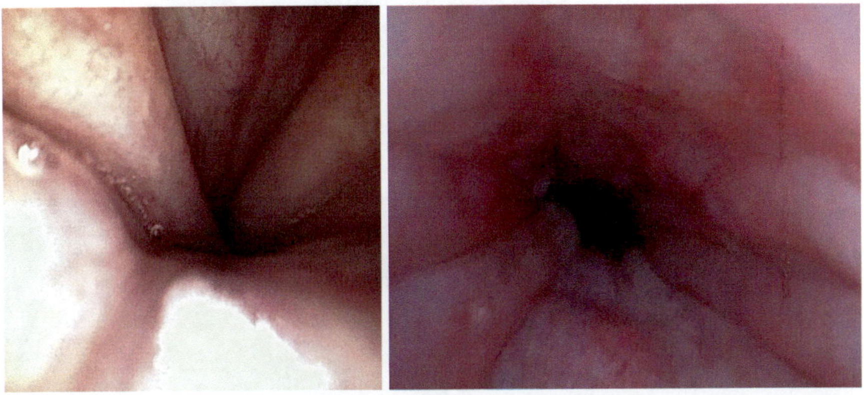

Fig. 2.6 Velum demonstrating complete concentric collapse (CCC)

Fig. 2.7 Velum demonstrating complete concentric obstruction with lymphoid hypertrophy

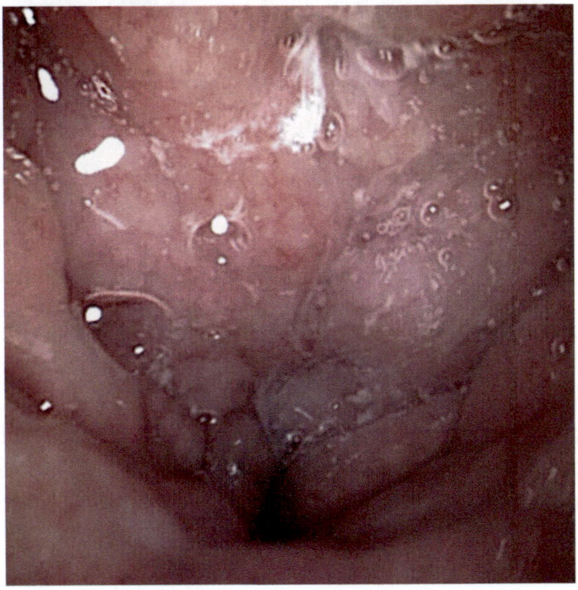

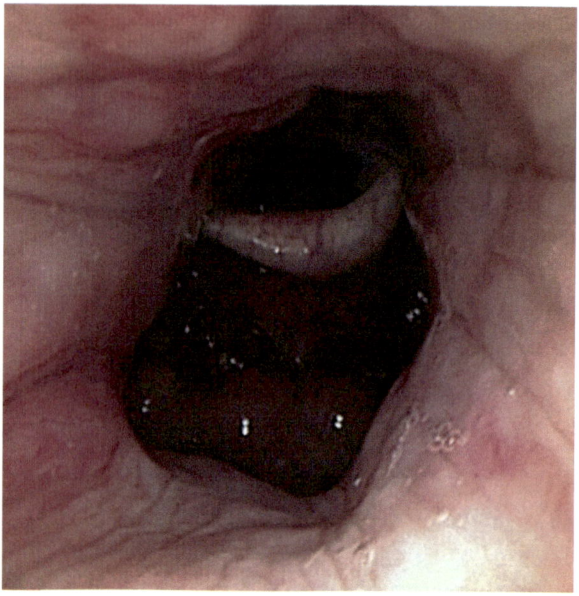

Fig. 2.8 Oropharynx showing normal patency

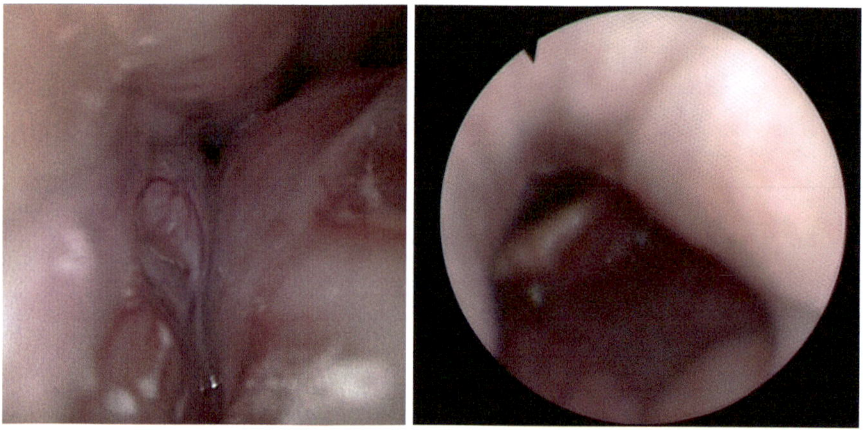

Fig. 2.9 Oropharynx: palatine tonsillar hypertrophy with complete lateral obstruction

- Patients should be observed in a recovery area with continuous monitoring of vital signs, oxygen saturation, and level of consciousness until the effects of sedation have sufficiently worn off. Supplemental oxygen may be administered during the early recovery phase, particularly in patients with moderate-to-severe OSA or preexisting cardiopulmonary comorbidities.
- *Airway and respiratory assessment*
- Airway patency s*houl*d be closely assessed, as residual sedation can predispose to desaturation or transient obstruction. Readiness for discharge requires stable respiratory effort, adequate oxygenation on room air, and protective airway reflexes intact.

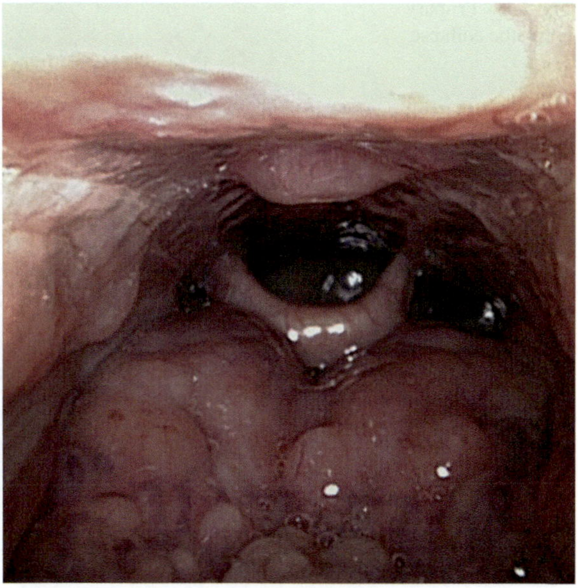

Fig. 2.10 Tongue base demonstrating lingual tonsillar hypertrophy

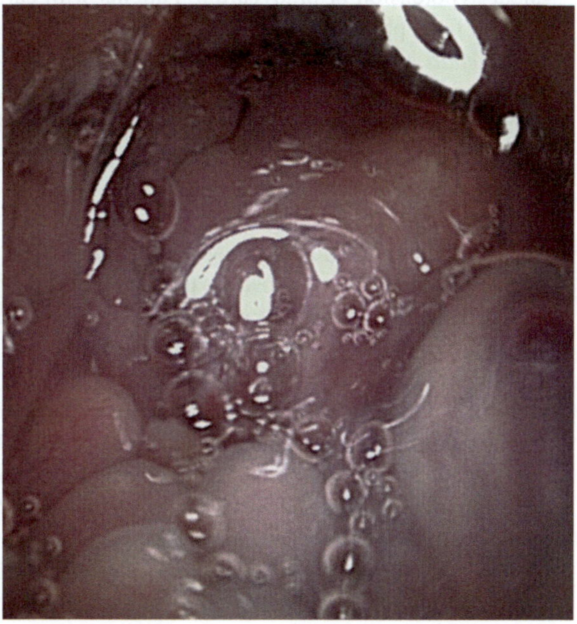

Fig. 2.11 Secondary epiglottic collapse with lingual tonsil hypertrophy

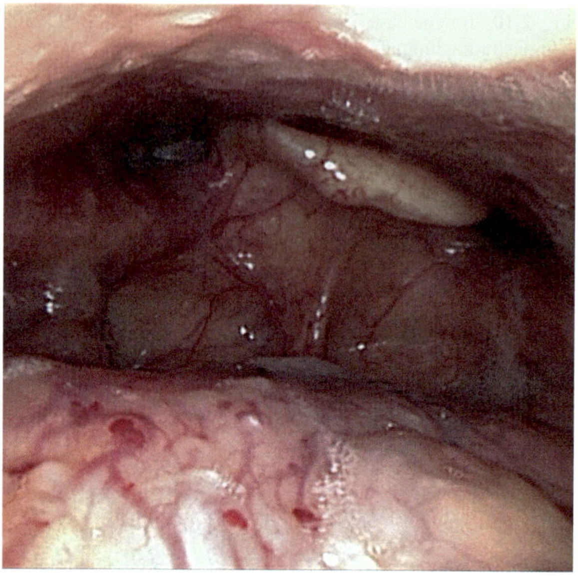

Fig. 2.12 Primary epiglottic collapse

- *Cardiovascular monitoring*
  Hemodynamic stability should be confirmed, as sedative agents may cause transient hypotension or bradycardia. Patients with cardiovascular risk factors may benefit from prolonged monitoring before discharge.
- *Post-sedation instructions*
  Clear instructions should be provided regarding the residual effects of sedatives. Patients must be advised against driving, operating heavy machinery, or making important decisions for at least 12–24 h post-procedure. A responsible adult escort is mandatory upon discharge.
- *Complications and management*
  Potential complications, though uncommon, include transient desaturation, minor epistaxis (from endoscope passage), laryngospasm, or prolonged sedation. These should be promptly recognized and managed according to institutional protocols. Documentation of any adverse events is essential for quality assurance.
- *Review of endoscopic video recordings*
  All DISE procedures should be recorded in their entirety. Videos are best reviewed after the procedure, once the patient is fully awake and stable. Ideally, the reviewing process should involve both the performing surgeon and, if available, members of the multidisciplinary sleep team. Reviewing the footage allows for careful assessment of dynamic airway collapse patterns, application of the VOTE classification, and identification of subtle findings that may have been missed during live endoscopy. Video review is also valuable for teaching, inter-rater reliability, and ensuring standardized documentation. Selected clips may later be shared with the patient during follow-up to enhance understanding of their condition and inform shared decision-making.
- *Communication and follow-up*

- Results of DISE should be reviewed with the patient during a dedicated consultation. Providing a clear explanation of findings, including VOTE classification and implications for management, ensures that the procedure translates into an actionable, personalized treatment plan.

2.3.10 Pearls and Pitfalls

Pearls

- *Standardized sedation protocol:* Use a consistent drug regimen (commonly propofol or dexmedetomidine) with careful titration to mimic natural sleep and avoid oversedation. Standardization enhances reproducibility and comparability of findings.
- *Optimal positioning:* Perform DISE with the patient supine, ideally replicating their usual sleep posture. Consider adding positional changes (e.g., lateral decubitus) in positional OSA patients.
- *Dynamic, not static, assessment:* Observe multiple respiratory cycles, noting changes during inspiration and expiration. This provides a more accurate depiction of collapse patterns.
- *Use of VOTE classification:* Apply structured frameworks such as VOTE (Velum, Oropharyngeal walls, Tongue base, Epiglottis) for systematic reporting. This improves interobserver reliability and facilitates communication among clinicians.
- *Video recording:* Always record the procedure. Reviewing videos post-procedure, ideally with colleagues, allows for detailed assessment, teaching opportunities, and incorporation into multidisciplinary discussions.

Pitfalls

- *Oversedation:* Excessive anesthetic depth may exaggerate airway collapse, producing findings that do not reflect natural sleep physiology.
- *Undersedation:* Inadequate sedation may prevent sufficient relaxation of pharyngeal musculature, leading to underestimation of obstruction.
- *Interobserver variability:* Without structured scoring, interpretation can be subjective. Reliance on classification systems and team review mitigates this.
- *Limited representation of REM sleep:* DISE replicates non-REM sleep more closely; clinicians should avoid assuming collapse patterns are identical in REM, where OSA often worsens.
- *Nasal route challenges:* In patients with significant septal deviation or turbinate hypertrophy, endoscope passage may be difficult and cause bleeding, compromising visualization.
- *Misinterpretation of epiglottic collapse:* Differentiate primary epiglottic collapse from secondary effects of tongue base prolapse, as surgical strategies differ.
- *Multilevel collapse complexity:* Collapse at several sites may obscure the dominant level of obstruction, requiring repeated review and careful correlation with clinical findings.

2.3.11 Conclusion

Drug-induced sleep endoscopy is an indispensable tool in the comprehensive management of OSA. When performed in a standardized and safe manner, DISE provides crucial insights into the dynamic behavior of the upper airway, guiding effective and tailored therapeutic interventions. Accurate documentation—using structured classifications like VOTE—ensures consistency, reproducibility, and collaborative decision-making in sleep surgery planning.

References

1. Azzopardi M, Parsons R, Cadby G, King S, McArdle N, Singh B, Hillman DR. Identifying risk of postoperative cardiorespiratory complications in OSA. Chest. 2024;166(5):1197–208.
2. Berezin L, Nagappa M, Poorzargar K, Saripella A, Ariaratnam J, Butris N, et al. The effectiveness of positive airway pressure therapy in reducing postoperative adverse outcomes in surgical patients with obstructive sleep apnea: a systematic review and meta-analysis. J Clin Anesth. 2023;84:110993.
3. Bolden N, Posner KL, Domino KB, Lee LA, Khan FA, Lorinc A, et al. Postoperative critical events associated with obstructive sleep apnea: results from the Society of Anesthesia and Sleep Medicine OSA registry. Anesth Analg. 2020;131(4):1032–41.
4. Ceban F, Yan E, Pivetta B, Hung KC, Tsang W, Wong J, et al. Perioperative adverse events in adult patients with obstructive sleep apnea undergoing ambulatory surgery: an updated systematic review and meta-analysis. J Clin Anesth. 2024;96:111464.
5. Cheong CSJ, Loke W, Thong MKT, Toh ST, Lee CH. The emerging role of drug-induced sleep endoscopy in the management of obstructive sleep apnea. Clin Exp Otorhinolaryngol. 2021;14(2):149–58.
6. Chung F, Nagappa M, Singh M, Mokhlesi B. CPAP in the perioperative setting: evidence of support. Chest. 2016;149(2):586–97.
7. Chung F, Waseem R, Wang CY, Nagappa M, Yang H, Kumar A, et al. Preoperative oximetry-derived hypoxemia predicts postoperative cardiovascular events in surgical patients with unrecognized obstructive sleep apnea. J Clin Anesth. 2022;78:110653.
8. Hung CJ, Kang BH, Lin YS, Su HH. Comparison of a home sleep test with in-laboratory polysomnography in the diagnosis of obstructive sleep apnea syndrome. J Chin Med Assoc. 2022;85(7):788–92.
9. Hung KC, Chuang MH, Kang FC, Chang YJ, Lin CM, Yu CH, et al. Prevalence and risk factors of difficult mask ventilation: a systematic review and meta-analysis. J Clin Anesth. 2023;90:111197.
10. Hwang M, Nagappa M, Guluzade N, Ismail S, Al-Abri A, Wong J, et al. Validation of the STOP-bang questionnaire as a preoperative screening tool for obstructive sleep apnea: a systematic review and meta-analysis. BMC Anesthesiol. 2022;22:366.
11. Kaw R, Bhateja P, Paz y Mar H, Hernandez AV, Ramaswamy A, Blackstone EH, et al. Postoperative complications in patients with unrecognized obesity hypoventilation syndrome undergoing elective noncardiac surgery. Chest. 2016;149(1):84–91.
12. Lam T, Nagappa M, Wong J, Singh M, Wong D, Chung F. Continuous pulse oximetry and capnography monitoring for postoperative respiratory depression and adverse events: a systematic review and meta-analysis. Anesth Analg. 2017;125(6):2019–29.
13. Ng KT, Lee ZX, Ang E, Teoh WY, Wang CY. Association of obstructive sleep apnea and postoperative cardiac complications: a systematic review and meta-analysis with trial sequential analysis. J Clin Anesth. 2020;62:109731.

14. Sharma V, Yadav HP, Prakash A, Yadav N, Kumar M, Abbas H. Assessment of different indices as predictors of difficult airway in obese patients. Cureus. 2024;16(2):e55005.
15. Suen C, Ryan CM, Mubashir T, Ayas NT, Abrahamyan L, Wong J, et al. Sleep study and oximetry parameters for predicting postoperative complications in patients with OSA. Chest. 2019;155(4):855–67.
16. Sun X, Yu J, Luo J, Xu S, Yang N, Wang Y. Meta-analysis of the association between obstructive sleep apnea and postoperative complications. Sleep Med. 2022;91:1–11.
17. Croft CB, Pringle M. Sleep nasendoscopy: a technique of assessment in snoring and obstructive sleep apnea. Clin Otolaryngol Allied Sci. 1991;16(5):504–9.
18. Bastier PL, Gallet de Santerre O, Bartier S, et al. Guidelines of the French society of ENT (SFORL): drug-induced sleep endoscopy in adult obstructive sleep apnea syndrome. Eur Ann Otorhinolaryngol Head Neck Dis. 2022;139(4):216–25.
19. Schwartz D, Schall C, Harders M, et al. Anesthesia for drug-induced sleep endoscopy (DISE). Curr Anesthesiol Rep. 2024;14:469–74.
20. Carrasco-Llatas M, Matarredona-Quiles S, De Vito A, Chong KB, Vicini C. Drug-induced sleep endoscopy: technique, indications, tips and pitfalls. Healthcare (Basel). 2019;7(3):93.
21. Shallik N. Anesthetic management for drug-induced sleep endoscopy. Middle East J Anaesthesiol. 2015;23(2):131–5.
22. De Vito A, Carrasco Llatas M, Ravesloot MJL, et al. European position paper on drug-induced sleep endoscopy: 2017 update. Clin Otolaryngol. 2018;43(6):1541–52.
23. Friedman M, editor. Sleep apnea and snoring: surgical and non-surgical therapy. 1st ed. Philadelphia: Saunders Elsevier; 2008.
24. Charakorn N, Kezirian EJ. Drug-induced sleep endoscopy. Otolaryngol Clin N Am. 2016;49(6):1359–72.
25. Martínez S, Lasa EM, Joral A, Infante S, Pérez R, Ibáñez MD. Childhood allergy committee, Spanish Society of Allergy and Clinical Immunology. Recommendations for the use of propofol in egg-allergic patients. J Investig Allergol Clin Immunol. 2019;29(1):72–4.
26. Hybášková J, Jor O, Novák V, Zeleník K, Matoušek P, Komínek P. Drug-induced sleep endoscopy changes the treatment concept in patients with obstructive sleep apnoea. Biomed Res Int. 2016;2016:6583216.
27. De Vito A, Carrasco Llatas M, Vanni A, et al. European position paper on drug-induced sedation endoscopy (DISE). Sleep Breath. 2014;18(3):453–65.
28. Soares D, Folbe AJ, Yoo G, Badr MS, Rowley JA, Lin HS. Drug-induced sleep endoscopy vs awake Müller's maneuver in the diagnosis of severe upper airway obstruction. Otolaryngol Head Neck Surg. 2013;148(1):151–6.
29. Sadaoka T, Kakitsuba N, Fujiwara Y, Kanai R, Takahashi H. The value of sleep nasendoscopy in the evaluation of patients with suspected sleep-related breathing disorders. Clin Otolaryngol Allied Sci. 1996;21(6):485–9.
30. Kim JS, Heo SJ. Test–retest reliability of drug-induced sleep endoscopy using midazolam. J Clin Sleep Med. 2020;16(5):675–8.
31. Chong KB, De Vito A, Vicini C. Drug-induced sleep endoscopy in treatment options selection. Sleep Med Clin. 2019;14(1):33–40.
32. Schwab RJ, Badr SM, Epstein LJ, Gay PC, Gozal D, Kohler M, Lévy P, Malhotra A, Phillips BA, Rosen IM, Strohl KP, Strollo PJ, Weaver EM, Weaver TE. An official American Thoracic Society statement: continuous positive airway pressure adherence tracking systems. The optimal monitoring strategies and outcome measures in adults. Am J Respir Crit Care Med. 2013;188(5):613–20. https://doi.org/10.1164/rccm.201307-1282ST.
33. Joshi GP, Ankichetty SP, Gan TJ, Chung F. Society for Ambulatory Anesthesia consensus statement on preoperative selection of adult patients with obstructive sleep apnea scheduled for ambulatory surgery. Anesth Analg. 2012;115(5):1060–68. https://doi.org/10.1213/ANE.0b013e318269cfd7.

34. Kapur VK, Auckley DH, Chowdhuri S, Kuhlmann DC, Mehra R, Ramar K, Harrod CG. Clinical practice guideline for diagnostic testing for adult obstructive sleep apnea: an American Academy of Sleep Medicine clinical practice guideline. J Clin Sleep Med. 2017;13(3):479–504. https://doi.org/10.5664/jcsm.6506.
35. Babak Mokhlesi, Juan Fernando Masa, Jan L. Brozek, Indira Gurubhagavatula, Patrick B. Murphy, Amanda J. Piper, Aiman Tulaimat, Majid Afshar, Jay S. Balachandran, Raed A. Dweik, Ronald R. Grunstein, Nicholas Hart, Roop Kaw, Geraldo Lorenzi-Filho, Sushmita Pamidi, Bhakti K. Patel, Susheel P. Patil, Jean Louis Pépin, Israa Soghier, Maximiliano Tamae Kakazu, Mihaela Teodorescu. Evaluation and Management of Obesity Hypoventilation Syndrome. An Official American Thoracic Society Clinical Practice Guideline. American Journal of Respiratory and Critical Care Medicine. 2019;200(3):e6–e24. https://doi.org/10.1164/rccm.201905-1071ST.
36. Verbraecken J, Hedner J, Penzel T. Pre-operative screening for obstructive sleep apnoea. Eur Respir Rev. 2017;26(143):160012. https://doi.org/10.1183/16000617.0012-2016.
37. Shahmoradi L, Rezaei N, Rezayi S, Zolfaghari M, Manafi B. Educational approaches for patients with heart surgery: a systematic review of main features and effects. BMC Cardiovasc Disord. 2022;22(1). https://doi.org/10.1186/s12872-022-02728-0.

Chapter 3
Nasal Surgery for Obstructive Sleep Apnea

Chu Qin Phua, Kugan Raman, Hui Yan Ong, Gagandeep Singh Mann, Chee Chean Lim, Prepageran Narayanan, Andrew Junior Charles Gomez, Song Tar Toh, and Liang Chye Goh

3.1 Radiofrequency Ablation of the Inferior Turbinates

Chu Qin PhuaKugan Raman, and Hui Yan Ong

3.1.1 Introduction

Radiofrequency volumetric tissue reduction (RFVTR) is a widely utilized thermal technique in otolaryngology for the treatment of upper airway obstruction and snoring. It is a minimally invasive, mucosal-sparing procedure performed on both the *inferior turbinates*, commonly in the setting of chronic nasal obstruction or sleep-disordered breathing [1]. In patients with obstructive sleep apnea (OSA),

C. Q. Phua (✉)
Department of Otorhinolaryngology, Sengkang General Hospital, Singapore, Singapore

K. Raman
Department of Otorhinolaryngology, Faculty of Medicine and Health Sciences, University Putra Malaysia (UPM), Seri Kembangan, Malaysia
e-mail: kugan@upm.edu.my

H. Y. Ong (✉) · G. Singh Mann (✉) · C. C. Lim · P. Narayanan · A. J. Charles Gomez · L. C. Goh (✉)
Department of Otorhinolaryngology, Faculty of Medicine, Universiti Malaya, Kuala Lumpur, Malaysia
e-mail: prepa@um.edu.my; acharles123@um.edu.my; juliusglc@um.edu.my

S. T. Toh (✉)
Department of Otorhinolaryngology-Head & Neck Surgery, Singapore General Hospital, Singapore, Singapore
e-mail: toh.song.tar@singhealth.com.sg

L. C. Goh, S. T. Toh (eds.), *Sleep Surgery in a Nutshell*,
https://doi.org/10.1007/978-981-95-9749-9_3

optimization of the nasal airway is a foundational element of a comprehensive, multilevel surgical strategy. Elevated nasal resistance can potentiate negative inspiratory pressures within the pharynx, increasing the likelihood of upper airway collapse. Moreover, nasal obstruction is recognized as a significant impediment to patient compliance with continuous positive airway pressure (CPAP) therapy.

In patients with OSA using CPAP, radiofrequency turbinate reduction has been shown to significantly improve CPAP adherence and tolerance. Randomized controlled trials demonstrate that reducing nasal resistance through turbinate reduction leads to improved CPAP compliance, and may reduce therapeutic pressure requirements, making this procedure particularly valuable for CPAP-intolerant patients with nasal obstruction [6, 7].

RFVTR provides a targeted method for submucosal tissue volume reduction while critically preserving the integrity and physiological function of the overlying respiratory mucosa. The technique employs *low-temperature, high-frequency energy* to generate precise submucosal lesions, which subsequently undergo fibrotic consolidation and tissue contraction, reducing turbinate volume and improving nasal patency.

Radiofrequency ablation (RFA) offers significant advantages including performance under local or general anesthesia, minimal intraoperative bleeding, short recovery times, and reproducible outcomes. It is especially valuable in patients who are not surgical candidates for more extensive resections [2].

3.1.2 Radiofrequency Ablation of the Inferior Turbinates

3.1.2.1 Indications

- Chronic nasal obstruction due to inferior turbinate hypertrophy (allergic and nonallergic rhinitis) [3]
- Failure of medical management
- Alternative to turbinate resection or microdebrider turbinoplasty [4]
- Sleep-disordered breathing patients with nasal obstruction and poor CPAP compliance or tolerance [6, 7]

3.1.2.2 Contraindications

- *Relative contraindications:*
  - Patients with cardiac pacemakers or implanted electronic devices (unless devices can be temporarily deactivated) [8]
  - Uncontrolled bleeding diathesis or coagulopathy
  - Active nasal or sinus infection
    Significant bony turbinate hypertrophy (RFA primarily targets soft tissue)

3.1.2.3 Advantages

- Minimally invasive with mucosal preservation
- Can be performed under local anesthesia
- Low complication rate [5]
- Effective relief up to 36 months [1]
- Approximately 80% of patients remain relapse-free at 36 months, with peak symptomatic improvement typically occurring at 3 months post-procedure [1, 9]
- Improves CPAP compliance and may reduce required therapeutic pressures in sleep apnea patients [6, 7]
- Repeatable if necessary

3.1.2.4 Mechanism of Action

RFA delivers thermal energy to the *submucosal layer* of the inferior turbinates via a needle-tip electrode. The resultant *thermal lesion* leads to *fibrosis and tissue contraction*, reducing the turbinate's submucosal volume while preserving surface mucosa.

RFA can be performed using monopolar or bipolar radiofrequency systems. Long-term efficacy is comparable between the two techniques, with no significant difference in nasal obstruction outcomes beyond the first few months [8, 10].

In the early postoperative period, bipolar systems may produce faster initial reduction in turbinate edema, while monopolar systems tend toward a slightly more gradual onset of improvement; neither approach has demonstrated a consistent advantage in postoperative pain [10]. Temperature-controlled systems typically target a submucosal temperature of 70–85°C (Fig. 3.1) [2, 8].

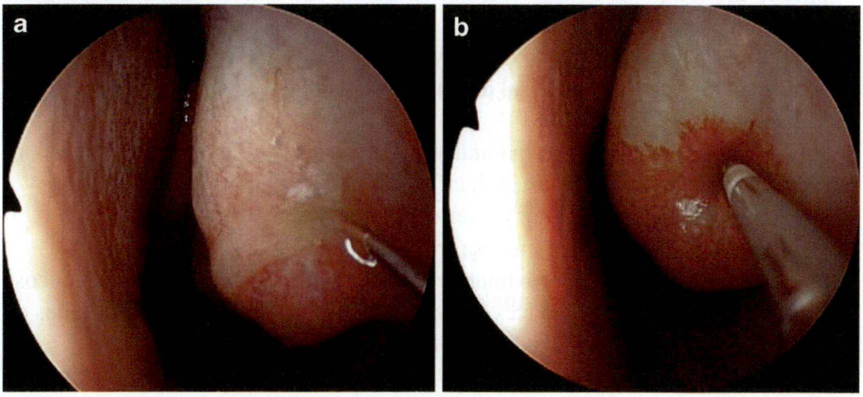

Fig. 3.1 (**a**) Local anesthesia being injected into left inferior turbinate (**b**) RF probe inserted into the anterior third of left inferior turbinate

3.1.3 Surgical Technique

The procedure can be done as an office procedure under local anesthesia or can be done under general anesthesia as part of multilevel surgery.

3.1.3.1 Preoperative Preparation

1. *Patient positioning*: The patient is placed in a supine or semireclined position.
2. *Nasal endoscopy*: Perform rigid nasoendoscopy to assess turbinate anatomy.

3.1.3.2 Local Anesthesia

- The nasal passages are prepared with patties soaked in a vasoconstrictor and topical anesthetic solution (e.g., 0.05% oxymetazoline and 4% lidocaine) and placed in the nasal cavity for 10–15 min.
- Infiltrate using a 27- or 30-gauge needle, approximately 1–2 mL of 1% lidocaine with 1:100,000 epinephrine is infiltrated into the submucosal plane of the anterior aspect (head) of each inferior turbinate. Adequate infiltration is confirmed by tissue blanching.
- Pack nasal cavities with *Co-Phenylcaine-soaked patties*.

3.1.3.3 Radiofrequency Application

1. Under endoscopic visualization, the tip of the RF probe is inserted into the head of the inferior turbinate, advancing posteriorly within the submucosal plane parallel to the long axis of the turbinate. Begin at the anterior third and progress posteriorly.
2. The probe is advanced approximately 10 mm along the long axis of the turbinate, maintaining a submucosal depth of approximately 5 mm below the mucosal surface.
3. It is crucial that the depth is maintained at around 5 mm to minimize the risk of damage to the surface mucosa, which could lead to ulcerations or sloughing.
4. Avoid penetrating medially or posteriorly through the turbinate.
5. Avoid damaging additional mucosa from surrounding tissue.
6. Energy is delivered for approximately 10–20 s per insertion, or until the mucosa begins to blanch. (Some devices comes with auto-stop function, which relies on 3D impedance feedback detected by the machine algorithm.)
7. The RF generator is activated. Typical energy parameters might include 350–500 J, 2–10 W, and 70–80 V, targeting a temperature of *70–85 °C (typically 80 °C)* per lesion. Energy is typically delivered until the target temperature is reached or for a predetermined duration, resulting in a contained zone of

coagulative necrosis. A common approach involves creating three to five separate lesions.

- *Lesion 1 (anterior):* The first lesion is created in the turbinate head.
- *Lesions 2–4 (body):* The probe is partially withdrawn and redirected to create subsequent lesions along the inferior and medial aspects of the turbinate body.
- *Lesion 5 (posterior):* A final lesion may be placed near the posterior aspect of the turbinate.

8. *Endpoint confirmation:* Successful ablation is often indicated by subtle tissue blanching around the probe entry point and increased tissue impedance noted by the RF generator. Each energy application typically lasts 10–20 s.
9. *Probe withdrawal:* After the final lesion is created, the probe is removed. Minimal to no bleeding is expected at the puncture sites.

3.1.3.4 Postoperative Care

- *Immediate care:* No nasal packing is required. The patient can typically be discharged shortly after the procedure.
- *Patient instructions:*
  - *Nasal saline:* Frequent use of isotonic saline nasal spray or irrigations is essential, starting the day after the procedure, to minimize crusting and facilitate healing.
  - *Activity:* Avoid strenuous activity and nose blowing for 3–5 days to minimize the risk of epistaxis.
    Analgesia: Over-the-counter analgesics such as acetaminophen are usually sufficient for managing mild discomfort.
- *Expected course:* Patients should be counselled to expect a period of increased nasal congestion and crusting for the first 1–2 weeks due to post-procedural edema and healing. Symptomatic improvement in nasal airflow is typically noticeable after 3–6 weeks as submucosal fibrosis and tissue contraction are completed.
- Long-term studies demonstrate that symptomatic benefit peaks at approximately 3 months post-procedure, with approximately 80% of patients maintaining improvement at 36 months. However, patients with allergic rhinitis may experience higher recurrence rates compared to those with nonallergic rhinitis and should be counseled regarding the potential need for repeat procedures or continued medical management [1, 9, 11]. In patients using CPAP for OSA, improvement in nasal patency typically correlates with enhanced CPAP tolerance and may allow for reduction in therapeutic pressure settings [6, 7].
- *Follow-up:* A follow-up visit is scheduled for 4–6 weeks postoperatively to assess healing and symptomatic improvement. For sleep apnea patients, CPAP pressure titration may be reassessed after complete healing to optimize therapy [6].

3.1.3.5 Complications

Early Complications

- *Pain and discomfort:* Mild to moderate nasal pain or pressure is common in the first few days following the procedure, usually managed with analgesics.
- *Bleeding (epistaxis):* Minor bleeding can occur intraoperatively or within the first 24–48 h. Significant hemorrhage is rare.
- *Edema and crusting:* Mucosal swelling and crust formation at the treatment site are expected during the initial healing phase, occasionally causing transient nasal obstruction.
- *Infection:* Though uncommon, secondary bacterial infection may manifest as increased pain, purulent discharge, or fever. Prompt antibiotic therapy is warranted.
- *Transient rhinorrhea or sneezing:* Irritation of the nasal mucosa may provoke watery discharge or sneezing, typically self-limiting.

Late Complications

- *Excessive scar formation or synechiae:* Adhesions between the inferior turbinate and nasal septum may develop, leading to persistent obstruction and requiring surgical release.
- *Atrophic changes:* Overreduction of turbinate tissue can result in dryness, crusting, or features of atrophic rhinitis, although this is far less common with RFA than with more aggressive resection techniques.
- *Empty nose syndrome (ENS):* Extremely rare but possible in cases of excessive tissue ablation, leading to paradoxical nasal obstruction despite a wide nasal cavity.
- *Persistent or recurrent obstruction:* Incomplete reduction of turbinate volume or tissue regrowth may cause recurrence of symptoms, sometimes necessitating repeat intervention. Recurrence rates are significantly higher in patients with allergic rhinitis compared to nonallergic rhinitis, particularly beyond 36 months post-procedure [1, 9].
- *Altered sensation:* Rarely, patients may report numbness or altered mucosal sensitivity in the treated area.

3.2 Endoscopic Septoplasty

Gagandeep Singh MannChee Chean Lim, and Prepageran Narayanan

3.2.1 Introduction

Septoplasty is a surgical procedure aimed at correcting deviations of the nasal septum to relieve nasal obstruction and improve nasal airflow. It is one of the most common procedures performed in otolaryngology. Deviations may involve the

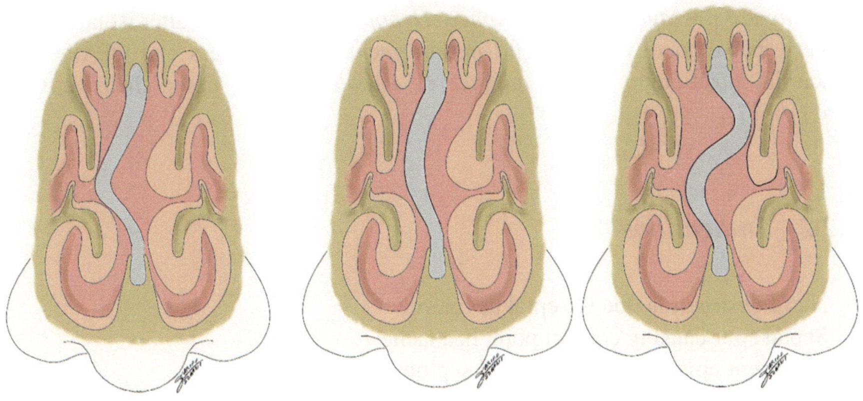

Fig. 3.2 Variations of nasal septal deviation

cartilaginous or bony septum and may present with symptoms such as nasal congestion, epistaxis, sinusitis, and contribute to sleep-disordered breathing. In patients with obstructive sleep apnea (OSA), optimizing nasal patency can improve tolerance to positive airway pressure therapy and alleviate nasal obstruction symptoms. There are various different types of septal deviations, depicted in Fig. 3.2 [18].

Septal deviation increases upstream nasal resistance and promotes unstable oronasal breathing during sleep. In OSA, this upstream load can amplify inspiratory suction forces on the pharyngeal airway, raising the likelihood of retropalatal and retroglossal collapse in predisposed phenotypes. Clinically, higher nasal resistance and mouth-opening are associated with *higher therapeutic CPAP pressures*, greater residual events when oronasal masks are used, and lower adherence—mechanistic and meta-analytic findings that explain why improving nasal patency benefits many patients even when it does not "cure" OSA. The nasal valve and inferior turbinates often compound septal deformity; a complete assessment therefore distinguishes fixed structural obstruction from dynamic valve collapse and mucosal disease (allergic/nonallergic rhinitis, CRS) [12–14].

Septoplasty corrects structural deviation of the nasal septum (cartilaginous and/or bony) to restore laminar nasal airflow. It is frequently combined with *inferior turbinate reduction* to address compensatory hypertrophy and with *valve support* (e.g., spreader or batten grafts) when internal or external valve compromise is contributory. By lowering nasal resistance, septoplasty aims to [12]:

- Reduce mouth breathing and inspiratory suction on collapsible pharyngeal segments;
- *decrease required CPAP pressures* and improve *mask comfort/adherence* in CPAP-intolerant patients;
- enhance tolerance of oral appliances and multilevel surgical plans by stabilizing the route of breathing;
- improve snoring and disease-specific nasal symptoms (e.g., NOSE scores) with corresponding gains in quality of life [19].

It is not primarily a curative operation for pharyngeal collapse. Meta-analyses show *modest average changes in Apnea–Hypopnea Index (AHI)* after isolated nasal surgery, but *clinically meaningful improvements* in sleepiness and CPAP use—hence its positioning as an *adjunct* or *enabler* within comprehensive OSA care [16, 17].

3.2.2 Indications

- Nasal obstruction due to septal deviation
- Septal spur causing contact point headache
- Recurrent epistaxis from deviated septum
- Access during endoscopic sinus surgery
- As part of rhinoplasty for nasal framework optimization
- Sleep-disordered breathing associated with nasal airflow limitation
- Poor tolerance or noncompliance with CPAP due to nasal blockage requiring high pressure for air delivery
- Failed medical management of nasal obstruction (e.g., intranasal corticosteroids, decongestants)

3.2.3 Contraindications

- Active nasal or sinus infection
- Uncontrolled systemic illness (e.g., uncontrolled diabetes, hypertension)
- Bleeding diathesis or use of anticoagulant therapy that cannot be stopped
- Suspicion of sinonasal malignancy requiring biopsy first

3.2.4 Surgical Technique

3.2.4.1 Anesthesia and Patient Positioning

- Procedure is typically performed under *general anesthesia.*
- Patient is positioned in *15–20° reverse Trendelenburg* to reduce venous congestion and bleeding.

3.2.4.2 Step-by-Step Procedure (Fig. 3.3)

1. *Local Infiltration*
    - Using a dental syringe, inject *1% lidocaine with 1:100,000 epinephrine* into the anterior one-third of the septum, in the *subperichondrial plane.*
    - This provides *hydrodissection*, vasoconstriction, and pain control.

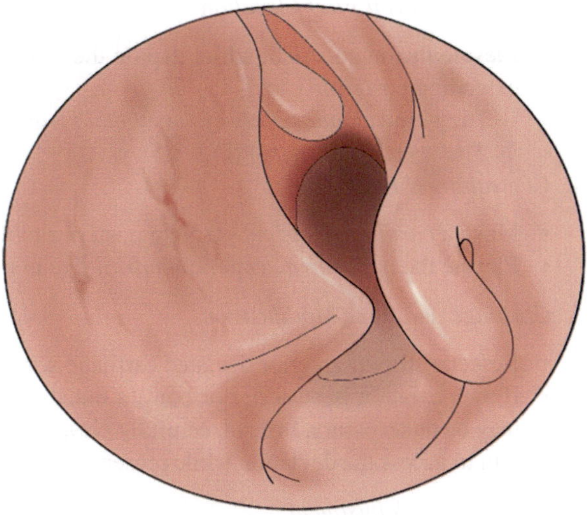

Fig. 3.3 Image depicting the left nasal cavity with a sided septal spur preoperatively

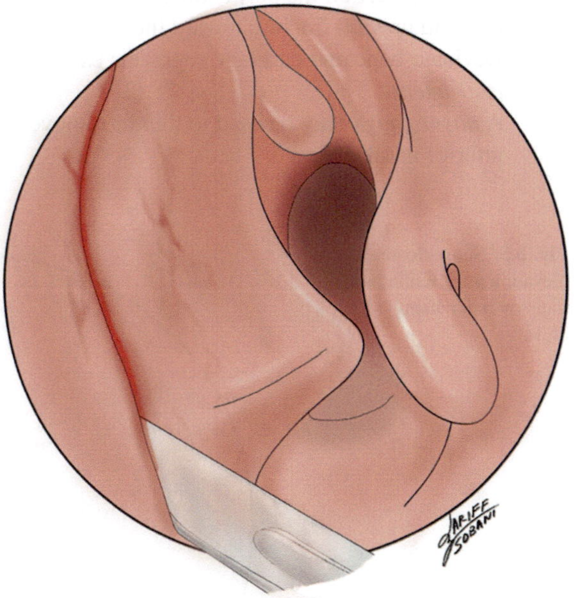

Fig. 3.4 Killian's incision made using a blade anterior to the deviated septum

2. *Killian Incision (*Fig. 3.4*)*

   - Make a *Killian's incision* with a No. 15 blade through the *mucosa and perichondrium* to the cartilage, approximately 1–2 cm posterior to the caudal septum.
   - Care should be taken to preserve at least *1 cm of the dorsal and caudal septal strut* to avoid destabilizing the nasal dorsum and tip (preventing *saddle nose deformity*).

3. *Subperichondrial Flap Elevation*
   - Elevate the mucoperichondrial flap on the same side using a *Cottle elevator*, extending posteriorly to:
     - The *perpendicular plate of the ethmoid* (superiorly)
       The *vomer* (inferiorly) (Fig. 3.5)
4. *Contralateral Flap*
   - Make a *cartilage incision* ~ 0.5 cm posterior to the mucosal incision.
   - Elevate the *opposite mucoperichondrial flap* in a similar fashion (Fig. 3.6).
5. *Cartilage and Bone Modification*
   - Resect a strip of anterior deviated cartilage with *Mayo scissors* if necessary.
   - If the deviation is posterior or bony, a mucosal incision on the opposite side may be unnecessary. Instead, carefully elevate mucosa from the posterior septum to access the deviation while preserving the anterior mucosal attachment.
6. *Bony Septum Adjustment*
   - Carefully section the *perpendicular plate of the ethmoid* with Mayo scissors to avoid upward fracture toward the skull base (Fig. 3.7).
   - Deviated bone and cartilage segments can be removed using *through-cutting instruments*.
   - A *nasal gouge* may be used to thin or remove the *maxillary crest*, improving inferior nasal airflow.

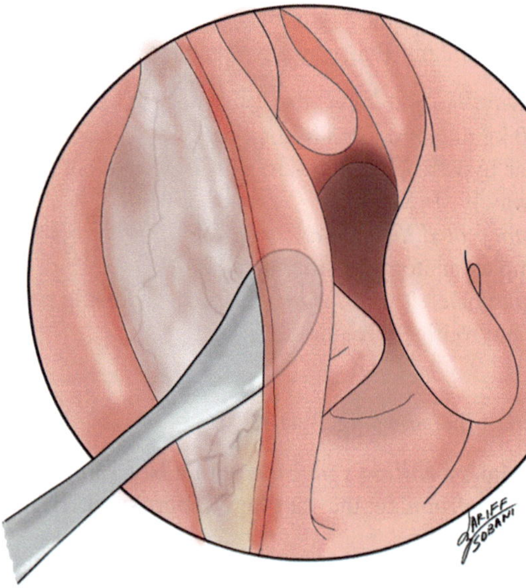

Fig. 3.5 Subperiosteal flap elevation after Killian's incision made using a freer elevator

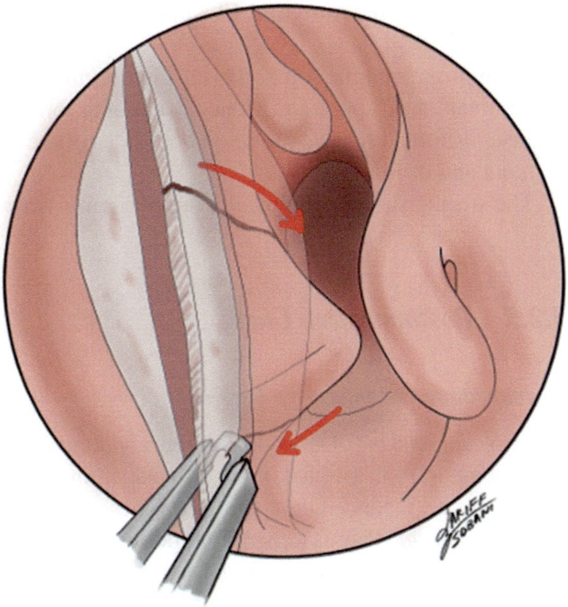

Fig. 3.6 Opposite subperiosteal flap raised after cartilage incision

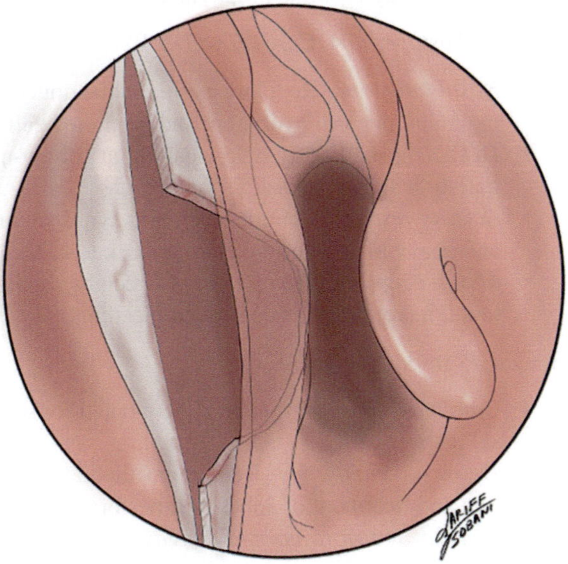

Fig. 3.7 Diseased septum removed using cutting instruments while preserving normal septal cartilage and bone

3.2.4.3 Reconstruction and Closure

- Re-approximate the septal flaps using *quilting sutures* with *4/0 Vicryl Rapide* to eliminate dead space and reduce hematoma formation.
- Insert trimmed *silastic sheets* on both sides of the septum to prevent *septal hematoma* and *intranasal synechiae.*
- The silastic sheets are typically removed on *postoperative day 10.*

3.2.5 Postoperative Care

1. *Immediate Postoperative Period*
   - *Nasal packing:* Depending on intraoperative bleeding or extent of correction, temporary nasal packing or silicone splints may be placed to stabilize septal flaps and reduce hematoma risk. These are usually removed within 24–72 h.
   - *Analgesia:* Pain is generally mild to moderate and well controlled with simple analgesics. Nonsteroidal anti-inflammatory drugs (NSAIDs) should be used cautiously in patients at risk of bleeding.
   - *Antibiotics:* Short courses may be prescribed if nasal packing or splints are in place, though routine prophylaxis remains debated.
2. *Early Postoperative Care (First 1–2 Weeks)*
   - *Nasal irrigation:* Regular isotonic saline douching or sprays help clear crusts, maintain mucosal hydration, and promote healing.
   - *Debridement:* Endoscopic cleaning at follow-up visits prevents crust accumulation and synechiae formation.
   - *Activity restriction:* Patients should avoid strenuous exercise, nose blowing, and heavy lifting during the first week to reduce bleeding risk.
   - *Monitoring for complications:* Clinicians should be vigilant for septal hematoma, infection, or uncontrolled bleeding.
3. *Late Postoperative Care*
   - *Continued saline irrigation:* Encouraged for several weeks to enhance mucosal recovery.
   - *Follow-up endoscopy:* Routine postoperative assessments allow early detection and treatment of adhesions, perforation, or persistent deviation.
   - *Gradual return to normal activity:* Most patients can resume full activities within 2–3 weeks, once healing is stable.
   - *Long-term outcomes:* Patient-reported nasal breathing improvement should be documented and correlated with endoscopic findings [19].

3.2.6 Complications

Early Complications [18]

- *Bleeding (epistaxis):* The most common complication, usually controlled with nasal packing or cauterization. Rarely, significant hemorrhage may require reexploration.
- *Septal hematoma:* Accumulation of blood between the septal flaps can cause pain, obstruction, and risk of cartilage necrosis if not promptly drained.
- *Infection:* Local infection or abscess formation is uncommon but possible, necessitating antibiotics and drainage when indicated.
- *Mucosal lacerations and flat Tears:* Intraoperative injury to the mucosa may impair healing, increase crusting, or predispose to synechiae formation.
- *Edema, crusting, and obstruction:* These are expected short-term sequelae of mucosal manipulation and generally resolve with saline irrigation and debridement.
- *Anosmia or hyposmia (rare):* Transient olfactory disturbance may occur due to mucosal trauma or edema.

Late Complications [18]

- *Septal perforation:* Can result from bilateral mucosal injury or unrecognized hematoma. Symptoms may include whistling, crusting, epistaxis, or nasal obstruction.
- *Synechiae formation:* Adhesions between the septum and turbinates may cause persistent obstruction, often requiring endoscopic lysis.
- *Saddle nose deformity:* Rare but serious, due to excessive resection or compromise of septal support leading to dorsal collapse.
- *Persistent or recurrent deviation:* Technical limitations, incomplete correction, or postoperative cartilage memory can result in residual obstruction requiring revision surgery.
- *Altered sensation or numbness:* Occasionally, patients report numbness of the upper incisors or palate due to traction or injury to nasopalatine nerve branches.

3.3 Microdebrider-Assisted Turbinoplasty

Chu Qin PhuaAndrew Junior Charles Gomez, and Prepageran Narayanan

3.3.1 Introduction

Inferior turbinate hypertrophy (ITH) is a prevalent cause of fixed nasal obstruction in adults with obstructive sleep apnea (OSA) [20, 21]. Elevated upstream nasal resistance promotes mouth breathing and increases downstream pharyngeal negative pressure, amplifying retropalatal and retroglossal collapse in susceptible phenotypes; it also drives higher therapeutic CPAP pressures and intolerance [21, 22]. In this context, *mucosa-preserving turbinate surgery* is often deployed to reduce resistance, restore comfortable nasal airflow, and improve adherence to positive airway pressure (PAP) or oral appliance therapy [10, 23]. Microdebrider-assisted turbinoplasty (MAT) achieves *submucosal debulking with epithelial preservation*, aiming to improve patency while minimizing bleeding, crusting, and long-term physiologic impairment [23, 24]. Contemporary meta-analytic evidence shows that MAT provides reductions in patient-reported nasal obstruction *comparable to submucosal resection, radiofrequency (RF), and laser*, with some advantages in operative efficiency over submucosal resection and a trade-off of slightly higher early postoperative bleeding versus RF [20, 25].

Typical candidates include adults with persistent nasal obstruction from ITH despite optimized medical therapy (saline, intranasal corticosteroids/antihistamines, allergy management), particularly when CPAP pressures are high or interface intolerance is prominent; patients planned for multilevel OSA surgery; and those with symptomatic snoring or mild OSA whose nasal resistance materially fragments sleep [21, 24]. Selection should differentiate *mucosal* from *bony* hypertrophy and identify any *nasal valve* compromise that may require concurrent graft-based support [22].

3.3.2 Surgical Principles and Technique

The defining features of MAT are *endoscopic visualization, submucosal tissue removal*, and *mucosal preservation* [23, 24]. After topical and infiltrative vasoconstriction (e.g., lidocaine with epinephrine), a *small anterior mucosal incision* is made at the head of the inferior turbinate. A *submucosal pocket* is created along the medial surface, and a *microdebrider blade* (commonly 2.0–2.9 mm) with integrated suction is advanced within this plane. Using gentle sweeping motions, *submucosal erectile tissue is debulked*; limited bony trimming can be performed where indicated, while *maintaining the medial mucosal envelope*. The incision is typically left open; bipolar spot hemostasis or short-duration packing may be used. Lateralization/outfracture may be added when the turbinate contour remains bulky [25].

Two families of technique are widely practiced:

- *Intraturbinoplasty (submucosal)*—the blade operates within a submucosal pocket; both medial and lateral mucosal layers remain intact. This is favored for predominantly *mucosal* hypertrophy and for tissue preservation.
- *Extraturbinoplasty/medial flap*—the lateral mucosa and erectile tissue are resected; *the medial mucosa is rotated laterally* to cover the resection bed ("medial flap" coverage). This approach is useful when the lateral soft tissue and/or bone contribute substantially to bulk.

Key technical pearls include: avoiding wide mucosal devitalization; conservative debulking at the *anterior head* (a frequent bottleneck); preserving the *inferior turbinate's physiologic role* (humidification, resistance modulation); and combining with *inferior turbinate outfracture* or *limited bony reduction* only as needed [23, 24].

3.3.3 Indications

1. *Chronic nasal obstruction with poor response to medical therapy [21] (corticosteroids, antihistamines, decongestant)*
   - *Chronic nasal block from patients account*
     - Objective assessment based on anterior rhinoscopy, nasoendoscopy
     - Drug-induced sleep endoscopy, radiological findings, and nasal airflow studies

     Allergic or vasomotor rhinitis with persistent turbinate swelling
2. *Concurrent procedures: MAT may be combined with:*
   - *Septoplasty (deviated nasal septum)*
   - *Functional endoscopic sinus surgery (FESS) for comorbid rhinosinusitis [22, 24]*

3.3.3.1 Mechanism of Action

The microdebrider's *rotary or oscillating blade* removes hypertrophic mucosal tissue in two manners [23]

- Submucosal removal of excess mucosal tissue oscillating blade and simultaneous suction
- Direct removal of inferior and lateral inferior turbinate mucosal tissue to facilitate inferior turbinate bone resection, while preserving medial mucosal layer to allow for better healing.

3.3.3.2 Contraindications

Bleeding disorders, untreated rhinitis medicamentosa, or active nasal infection.

3.3.4 Advantages

Advantages over conventional techniques [10, 23, 24]

Technique	Key benefits of MAT
Electrocautery	Less postoperative crusting and faster mucosal healing due to reduced thermal spread
Laser ablation	Superior preservation of mucociliary transport function
Total turbinectomy	Lower risk of empty nose syndrome through structural and mucosal conservation

Limitations

- More invasive compared to radiofrequency of inferior turbinate reduction Requires formal incision and submucosal dissection
- Requires operation under general anesthesia in most cases unlike office based radiofrequency
- Requires *training and familiarity* with microdebrider use and technique
- Risk of *inadequate tissue reduction* if performed superficially
- Recurrence is possible without *allergy control*

Other instruments

- 0° rigid nasal endoscope
- Cottle elevator, sickle knife
- Decongestant-soaked nasal patties (e.g., cophenylcaine, oxymetazoline)
- Local anesthetic with epinephrine
- Nasal packing

3.3.5 Surgical Technique

Preoperative Preparation

1. Patient selection: Candidates include those with inferior turbinate hypertrophy unresponsive to medical therapy.
2. Imaging: Nasal endoscopy confirms hypertrophic turbinates; CT may rule out concurrent sinus pathology.
3. Stop antiplatelet/anticoagulant prior to surgery, e.g., aspirin, clopidogrel, warfarin, and rivaroxaban.
4. Check for supplements that might increase bleeding risks and stop prior to surgery (e.g., cordyceps, ginkgo biloba, and lingzhi).

Anesthesia and Exposure

- General anesthesia

Topical decongestion with oxymetazoline/cophenylcaine
Local infiltration with 2% lignocaine +1:80,000 adrenaline

Local Anesthesia and Nasal Decongested

- Moffett's solution/modified Moffett's solution applied

Nasal patties with 1:100,000 epinephrine are placed for 5–10 min.
Infiltrate 0.5% Marcaine with adrenaline into the turbinate/lateral nasal wall to reduce bleeding. (Fig. 3.8)

Incision and Procedure

1. Use 0° endoscope to visualize the inferior turbinate. (Fig. 3.9)
2. *Incision:* A vertical mucosal incision is made at the anterior head of the inferior turbinate. Superior and inferior flaps are made (Fig. 3.10).
3. *Two approaches are available* (Fig. 3.11)

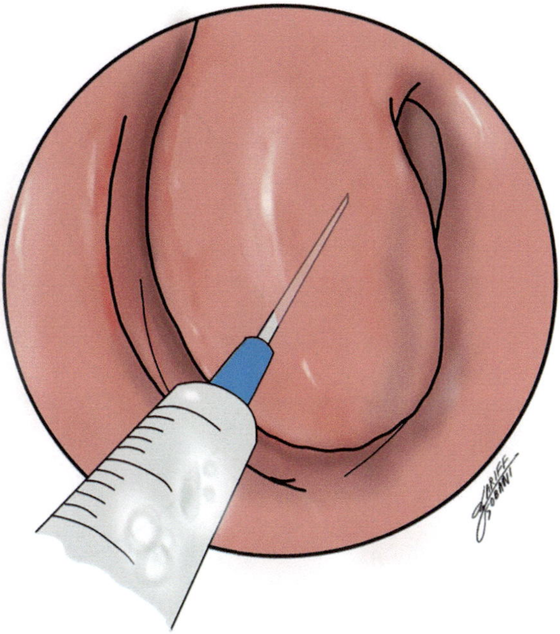

Fig. 3.8 Local anesthesia infiltrated into the anterior end of the turbinate

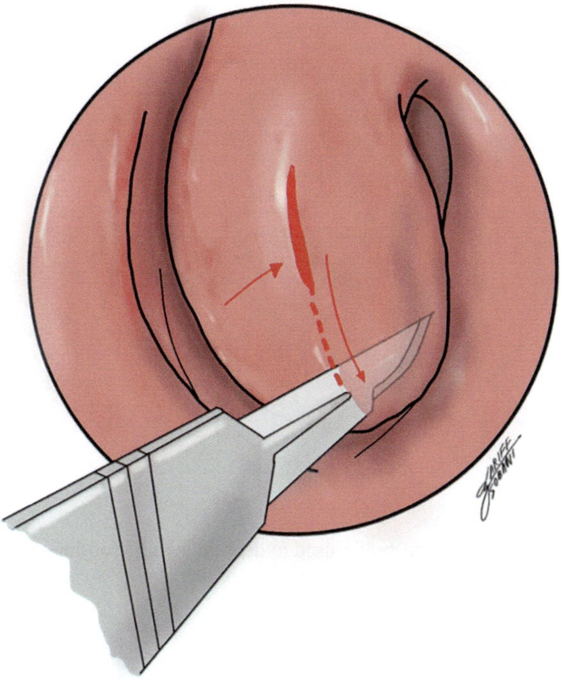

Fig. 3.9 A vertical mucosal incision made at the anterior end of the inferior turbinate

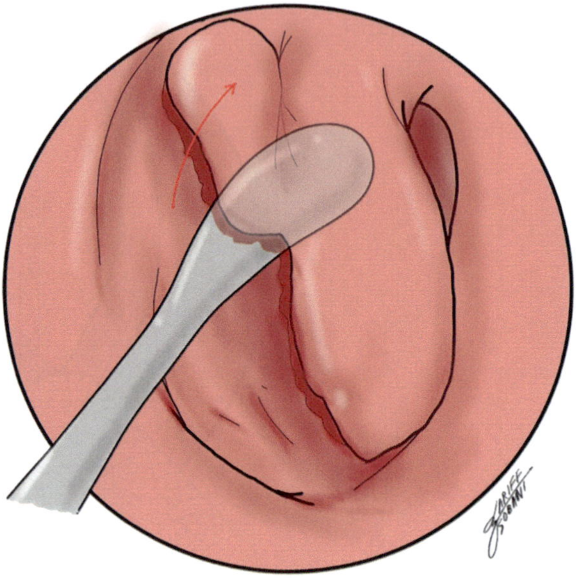

Fig. 3.10 Superior and Inferior Flaps are made after incision is made

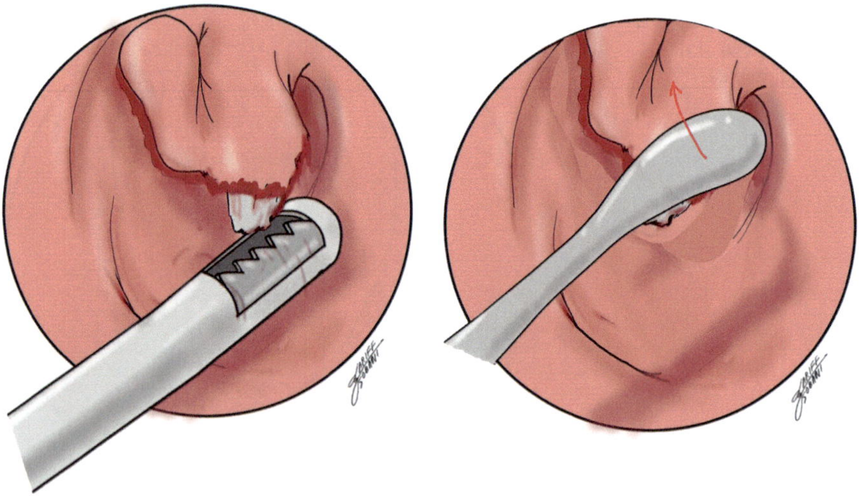

Fig. 3.11 Microdebrider used to debride the inferior flap till bony tissue is felt. This is followed by outfracture of the inferior portion of the flap

1. *Submucosal dissection:* Make a small anterior mucosal incision at head of inferior turbinate, insert microdebrider blade submucosally, begin slow shaving in anterior-to-posterior direction to remove excess submucosal soft tissue. Outfracture the inferior turbinate bone if necessary (Fig. 3.12).
2. *Direct dissection:* Microdebrider to debride inferior and lateral mucosa, raise medial mucosa with Freer/Cottle's elevator, in-fracture the inferior turbinate bone, resect the bone, replace the medial mucosal flap, and out-fracture it laterally.
3. *Microdebrider insertion:* A 2.0–3.5 mm microdebrider blade is used depending on the extent of tissue and approach used, (set at 1500–3000 rpm) is introduced to resect hypertrophic soft tissue while sparing mucosa. (Fig. 3.13)

4. *Hemostasis:* Light electrocautery or nasal packing (absorbable hemostatic agents) is applied if needed (Fig. 3.14).
5. *Closure:* The mucosal flap is repositioned; a suture may be required.

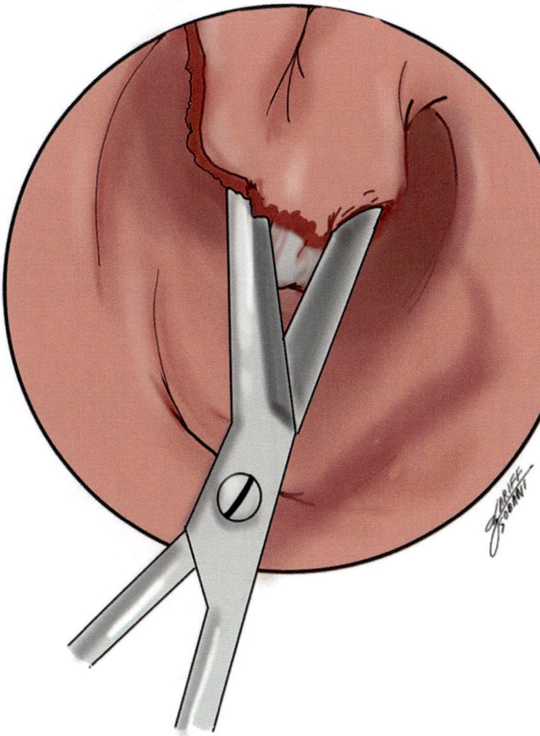

Fig. 3.12 Inferior turbinate incised using a turbinate scissors

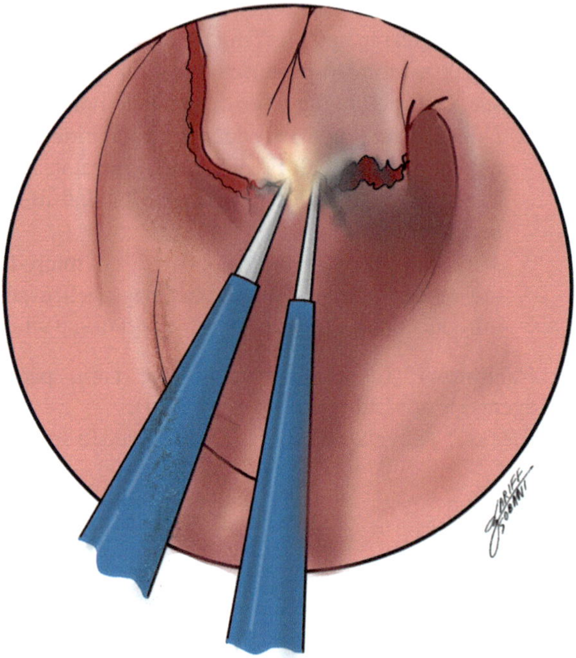

Fig. 3.13 Hemostasis made using low powered bipolar diathermy

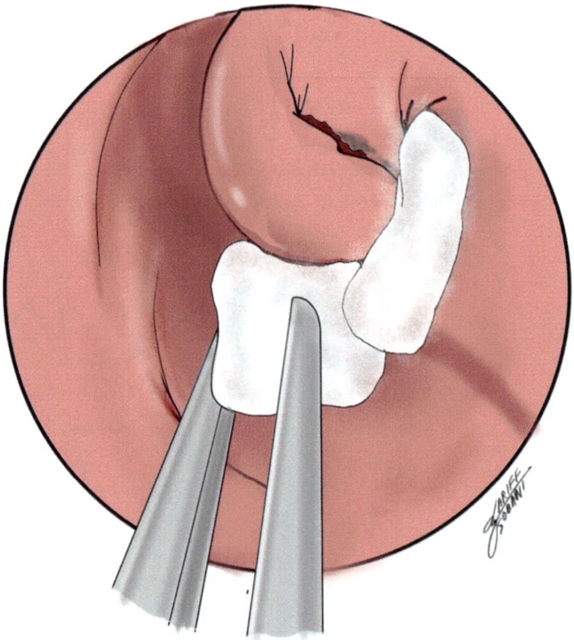

Fig. 3.14 Absorbable hemostatic agents used to pack the superior flap close to the inferior flap

Adjunct Consideration

- When performed with procedures such as septoplasty in which two opposing mucosal surfaces are raw and may come in contact resulting in a synechiae formation, the placement of silastic sheets to avoid synechiae formation may be used.

3.3.6 Postoperative Care

1. Immediate Postoperative Period
   - *Nasal packing or splints*: In most cases, packing is unnecessary due to the limited mucosal trauma associated with the technique. If placed for hemostasis, packing or splints are usually removed within 24–48 h.
   - *Hemostasis and observation*: Patients should be observed for early bleeding or hematoma formation, though significant hemorrhage is rare.
   - *Pain control*: Discomfort is typically mild and managed with simple analgesics.
2. Early Postoperative Care (First 1–2 Weeks)
   - *Saline irrigation (FloSinus or Neilmed)*: Regular isotonic saline douching is strongly recommended to minimize crust formation, maintain mucosal hydration, and promote epithelialization of the turbinate surface.
   - *Nasal debridement*: Endoscopic cleaning during follow-up visits helps remove crusts, coagulum, and debris that could impair healing or cause synechiae.
   - *Activity precautions*: Patients should avoid nose blowing, vigorous exercise, and bending forward during the early recovery phase to reduce bleeding risk.
   - *Medication support*: Topical decongestants are generally avoided to prevent mucosal ischemia, though short courses of topical steroids may be prescribed in selected cases to control postoperative inflammation.
3. Late Postoperative Care
   - *Continued irrigation*: Ongoing saline irrigation for several weeks enhances mucosal recovery and reduces long-term crusting.
   - *Monitoring for complications*: Regular endoscopic evaluation allows early detection of rare complications such as turbinate synechiae, excessive scarring, or persistent hypertrophy.
   - *Symptom assessment*: Long-term follow-up should document improvements in nasal obstruction and patient quality of life. In some cases, adjunctive medical therapy (e.g., topical corticosteroids for allergic rhinitis) may be needed to sustain results.

3.3.6.1 Complications

Early

- *Bleeding*
- *Cause*: Incomplete hemostasis, trauma to posterior turbinate vasculature.
  Management: Nasal packing, topical tranexamic acid, or electrocautery.
- *Pain/discomfort*
  - Typically mild; resolves within 48 h with analgesics (e.g., acetaminophen).
- *Edema and crusting*
  - *Cause*: Mucosal trauma during dissection.
  - *Prevention*: Saline irrigation starting at 24 h post-op.
- *Infection*

  Rare; may present as purulent rhinorrhea. Prophylactic antibiotics are not routinely recommended.
- *Adhesions/synechiae*
  - *Risk factors*: Concurrent septoplasty, excessive mucosal damage.
  - *Prevention*: Silicone spacers or early nasal debridement.

Late

- Persistent nasal obstruction
- *Causes*: Inadequate resection, scar formation, or unresolved mucosal inflammation.
  Management: Revision surgery or steroid sprays.
- Empty nose syndrome
  - *Cause*: Over-resection of turbinate tissue
  - *Prevention*: Conservative submucosal resection preserving structural support.
- Atrophic rhinitis
  - *Features*: Dryness, foul-smelling crusts.
  - *Management*: Humidification, nasal emollients
- Olfactory dysfunction
  - Usually temporary due to postoperative edema.

3.3.7 Conclusion

Inferior turbinate hypertrophy is a leading cause of chronic nasal obstruction, often refractory to medical management. MAT is appropriate for patients with persistent turbinate hypertrophy unresponsive to medical therapy, particularly where mucosal preservation and avoidance of empty nose syndrome are priorities. It can be performed as an isolated procedure or combined with septoplasty and FESS within a multilevel nasal correction.

3.4 Nasal Valve Stabilization

Song Tar Toh and Liang Chye Goh

3.4.1 Introduction

The nasal valve—encompassing the internal nasal valve (junction of the upper lateral cartilage and septum, with the head of the inferior turbinate and caudal septum) and the external nasal valve (alar rim/soft triangle)—is the narrowest segment of the nasal airway and a principal resistor of inspiratory flow. Small geometric changes at this segment have disproportionate impact on resistance, especially during inspiratory acceleration typical of sleepsleep and snoring [14]. With rising negative intraluminal pressure, compliant lateral walls can be drawn medially, producing dynamic collapse that increases upstream load, encourages mouth-breathing, and raises downstream pharyngeal suction forces.

In patients with obstructive sleep apnea (OSA), this upstream instability often worsens snoring, exacerbates pharyngeal collapsibility, and undermines CPAP tolerance [12, 13] by increasing required pressures and leak [12, 13]. Clinical consensus emphasizes that valve compromise is a distinct entity that must be identified and treated directly—medical therapy alone rarely corrects a structurally weak or malpositioned lateral wall.

Nasal valve collapse is a frequently overlooked but important cause of nasal obstruction, particularly in patients with dynamic inspiratory collapse. The *internal nasal valve*—the narrowest portion of the nasal airway—is particularly susceptible to inspiratory negative pressure, especially in individuals with weak or malpositioned upper lateral cartilages [26].

Nasal valve stabilization is a targeted surgical technique designed to *reinforce the upper lateral cartilage (ULC)* using *suture suspension to the bony piriform aperture*. This technique offers a minimally invasive and effective means of correcting *dynamic nasal valve collapse (DNVC)*, and may be used as a *standalone procedure* or in conjunction with other functional or cosmetic nasal surgeries [14, 26, 27].

3.4.2 Principle [27–29] (Fig. 3.15)

- Nasal valve stabilization is based on *anchoring the upper lateral cartilage* to the *bony piriform rim* using sutures to *prevent lateral wall collapse during inspiration*.
- The procedure addresses *dynamic* collapse rather than static narrowing and does *not alter the external nasal contour*.
- The *piriform aperture* serves as a rigid anchor point, enabling effective medialization and stabilization of the upper lateral cartilage.
- *Clinical evaluation* with the *Cottle's maneuver* and *modified Cottle's maneuver* aids in diagnosis and patient selection.

3.4.3 Indications

Nasal valve stabilization is indicated in the following scenarios:

1. *Dynamic Nasal Valve Collapse (DNVC)*
    - Patients experiencing *inspiratory nasal obstruction* worsened with deep inhalation or exercise
    - Positive response to *Cottle's maneuver* (improvement of airflow when cheek is pulled laterally)
    - Dynamic collapse of the *upper lateral cartilage* observed on anterior rhinoscopy or nasal endoscopy

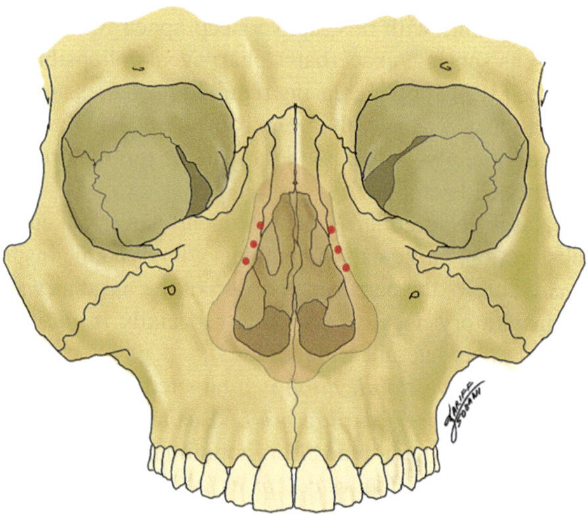

Fig. 3.15 Illustration showing puncture sites for suspension points

2. *Structural Weakness or Trauma*

   - Post-rhinoplasty patients with upper lateral cartilage weakening or excessive resection
   - Congenital or acquired cartilage malformation
   - Post-traumatic nasal deformity causing nasal valve incompetence

3. *Adjunct to Other Procedures*

   - Functional rhinoplasty or septoplasty where internal valve compromise is noted
   - Revision rhinoplasty with persistent valve collapse
   - Combined procedures for snoring or sleep apnea in which nasal airflow is optimized preoperatively

Contraindications
- Static nasal valve narrowing due to bony or mucosal hypertrophy (address with alternative techniques)
- Severe external nasal deformity requiring structural grafting
- Active infection at the surgical site

Preoperative Preparation
- Topical *nasal decongestant* (e.g., oxymetazoline) is applied to reduce mucosal congestion.
- Local infiltration with *1% lignocaine and 1:100,000 adrenaline* is administered along the incision site over the *piriform rim.*
- The procedure can be performed under *local or general anesthesia*, depending on patient and surgical context.

3.4.4 Surgical Technique

1. *Incision and Exposure* (Figs. 3.16 and 3.17)

   - Under *anterior rhinoscopy*, a *small incision* is made over the *piriform rim* using a *needle-tip electrocautery.*
   - *Subperiosteal dissection* is carried out both medially and laterally to expose *5–10 mm of the bony piriform rim.*

2. *Creation of Anchor Points* (Fig. 3.18)

   - Using a *short, fine drill bit* (e.g., *0.76 mm diameter, 6 mm length*), *three to four holes* are drilled into the *bony piriform rim*, spaced *3 mm from the edge.*

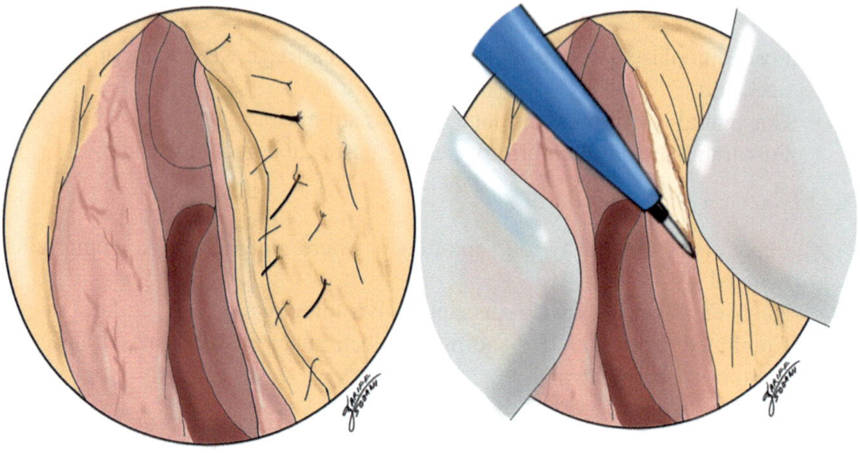

Fig. 3.16 Incision (yellow arrow) made with needle point diathermy on left pyriform rim

Fig. 3.17 Subperiosteal dissection over pyriform rim (red arrow) performed

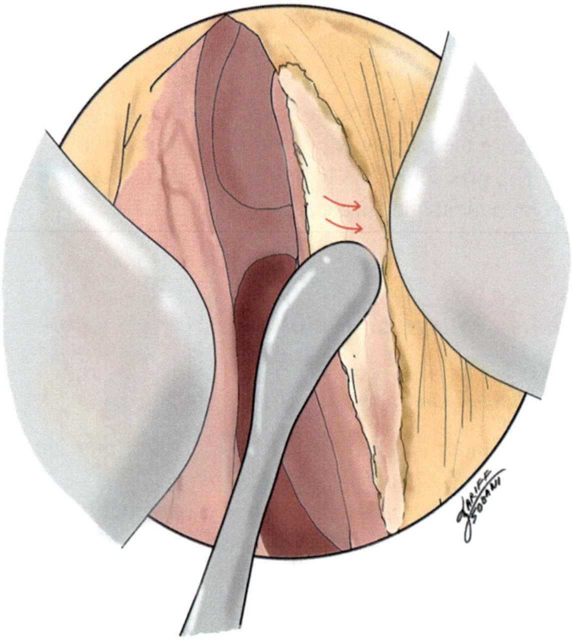

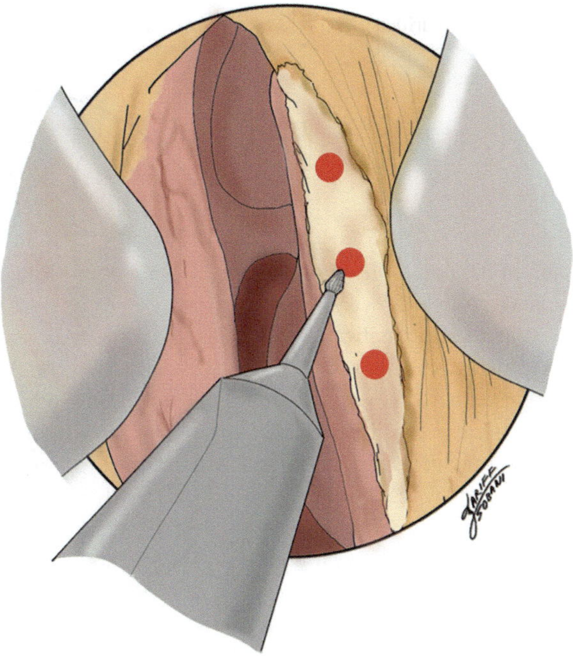

Fig. 3.18 Three to four holes drilled 3 mm from bony rim (yellow dots in picture)

3. *Suture Placement* (Fig. 3.19)
   - A *2–0 absorbable polyglactin suture (Vicryl)* is passed:
     - Through the *top drill hole*, from lateral to medial
     - Then through the *upper lateral cartilage*, from the external surface into the nasal cavity
     - The suture is then redirected back through the cartilage into the surgical wound
     - Finally, the suture is *tied securely*, stabilizing the cartilage to the bone
4. *Additional Sutures* (Fig. 3.20)
   - This technique is repeated for the remaining holes to create *multiple fixation points*, ensuring stable and symmetric lateralization of the ULC.
5. *Closure* (Figs. 3.21 and 3.22)
   - The *mucosal incision is closed* using a *fine absorbable 5–0 suture*, maintaining a clean internal nasal contour and avoiding mucosal redundancy.

Fig. 3.19 Vicryl suture passed through drilled bony hole

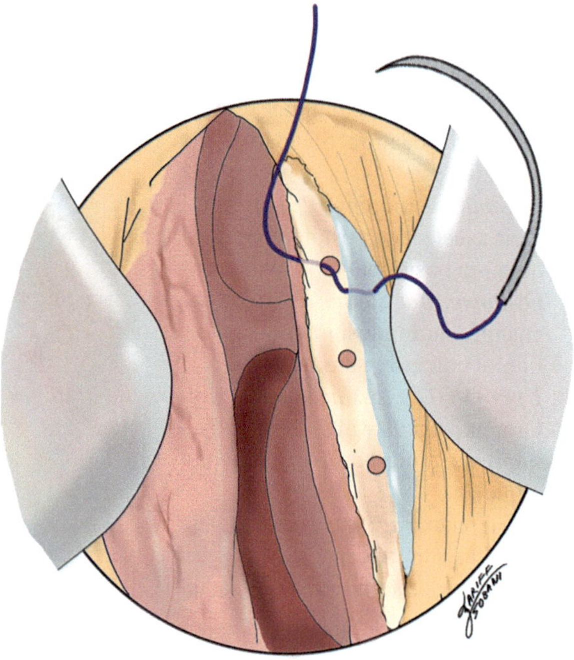

Fig. 3.20 All three sutures tied down on bony rim

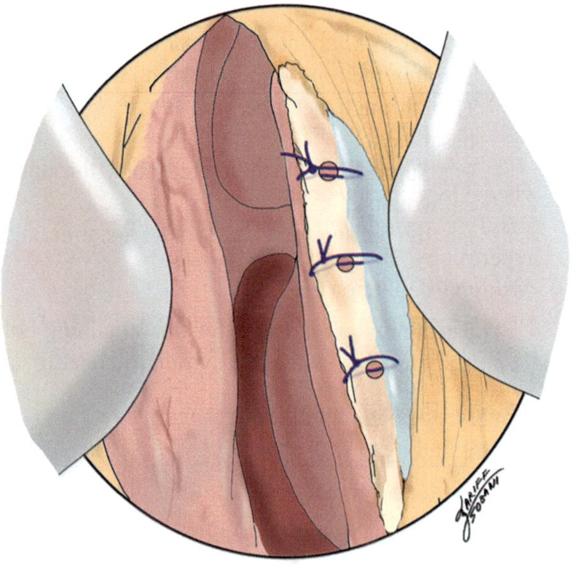

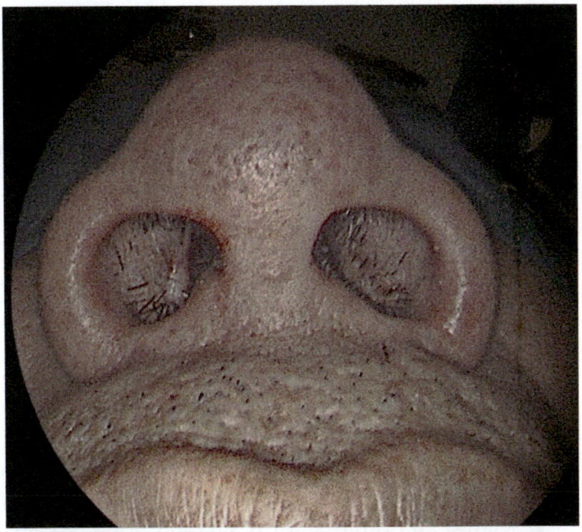

Fig. 3.21 Before nasal valve suspension

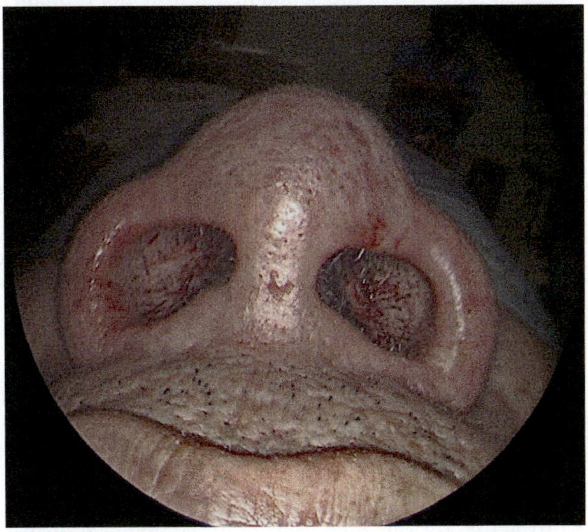

Fig. 3.22 Post-nasal valve suspension—bilateral

3.4.5 *Postoperative Care [27–29]*

1. *Immediate Postoperative Period*

   - *Stabilization and dressing:* External nasal splints or tapes may be applied to support the nasal framework and minimize edema. Sutures are usually left in place for 5–7 days, and absorbable sutures, if used, require no removal.

- *Hemostasis and monitoring:* Mild oozing or bruising around the operated site is common; however, significant bleeding is rare. Patients should be observed for early hematoma or excessive swelling.
- *Analgesia and cold compresses:* Pain is typically mild to moderate and can be managed with oral analgesics. Intermittent cold compresses reduce edema and ecchymosis.

2. *Early Postoperative Care (First 1–2 Weeks)*
   - *Nasal hygiene:* Gentle saline irrigation may be initiated after the first few days to keep the nasal cavity moist, minimize crusting, and aid mucosal healing.
   - *Activity restriction:* Patients should avoid nose blowing, heavy lifting, contact sports, or any activity that could increase intranasal pressure or disrupt the suspension sutures.
   - *Edema and bruising management:* Patients should be counseled that swelling and discoloration are expected but generally resolve within 1–2 weeks.
   - *Suture and splint care:* If external splints or sutures are present, they should be removed at the scheduled follow-up, typically within a week.
3. *Late Postoperative Care*
   - *Follow-up endoscopy:* Early endoscopic review ensures proper healing, absence of synechiae, and stability of the suspension.
   - *Monitoring for complications:* Rare complications include suture extrusion, localized infection, persistent edema, or asymmetry. These should be identified early and managed appropriately.
   - *Long-term results:* Patients should be reassessed for improvement in nasal airflow and quality-of-life measures. Residual obstruction may occasionally require adjunctive procedures or revision surgery.

Advantages of Nasal Valve Stabilization
- Minimally invasive; preserves native cartilage
- Reversible and modifiable
- Avoids external scars or grafts
- Can be performed in-office under local anesthesia
- Effective for selected cases of dynamic nasal obstruction

3.4.6 Complications to Watch for [27–29]

Early Complications
- *Bleeding and hematoma:* Minor oozing or ecchymosis at the suspension site is common, but significant hemorrhage is rare.
- *Edema and bruising:* Swelling and periorbital bruising may occur due to manipulation of soft tissues, typically resolving within 1–2 weeks.

- *Infection:* Local infection at the suture entry site is uncommon but possible; it usually responds to antibiotics.
- *Discomfort or pain:* Temporary pain or tenderness along the suspension track can occur, generally managed with oral analgesics.

Late Complications

- *Suture extrusion or visibility:* The suspension suture may become palpable or visible under thin skin, or rarely, extrude through the mucosa or skin.
- *Asymmetry or irregular contour:* Uneven suspension tension can lead to nasal asymmetry or subtle contour deformities.
- *Persistent or recurrent obstruction:* In some cases, airflow improvement may be inadequate, or obstruction may recur over time, necessitating revision or adjunctive procedures.
- *Overcorrection or valve stiffness:* Excessive suspension may create an unnatural appearance, valve rigidity, or altered nasal airflow sensation.
- *Scar formation:* Subtle scar tissue can form along the suspension track, though this is typically of little functional consequence.

3.4.7 Conclusion

Nasal valve stabilization offers a safe and reliable method to treat *dynamic inspiratory nasal obstruction* due to upper lateral cartilage collapse. By anchoring the ULC to stable bony landmarks, this technique achieves physiological restoration of valve function with minimal morbidity. Proper *diagnosis*, *surgical execution*, and *postoperative care* are essential to maximize functional outcomes.

3.5 Transoral Endoscopic Adenoidectomy

Liang Chye Goh

3.5.1 Introduction

Adenoidectomy remains one of the most frequently performed surgeries for obstructive sleep apnea. Traditional blind curettage has significant limitations in visualization, often resulting in residual tissue and injury to adjacent structures. The *transoral endoscopic adenoidectomy* method addresses these issues by providing magnified, direct visualization of the nasopharynx, enabling precise tissue removal [30–32].

Adenoidal hypertrophy contributes to pediatric nasal obstruction, snoring, sleep-disordered breathing and obstructive sleep apnea (OSA), and to Eustachian tube dysfunction (ETD) and otitis media with effusion (OME). Adenotonsillectomy remains first-line therapy for childhood OSA with meaningful improvements in symptoms and polysomnography in appropriately selected children. In this context, *transoral endoscopic adenoidectomy (TEA)* applies rigid endoscopy through the oral cavity to perform a complete, hemostatic, and *anatomy-sparing* removal under direct vision. Compared with blind curettage, TEA offers precise clearance around the *choanae, torus tubarius, fossa of Rosenmüller*, and *Passavant ridge*, reducing residual tissue and iatrogenic injury while permitting tailored conservative resections in patients at risk for velopharyngeal insufficiency (VPI) [30, 31, 33–36].

Indications for TEA mirror those for adenoidectomy (nasal obstruction, recurrent rhinopharyngitis, chronic adenoiditis, OME/ETD refractory to medical therapy), with added value where visualization matters: *peritubaric disease*, revision surgery after curettage, syndromic airways, and *palatal anomalies* where partial (conservative) adenoidectomy is desired [32, 37].

3.5.2 Preoperative Assessment

History focuses on *nocturnal symptoms* (snoring, witnessed apneas), daytime obstruction, rhinosinusitis burden, and *otologic history*. Examine the palate for *submucous cleft stigmata* (bifid uvula, zona pellucida, posterior notch) and assess speech resonance. *Flexible nasopharyngoscopy* establishes adenoid grade and documents peritubaric extension; a *NOSE-like* symptom score and tympanometry/baseline audiology are useful in OME. Children with suspected OSA should be evaluated for adenotonsillar hypertrophy and comorbidities; polysomnography is reserved for high-risk phenotypes or diagnostic uncertainty.

Cleft palate (repaired or submucous) requires special planning. In these patients the adenoid pad may augment velopharyngeal closure; thus, *partial adenoidectomy* is preferred, removing choanal-obstructing tissue while *preserving the inferior adenoid "velar shelf."* Contemporary series indicate that *transoral endoscopic partial adenoidectomy* does *not* worsen speech outcomes when performed with strict visualization of the velopharyngeal valve [38].

3.5.3 Surgical Indications

- Pediatric or adult *obstructive sleep apnea (OSA)* due to adenoidal hypertrophy
- *Chronic nasal obstruction* with radiological evidence of adenoidal hypertrophy
- *Eustachian tube dysfunction* secondary to adenoidal impingement
- Recurrent or chronic *adenoiditis*
- Failure of previous adenoidectomy (*residual or regrowth cases*)
- Adenoidal mass requiring histopathological evaluation

3.5.4 Detailed Surgical Anatomy

Understanding nasopharyngeal anatomy is critical to avoid inadvertent injury:

- *Adenoidal pad*: Occupies the posterior wall and roof of the nasopharynx.
- *Eustachian tube orifices*: Located laterally within the *torus tubarius*; critical to preserve.
- *Fossa of Rosenmüller*: Lateral recess behind the torus tubarius; a potential site for residual adenoids.
- *Velopharyngeal musculature*: Located inferiorly; trauma risks postoperative velopharyngeal insufficiency.
- *Choanae*: Posterior openings of the nasal cavity into the nasopharynx.

3.5.5 Instrumentation and Equipment

Surgeon may choose between Coblator, microdebrider, or suction diathermy.

- *Rigid Endoscope*: 4 mm 30° or 70° for adults
- *Camera and Display Unit*: High-definition preferred
- *Mouth Gag*: Boyle–Davis or Dingman with tongue blade
- *Coblator Wand* (e.g., Smith & Nephew EVac 70°, EVac 90°)
- *Coblation Control Unit* (plasma ablation and coagulation settings)
- *Suction Monopolar Electrocautery* or *Microdebrider* with adenoid blade
- *Suction Cannula* and *Irrigation Set*
- *Headlight* (as backup)

3.5.6 Preoperative Preparation

- General anesthesia with endotracheal intubation
- Adequate mouth opening using Boyle–Davis gag, suspended on Mayo stand
- Neck extended; table in reverse Trendelenburg for optimal visualization
- Preoperative prophylactic antibiotics based on institutional protocol

3.5.7 Step-by-Step Surgical Technique

3.5.7.1 Endoscope Introduction

- Introduce the rigid endoscope (30° or 70°) *transorally* over the tongue.
- Direct the endoscope superiorly to visualize the adenoidal pad in the nasopharynx.
- Adjust light intensity to minimize glare.

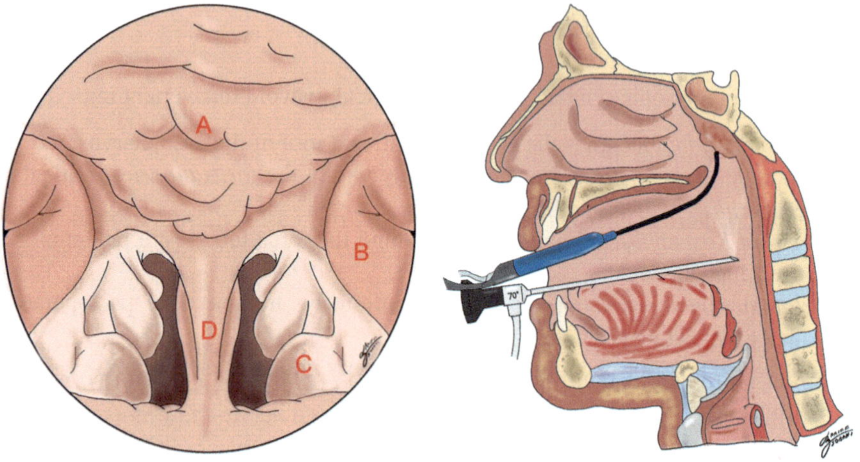

Fig. 3.23 Trans-oral endoscopic view of the adenoids. A = adenoid tissue, B = tubal elevation with fossa of Rosenmülle, C = inferior turbinates, D = posterior nasal septum

3.5.7.2 Visualization and Mapping (Fig. 3.23)

- Identify:
  - Midline adenoidal tissue
  - Bilateral torus tubarius and Eustachian tube openings
  - Fossa of Rosenmüller
  - Posterior choanae
- Assess for any aberrant vasculature or anomalous tissue growth.

3.5.7.3 Adenoidal Tissue Removal

- Using *suction monopolar cautery*, *microdebrider, or Coblator*:
  - If Coblator
    - *Ablation mode*: 5–7
      Coagulation mode: 3–5
  - Start *from the midline superior adenoidal pad.*
  - Progressively clear tissue *inferiorly and laterally*, avoiding aggressive lateral dissection.
  - Exercise extreme caution near the *Eustachian tubes* and *fossa of Rosenmüller*.
- Employ *continuous suction* to evacuate smoke plume and blood.
- In large adenoidal masses, *piecemeal removal* may be necessary.

3.5.7.4 Hemostasis

- Control bleeding via:
  - Coagulation function from Coblator.
  - Suction monopolar cautery at low power settings (20–25 W).
  - Avoid deep cauterization to prevent mucosal scarring.
- Inspect for:
  - Bleeding points near choanae.
  - Oozing around Eustachian tube orifices.

3.5.7.5 Final Inspection

- Reexamine:
  - Lateral recesses for residual tissue.
  - Choanae for obstruction.
  - Torus tubarius for edema or injury.
- Use saline irrigation to clear the field during inspection.

3.5.8 Surgical Tips and Pearls

- *Endoscopic holder* allows solo operation with both hands free.
- Continuous *saline irrigation* optimizes visualization and reduces tissue desiccation.
- Avoid suction directly over torus tubarius to prevent mechanical trauma.
- *Microdebrider* provides precise tissue shaving with minimal thermal injury.
- If Coblator is used, it allows controlled ablation of tissue with low temperature. This allows easy ablation and controlled bleeding.
- Avoid over-resection inferiorly to preserve velopharyngeal closure mechanism.

3.5.9 Postoperative Care

1. *Immediate Postoperative Period*
   - *Observation:* Patients should be monitored in the recovery area until fully awake, with close attention to airway patency and bleeding. Mild blood-stained saliva is common, but active bleeding warrants prompt evaluation.

- *Analgesia:* Pain is typically mild, localized to the throat or nasal cavity, and well managed with paracetamol or etoricoxib. Stronger analgesics are rarely required.
- *Hydration:* Early oral fluids are encouraged to prevent dehydration and soothe the throat.

2. *Early Postoperative Care (First 1–2 Weeks)*

- *Diet:* A soft, cool diet is recommended for the first few days to minimize discomfort. Spicy or acidic foods should be avoided.
- *Activity restriction:* Strenuous exercise and vigorous nose blowing should be avoided for at least 1 week to reduce bleeding risk.
- *Nasal hygiene:* Gentle saline irrigation or sprays may be prescribed to clear crusts and aid mucosal healing, especially in older children or adults.
- *Antibiotics:* Routine antibiotics are not universally required but may be considered in cases with concurrent infection or middle ear disease.
- *Follow-up:* Endoscopic examination at 1–2 weeks helps assess healing, detect crusting, and exclude residual adenoid tissue [32, 34–37, 39].

3. *Late Postoperative Care*

- *Symptom monitoring:* Caregivers should observe for signs of nasal obstruction, persistent snoring, or otitis media, which may suggest residual or regrown adenoidal tissue [32, 37, 39].
- *Complication surveillance:* Rare complications include velopharyngeal insufficiency, nasopharyngeal scarring, or eustachian tube dysfunction [37, 38, 40].
- *Return to normal activity:* Most children resume normal diet and activities within 7–10 days, with full recovery expected in 2–3 weeks.

3.5.10 Complications and Management

Complication	Prevention	Management
Residual adenoidal tissue	Careful endoscopic mapping	Revision surgery if symptomatic
Bleeding (intra/postoperative)	Meticulous hemostasis	Cautery; nasal packing rarely needed
Eustachian tube injury	Avoid deep lateral dissection	Conservative; myringotomy if required
Velopharyngeal insufficiency	Preserve inferior margin	Usually temporary; speech therapy

3.5.11 Advantages Over Traditional Curettage

- Complete adenoidal removal under direct vision [31, 32, 34–36]
- Preservation of surrounding structures [31, 32, 34–36]
- Reduced intraoperative bleeding [32, 34, 35, 37]
- Lower revision surgery rates [32, 34–37, 39]
- Better outcomes in revision cases [32, 37, 39]

References

1. De Corso E, Bastanza G, Di Donfrancesco V, Guidi ML, Morelli Sbarra G, Passali GC, et al. Radiofrequency volumetric inferior turbinate reduction: long-term clinical results. Acta Otorhinolaryngol Ital. 2016;36(3):199–205.
2. Chaudhry S, Maresco-Pennisi D, Cervin A. Radiofrequency ablation in the treatment of inferior turbinate hypertrophy. Aust J Otolaryngol. 2021;4:5.
3. Türk B, Korkut AY, Kaya KS, Salepçi E, Ünsal Ö, Coşkun BU, et al. Results of radiofrequency ablation of inferior turbinate hypertrophy in patients with allergic and non-allergic rhinitis. Sisli Etfal Hastan Tip Bul. 2018;52(4):296–301.
4. Akagün F, İmamoğlu M, Çobanoğlu HB, Ural A. Comparison of radiofrequency thermal ablation and microdebrider-assisted turbinoplasty in inferior turbinate hypertrophy: a prospective, randomized, and clinical study. Turk Arch Otorhinolaryngol. 2016;54(3):118–23.
5. Means C, Camacho M, Capasso R. Long-term outcomes of radiofrequency ablation of the inferior turbinates. Indian J Otolaryngol Head Neck Surg. 2016;68(4):424–8.
6. Powell NB, Zonato AI, Weaver EM, Li K, Troell R, Riley RW, Guilleminault C. Radiofrequency treatment of turbinate hypertrophy in subjects using continuous positive airway pressure: a randomized, double-blind, placebo-controlled clinical pilot trial. Laryngoscope. 2001;111(10):1783–90.
7. Sugiura T, Noda A, Nakata S, Yasuda Y, Soga T, Miyata S, et al. Influence of nasal resistance on initial acceptance of continuous positive airway pressure in treatment for obstructive sleep apnea syndrome. Respiration. 2007;74(1):56–60.
8. Banhiran W, Assanasen P, Tantilipikorn P, Nujchanart N, Voraprayoon S, Bunnag C. A randomized study of temperature-controlled versus bipolar radiofrequency for inferior turbinate reduction. Eur Arch Otorrinolaringol. 2015;272(10):2877–84.
9. Hytönen ML, Bäck LJ, Malmivaara AV, Roine RP. Radiofrequency thermal ablation for patients with nasal symptoms: a systematic review of effectiveness and complications. Eur Arch Otorrinolaringol. 2009;266(8):1257–66.
10. Cavaliere M, Mottola G, Iemma M. Monopolar and bipolar radiofrequency thermal ablation of inferior turbinates: 20-month follow-up. Otolaryngol Head Neck Surg. 2007;137(2):256–63.
11. Coste A, Yona L, Blumen M, Louis B, Zerah F, Rugina M, et al. Radiofrequency is a safe and effective treatment of turbinate hypertrophy. Laryngoscope. 2001;111(5):894–9.
12. Andrade RGS, Viana FM, Nascimento JA, Drager LF, Moffa A, Genta PR, et al. Nasal vs oronasal CPAP for obstructive sleep apnea: a meta-analysis. Chest. 2018;153(3):665–74.
13. Deshpande S, Joosten SA, Turton A, Landry S, Mann DL, Carberry JC, et al. Oronasal masks require a higher pressure than nasal and nasal pillow masks for the treatment of obstructive sleep apnea. J Clin Sleep Med. 2016;12(9):1263–8.
14. Rhee JS, Weaver EM, Park SS, Baker SR, Hilger PA, Kriet JD, et al. Clinical consensus statement: diagnosis and management of nasal valve compromise. Otolaryngol Head Neck Surg. 2010;143(1):48–59.

15. Stewart MG, Witsell DL, Smith TL, Weaver EM, Yueh B, Hannley MT. Development and validation of the nasal obstruction symptom evaluation (NOSE) scale. Otolaryngol Head Neck Surg. 2004;130(2):157–63.
16. Ishii LE, Roxbury CR, Godoy A, Ishman SL, Ishii M, Gourin CG, et al. Isolated nasal surgery for obstructive sleep apnea: a systematic review and meta-analysis. Otolaryngol Head Neck Surg. 2015;153(3):326–33.
17. Wu J, Zhao G, Li Y, Zang H, Wang T, Wang D, et al. Apnea–hypopnea index decreased significantly after nasal surgery for obstructive sleep apnea: a meta-analysis. Medicine (Baltimore). 2017;96(5):e6008.
18. Pons Y, Champagne C, Genestier L, Ballivet de Régloix S. Endoscopic septoplasty: tips and pearls. Eur Ann Otorhinolaryngol Head Neck Dis. 2015;132(6):353–6.
19. Gandomi B, Bayat A, Kazemei T. Outcomes of septoplasty in young adults: the nasal obstruction septoplasty effectiveness (NOSE) study. Am J Otolaryngol. 2010;31(3):189–92.
20. Kanesan N, Norhayati MN, Sheikh Abdul Hamid S, Abdullah B. Microdebrider-assisted inferior turbinoplasty versus other surgical techniques: a meta-analysis. Acta Otorhinolaryngol Ital. 2022;42(5):415–26.
21. Abdullah B, Singh S. Surgical interventions for inferior turbinate hypertrophy: a comprehensive review of current techniques and technologies. Int J Environ Res Public Health. 2021;18(7):3441.
22. Berger G, Gassner I, Steiner A, Moser G, Stammberger H. Histopathology of the inferior turbinate with compensatory hypertrophy in patients with deviated nasal septum. Laryngoscope. 2000;110(12):2100–5.
23. Romano A, Orabona GD, Salzano G, Abbate V, Iaconetta G, Califano L. Comparative study between partial inferior turbinotomy and microdebrider-assisted inferior turbinoplasty. J Craniofac Surg. 2015;26(3):e235–8.
24. Harju T, Numminen J, Kivekäs I, Rautiainen M. A prospective, randomized, placebo-controlled study of inferior turbinate surgery. Laryngoscope. 2018;128(9):1997–2003.
25. Rajeev R, Lathadevi HT, Karadi RN, Shashikumar T, Ajur S. Microdebrider-assisted turbinoplasty versus the coblation method of turbinoplasty: a comparative study. Cureus. 2025;17(4):e82422.
26. Most SP. Analysis of outcomes after functional rhinoplasty using a disease-specific quality-of-life instrument. Arch Facial Plast Surg. 2006;8(5):306–9.
27. Lianou AD, Zarachi A, Markou K, Kastanioudakis I, Psychogios G. Nasal valve management in rhinoseptoplasty. Maedica (Bucur). 2022;17(4):921–4.
28. Spielmann PM, White PS, Hussain SS. Surgical techniques for the treatment of nasal valve collapse: a systematic review. Laryngoscope. 2009;119(7):1281–90.
29. Weaver EM. Nasal valve stabilization. Oper Tech Otolaryngol Head Neck Surg. 2012;23(1):67–71.
30. Marcus CL, Moore RH, Rosen CL, et al. A randomized trial of adenotonsillectomy for childhood sleep apnea (CHAT). N Engl J Med. 2013;368(25):2366–76.
31. El-Badrawy A, Abdel-Aziz M. Transoral endoscopic adenoidectomy. Int J Otolaryngol. 2009;2009:949315.
32. Yang L, Shan Y, Wang S, Cai C, Zhang H. Endoscopic assisted adenoidectomy versus conventional curettage adenoidectomy: meta-analysis of randomized controlled trials. Springerplus. 2016;5:426.
33. Capaccio P, Torretta S, Marciante GA, Marchisio P, Forti S, Pignataro L. Endoscopic adenoidectomy in children with otitis media with effusion and mild hearing loss. Clin Exp Otorhinolaryngol. 2016;9(1):33–8.
34. Juneja R, Meher R, Raj A, Rathore P, Wadhwa V, Arora N. Endoscopic assisted powered adenoidectomy versus conventional adenoidectomy: a randomised controlled trial. J Laryngol Otol. 2019;133(4):289–93.
35. Ozturk O, Polat S. Comparison of transoral power-assisted endoscopic adenoidectomy to curettage adenoidectomy. Adv Ther. 2012;29(8):708–21.

36. Yaman H, Memis M, Ilhan E. Comparison of transoral/transnasal endoscopic-guided adenoidectomy with endoscopic nasopharyngeal inspection at the end of curettage adenoidectomy. Indian J Otolaryngol Head Neck Surg. 2015;67(2):124–7.
37. Malas M, Althobaiti AA, Sindi A, et al. Comparison of the efficacy and safety of conventional curettage adenoidectomy with those of other adenoidectomy surgical techniques: a systematic review and network meta-analysis. J Otolaryngol Head Neck Surg. 2023;52(1):21.
38. Abdel-Aziz M, El-Badrawy A. Trans-oral endoscopic partial adenoidectomy does not worsen speech after cleft palate repair. Braz J Otorhinolaryngol. 2016;82(1):70–6.
39. Wang L, Ji K, Tu J. Comparative outcomes of microdebrider adenoidectomy, curettage adenoidectomy through oral cavity under 70-degree endoscope, and endoscopic transoral low-temperature ablation for adenoid hypertrophy. Int J Pediatr Otorhinolaryngol. 2024;186:112143.
40. Heras HA, Koltai PJ. Safety of powered instrumentation for adenoidectomy. Int J Pediatr Otorhinolaryngol. 1998;44(2):149–53.

Chapter 4
Palatal and Oropharyngeal Surgery for Obstructive Sleep Apnea

John Ming Ren Loh, Chu Qin Phua, Hui Yan Ong, Song Tar Toh, Liang Chye Goh, Claudio Vicini, Stephen Shih-Teng Kao, and Mackay Stuart Grayson

J. M. R. Loh
Department of Otorhinolaryngology, Changi General Hospital, Singapore, Singapore
e-mail: john.loh.m.r@singhealth.com.sg

C. Q. Phua
Department of Otorhinolaryngology, Sengkang General Hospital, Singapore, Singapore

H. Y. Ong (✉) · L. C. Goh (✉)
Department of Otorhinolaryngology, Faculty of Medicine, Universiti Malaya, Kuala Lumpur, Malaysia
e-mail: graceong155@um.edu.my; juliusglc@um.edu.my

S. T. Toh
Department of Otorhinolaryngology-Head & Neck Surgery, Singapore General Hospital, Singapore, Singapore
e-mail: toh.song.tar@singhealth.com.sg

C. Vicini
Department of Head-Neck Surgery, Otolaryngology, Head-Neck and Oral Surgery Unit, Morgagni Pierantoni Hospital, Azienda USL Della Romagna, Forlì, Italy
e-mail: claudio@claudiovicini.com

S. S-T. Kao
Department of ENT Head and Neck Surgery, Wollongong Hospital, Wollongong, NSW, Australia

Department of ENT Head and Neck Surgery, Lyell McEwin Hospital, Adelaide, SA, Australia
e-mail: stephen.kao@sa.gov.au

M. Stuart Grayson
Department of ENT Head and Neck Surgery, Wollongong Hospital, Wollongong, NSW, Australia
e-mail: sgmackay@ozemail.com.au

L. C. Goh, S. T. Toh (eds.), *Sleep Surgery in a Nutshell*,
https://doi.org/10.1007/978-981-95-9749-9_4

4.1 Palatal Surgery for Obstructive Sleep Apnea

John Ming Ren Loh

4.1.1 Introduction: History and Evolution of Palatal Surgery

Palatal surgery for snoring was first developed by Dr. Takenosuke Ikematsu in 1952 to treat a woman who was divorced due to her loud snoring [1]. He subsequently published his technique in Japanese literature in 1964. The technique focused on trimming and shortening the free edge of the soft palate. Though initially described for snoring, the surgical technique uvulopalatopharyngoplasty (UPPP) was subsequently adapted for obstructive sleep apnea and popularized in the United States by Fujita and published in English literature in 1981 [2].

Since its original description, many pioneers of sleep surgery described refinements and modifications of UPPP over the years. Powell and Riley described the uvulopalatal flap in 1996 as a technique designed to reduce the risk of velopharyngeal insufficiency (VPI) and allow reversal of the procedure should VPI occur [3]. Fairbanks described his technique in 1996, in which excision at the mid palate and uvula was minimized, uvulopalatal webbing incisions were created for mobilization, and emphasis placed on posterior pillar advancement in a cephalo-lateral (upward and outward) direction [4]. The general trend across the following decades was an emphasis on mobilization and advancement or rotation of tissues, while minimizing muscle and mucosa excision. Cahali in 2003 described the lateral pharyngoplasty in which the posterior pillar and superior constrictor muscles were dissected and mobilized to allow lateralization of the muscles [5]. Friedman described the Z-palatoplasty in 2004 in which only anterior uvula and soft palate mucosa was removed, without any muscle excision [6]. The uvula and soft palate are then partially divided in the midline and stitched anterolaterally. In the same year, Han described his technique advocating submucosal soft palate adipose tissue removal through inverted V-shaped incisions in the palate and uvula preservation [7].

Pang and Woodson described the expansion pharyngoplasty in 2007 in which the posterior pillars were transected inferiorly, mobilized and stitched toward the pterygoid hamulus [8]. Li described the relocation pharyngoplasty in 2009 with an emphasis on cephalo-lateral rotation of the posterior pillar toward a superior-lateral counterpoint at the soft palate superiorly and the superior constrictor inferiorly. Li published an updated technique of palatal hybrid surgery in 2023 combining suspension of the posterior pillar to the pterygoid hamulus and relocation toward the superior constrictor [9, 10]. In 2012, Mantovani described the velo-uvulo-pharyngeal lift "Roman blind" technique in which the soft palate and posterior pillars were anchored with three separate sutures toward the hard–soft palate junction and pterygoid hamulus bilaterally [11]. A year later, Mantovani described doing the same procedure but using barbed suture as a knotless method, which distributed tension along the entire length of suture [12]. Vicini later described the barbed reposition pharyngoplasty that combined the anterior suspension of the soft palate to the hard palate junction, and Li's relocation vectors of the posterior pillars, while using a knotless barbed suture [13].

Robinson and Mackay described the Australian Modified UPPP in 2013, which encompassed dissection of the supra-tonsillar fat pad, incision of the posterior pillar muscle at the upper third portion, and advancement of the muscle toward the pterygomandibular raphe [14]. These named techniques play an important role in understanding the historical basis and rationale of palatal surgery. Choosing a single technique provides consistency, which is important for teaching the techniques in a step-by-step approach, as well as in the research realm to standardize surgical techniques to show an outcome. However, with a gamut of techniques to choose from, how should one make sense of which technique to learn?

4.1.2 Rethinking Palatal Surgery

Rather than thinking of UPPP or its modifications as a single surgery with fixed steps, palatal surgery can be thought of as an umbrella term for a combination of different palatal maneuvers, akin to rhinoplasty in which different approaches, incisions, grafts, and sutures techniques are used in an individualized manner.

Even from the early years of palatal surgery, Ikematsu had described 15 different variations of palatal anatomy [1]. As with rhinoplasty where no two noses are identical, each patient's pharynx and palate have subtle variations, which may require selection, adjustment, and modification of different techniques.

Palatal techniques can be broadly classified into:

- Tissue excision/ablation
- Relaxing and releasing techniques
- Posterior pillar lateralization
- Suspension techniques
- Advancement techniques

4.1.2.1 Tissue Excision

Palatine Tonsils

In surgically naïve patients, tonsillectomy is a routine step prior UPPP to reduce soft tissue volume and expose the palatoglossus and palatopharyngeus muscles. Friedman showed that in patients with large Brodsky Grade 3 and 4 tonsils together with a favorable tongue position, tonsillectomy with UPPP had success rates greater than 80%, but success rates were poorer in patients with smaller tonsil size [15].

In the TEAM-UP randomized clinical trial, patients had similar improvements in Apnea–Hypopnea Index (AHI) at the 6 months whether tonsillectomy alone or tonsillectomy was done together with modified UPPP in patients with grades 2–4 tonsils [16]. This demonstrates the importance of volume removal in patients with large tonsils and opens up a discussion if palatoplasty is necessary in patients with larger tonsils. However, in patients with small palatal tonsils and mainly anterior–posterior collapse on drug-induced sleep endoscopy, Chiu et al. showed that tonsillectomy can be avoided during UPPP with equally favorable outcomes, thus demonstrating the effectiveness of UPPP without tonsillectomy [17].

During tonsillectomy, excision of the anterior and posterior tonsillar pillars (palatoglossus and palatopharyngeus muscles) should be avoided.

Supratonsillar Fat Pad

The supratonsillar fat pad lies within the lateral palatal space, bounded by the palatopharyngeus muscles Posteriorly, the superior constrictor muscles laterally, the Superior pole of the tonsil laterally, and the palatoglossus muscle and soft palate mucosa anteriorly.

The supratonsillar fat pad can be accessed through a variety of approaches. The Australian-modified UPPP technique describes an oblique incision made lateral to the base of the uvula toward the pterygomandibular raphe, then elevating a triangular flap of mucosa to expose the supratonsillar fat. Excising an inverted V- or U-shaped area of mucosa can give similar exposure to the peritonsillar fat pad. The incision or excised area is often closed with mobilization of the posterior pillar.

Supratonsillar fat pad excision can be considered in patients with a thicker palate associated with a greater body mass index (Figs. 4.1 and 4.2).

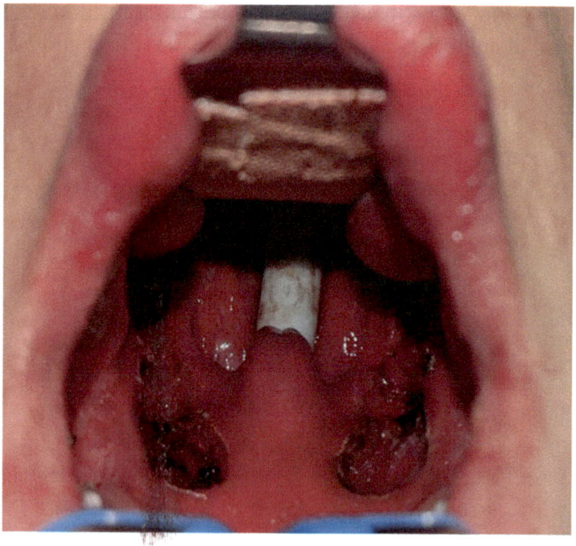

Fig. 4.1 Soft palate after removal of supratonsillar fat pad

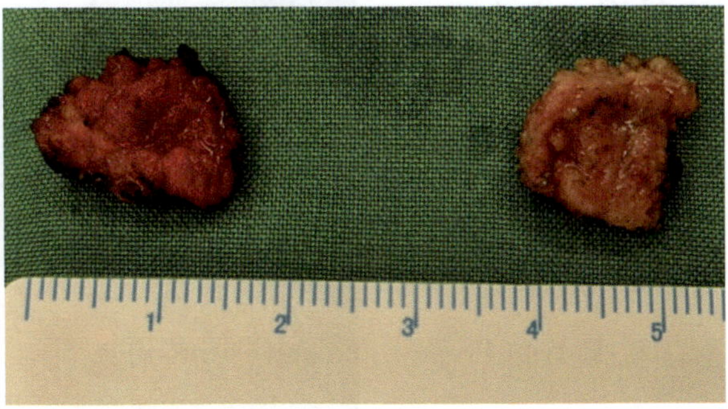

Fig. 4.2 Supratonsillar fat

Uvula

The uvula consists of the paired muscularis uvulae, covered by mucosa and minor salivary glands. During swallowing, the uvula sweeps against the posterior pharyngeal wall, providing lubrication to the pharynx. Excision of the uvula (uvulectomy) has been performed since ancient times in some cultures in Africa and the Middle East. In Ikematsu's original description of UPPP, the uvula was completely resected. Total uvulectomy may result in throat dryness and globus sensation. Nearly all modern UPPP techniques avoid complete resection of the uvula or avoid any resection of uvula at all. Partial uvulectomy of the distal half or third of the uvula may still be considered especially in long redundant uvulas, or when vibrations or prolapse of the uvula into the velopharynx is seen during sleep endoscopy.

4.1.2.2 Relaxing and Releasing Techniques

Relaxing and releasing techniques are mostly focused on the posterior pillar (palatopharyngeus) muscles. Prior to performing any releasing incisions or mobilization, the native mobility and pliability of the muscles and mucosa should be checked by grasping the muscle with forceps and moving it to its intended position. If there is good mobility without excessive tension, releasing incision and additional mobilization may not be required. If there is excessive tension, relaxing incisions or mobilization can be considered (Figs. 4.3 and 4.4).

Relaxing Incisions

Relaxing incision can be made along the posterior pillar at the upper third junction, mid-point, or lower third junction. The incision can be made partially to the medial portion of the muscle bundle, instead of a complete transection, to avoid excessive laxity (Fig. 4.5).

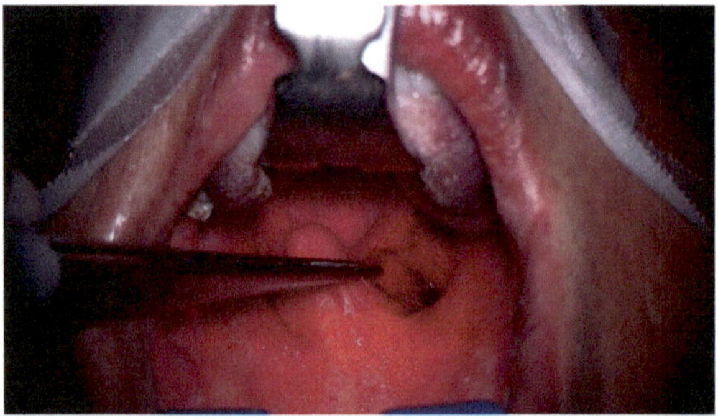

Fig. 4.3 Grasping the palatopharyngeus muscle

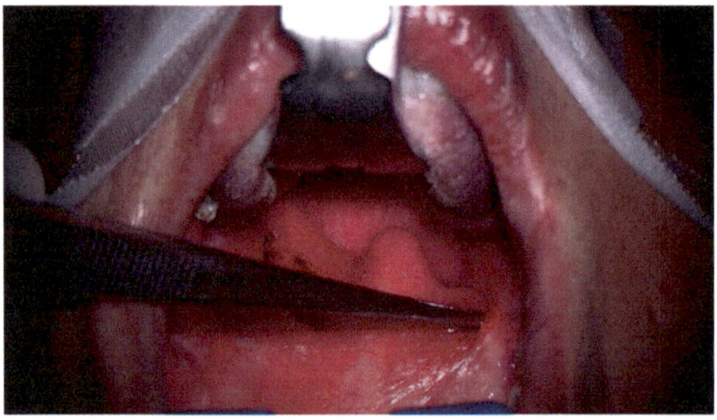

Fig. 4.4 Checking the mobility and tension of the palatopharyngeus

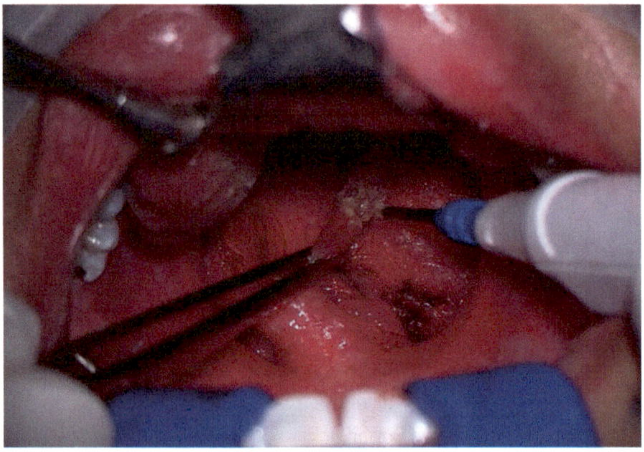

Fig. 4.5 Creating a relaxing incision of the palatopharyngeus

4.1.2.3 Releasing Techniques

Mobilization techniques involve dissecting and freeing the posterior pillar off its inferior attachment, or from the superior constrictor muscles to gain more mobility. Dissection between the palatopharyngeus and superior constrictor, and between the superior constrictor and buccopharyngeal fascia, can allow for better mobility of these muscles to allow for movement and lateralization. However, care must be taken to avoid dissecting lateral to the buccopharyngeal fascia and stylohyoid ligament to avoid injury to the glossopharyngeal nerve. Updated versions of Cahali's lateral pharyngoplasty limited the dissection of the superior constrictor muscle to the superior 1 cm within the tonsillar fossa.

Partial or complete transection of the palatopharyngeus muscle bundle at its inferior third, with dissection of the muscle off the underlying superior constrictor allows for superior mobility of the muscle bundle and to redirect the fibers from a superior–inferior direction to an anterior–lateral direction (Figs. 4.6 and 4.7).

4.1.2.4 Suspension Techniques

Suspension techniques focus on using sutures to hitch the palatopharyngeus muscle to a bony or fibrous anchor point. Commonly used lateral anchor points are the pterygoid hamulus and pterygomandibular raphe. The pterygoid hamulus is a hook-like structure arising from the medial pterygoid plate, which can be palpated intraorally posterior to the posterior–medial aspect of the maxillary alveolar ridge. The tensor veli palatini, superior constrictor, and buccinator muscles attached to the hamulus.

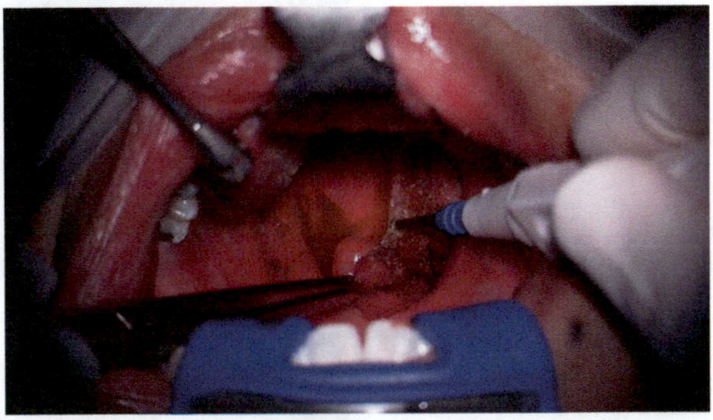

Fig. 4.6 Releasing the medial fibers of the palatopharyngeus

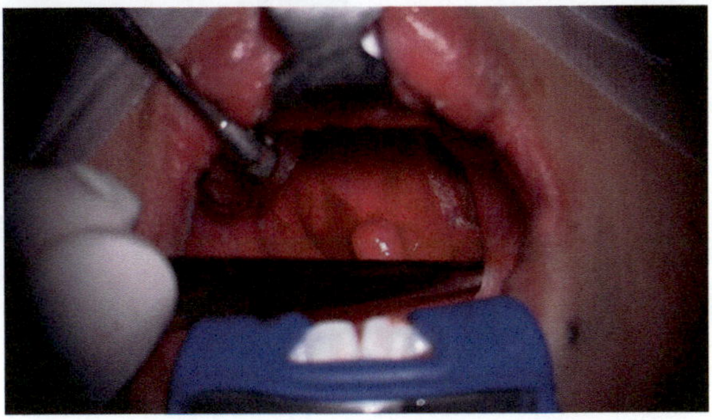

Fig. 4.7 Redirecting the fibers of the palatopharyngeus anterior-superiorly (expansion pharyngoplasty maneuver)

The pterygomandibular raphe is a condensation of muscular and fibrous tissue from the buccinator, deep temporalis tendon, and superior constrictor that runs from the pterygoid hamulus to the posterior mylohyoid ridge or retromolar trigone inferiorly. This can be palpated intra-orally like a guitar string beneath the mucosa. In cadaveric studies, the pterygomandibular raphe can be absent in up to 13% of individuals [18].

The hamulus itself, or the fibrous tendons of these muscles near the hamulus, or the pterygomandibular raphe, can provide an anchor point for sutures, which pull the palatopharyngeus in a superior–anterior–lateral direction. These anchor points can either be identified with an incision and dissection to expose the structure or by simple palpation without dissection. Suspension techniques can also be used in the midline, in order to hitch the soft palate anterior-superiorly toward the posterior nasal spine. Suspension can be done with either strong resorbable polyglactin sutures, or with barbed sutures, to achieve similar vectors of pull (Figs. 4.8 and 4.9).

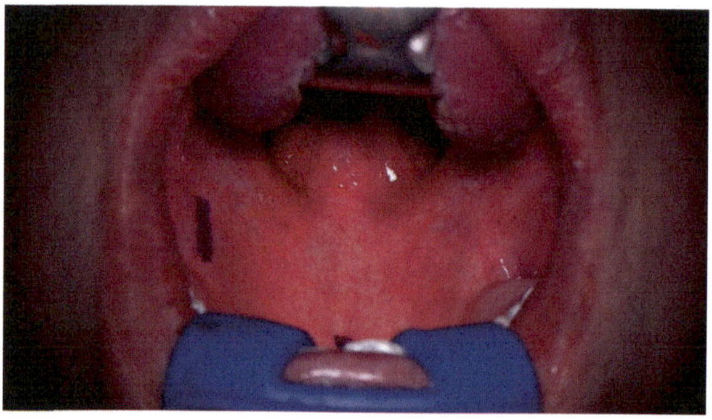

Fig. 4.8 Surface marking of the left pterygomandibular raphe

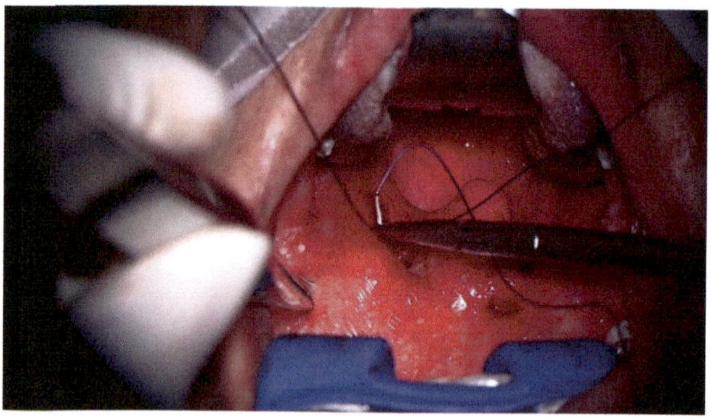

Fig. 4.9 Suture being passed toward the pterygomandibular raphe

4.1.2.5 Lateralization Techniques

Lateralization may be considered in patients with lateral wall collapse, as well as thicker, bulkier palatopharyngeus muscles. After adequate mobilization of the palatopharyngeus muscles and/or superior constrictor muscles, the muscle bundle can be stitched laterally to the palatoglossus muscles. This can be done in isolation or in combination with suspension techniques.

4.1.2.6 Advancement Techniques

Soft palate advancement techniques can be considered in patients with a long redundant soft palate. Advancement of the palate is typified by the anterior palatoplasty technique, in which a horizontal rectangular area of mucosa is denuded off the proximal soft palate, avoiding any incisions to the free edge of the soft palate. The denuded area and underlying muscle are then closed in an anterior–posterior direction, thus pulling the palate anteriorly.

The advancement concept can also be used to shorten the muscularis uvulae within the proximal soft palate, thereby shortening the uvula without the need to excise the free edge of the uvula.

4.1.3 Conclusion

Modern palatal surgery has progressed over the last several decades. By understanding every technique, the contemporary surgeon can pick and combine maneuvers to best suit their patient's anatomy.

4.2 Radiofrequency Ablation of the Soft Palate

Chu Qin Phua and Hui Yan Ong

4.2.1 Introduction

Vibratory snoring and a proportion of *mild obstructive sleep apnea (OSA)* arise from *retropalatal flutter* and/or anteroposterior soft-palate collapse during sleep. Temperature-controlled radiofrequency (TCRF) applies submucosal thermal energy to the soft palate to induce *volumetric tissue reduction* and *collagen remodeling*, thereby *stiffening* the palatal lamina and reducing flutter and collapsibility with *minimal mucosal injury* [19, 20]. The technique is designed as a *mucosa-preserving*, office-based intervention that can be delivered in staged sessions. Unlike resective palatoplasty, TCRF seeks to *reduce compliance* rather than excise tissue, preserving velopharyngeal function and lowering perioperative morbidity.

Ideal candidates are adults with *primary snoring* or *mild OSA* (AHI typically ≤15 events/h) [21, 22], *low–moderate BMI*, and drug-induced sleep endoscopy (DISE) or awake phenotyping that shows *retropalatal flutter/AP collapse* without dominant lateral pharyngeal wall or tongue-base failure. Small or absent tonsils, a favorable Friedman palate/tongue position, and the absence of *complete concentric palatal collapse* favor response, whereas multilevel collapse, morbid obesity, and severe OSA predict limited efficacy. Screen for *palatal anomalies* (submucous cleft, prior scarring), velopharyngeal symptoms, and prominent nasal/valve obstruction that may require treatment first. Concomitant nasal optimization (medical or surgical) improves comfort and facilitates positive airway pressure (PAP) if needed later [22].

Baseline outcomes should include *bed-partner snoring VAS*, *Epworth Sleepiness Scale (ESS)*, targeted quality-of-life instruments, and (for OSA) polysomnography or technically adequate HSAT with consistent scoring. In equivocal anatomy, *DISE* clarifies the palatal contribution and screens for lateral wall or epiglottic phenotypes that TCRF will not correct.

4.2.2 Indications

- Primary snoring caused by palatal collapse
- Mild obstructive sleep apnea caused by palatal collapse
- As part of multilevel sleep apnea surgery following CPAP failure
- Patients seeking minimally invasive surgery compared to traditional ablative/invasive uvulopalatoplasty
- Patients who are unfit for general anesthesia

Advantages
- Minimally invasive
- Less painful compared to other resective/ablative palatal procedures for OSA
- Shorter recovery time and less complications compared to other resective/ablative palatal procedures for OSA
- Can be done as an in-office procedure
- Can be repeated easily

Limitations
- May be less effective for patients with severe OSA or significant palatal collapse
- Multiple sessions may be needed to achieve optimal results
- Long-term outcome is still to be established.
- Requires careful patient selection and expectation management

4.2.3 Mechanism of Action [22, 23]

Delivery of radiofrequency energy to specific points of the soft palate causes a controlled thermal injury. This induces submucosal fibrosis, leading to volume reduction and stiffening of the soft palate as it heals. This therefore reduces vibration and collapsibility of the soft palate during sleep.

4.2.4 Instruments Required

A few of the soft palate wands (as below) are available for purposes of radiofrequency ablation of soft palate

- Reflex Ultra 55 Soft palate wand (Smith and Nephew)
- Celon ProSleep Wand (Olympus)
- Ravor bipolar electrode (Sutter)
- Topical anesthetic spray (e.g., 10% lidocaine)
- 2% lidocaine with 1:80,000 epinephrine for local infiltration
- Oral retractor and tongue depressor
- Suction apparatus

4.2.4.1 Surgical Technique (Fig. 4.10)

Preoperative Precautions

1. Stop antiplatelet/anticoagulant prior to surgery, e.g., aspirin, clopidogrel, warfarin, and rivaroxaban.
2. Check for supplements that might increase bleeding risks and stop prior to surgery (e.g., cordyceps, ginkgo biloba, and lingzhi).

Anesthesia and Exposure

- General anesthesia is preferred.
- Insert a *Boyle–Davis mouth gag* for exposure.
- Place *throat pack* to elevate the palate and protect posterior pharyngeal wall.

Local Anesthesia

- Spray soft palate with *topical lignocaine*.
- Infiltrate *0.5% Marcaine with adrenaline* into treatment areas to reduce bleeding and identify submucosal planes.
- Infiltration with local anesthesia (e.g., lidocaine 2% with 1:80,000 adrenaline, according to weight and dosage), at about 5–8 points, around the target entry point of RF probe.
- Insert radiofrequency probe into soft palate and apply radiofrequency energy (Celon: setting 8–10 W) (Reflex ultra 55: setting ablate 5, coag 4) (Ravor, setting Power 2)

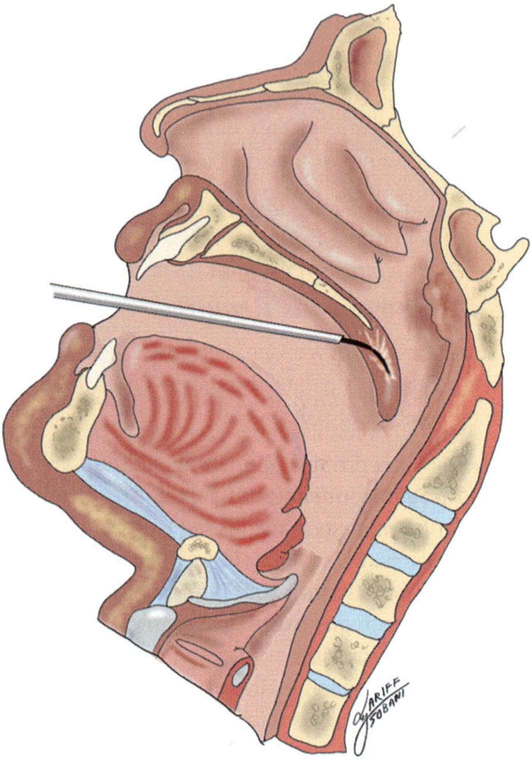

Fig. 4.10 Sagittal view of radiofrequency being used at the soft palate

Radiofrequency Application (Fig. 4.11)

1. Insert the probe into the *junction of the hard and soft palate*.
2. Treat along *midline and paramedian zones*, 1 cm apart.
3. Additional applications at the *base of the uvula* and *tonsillar pillars* as needed.
4. Do *not blanch the mucosa* or exit posteriorly.
5. Use a *thermally shielded probe*, exposing only the tip to prevent surface burns.
6. Reduce energy setting at the uvular base to minimize pain and edema (Figs. 4.12 and 4.13).

Note Avoid lateral soft palate or excessive application in thin tissues to prevent complications such as *palatal fistula (Fig. 4.14)*.

Adjunct Consideration

- Muscular or bulky palates may require *laser-assisted uvulopalatoplasty (LAUP)* or *uvulopalatopharyngoplasty (UPPP)*.
- Best results are seen when combined with *multilevel airway procedures*.

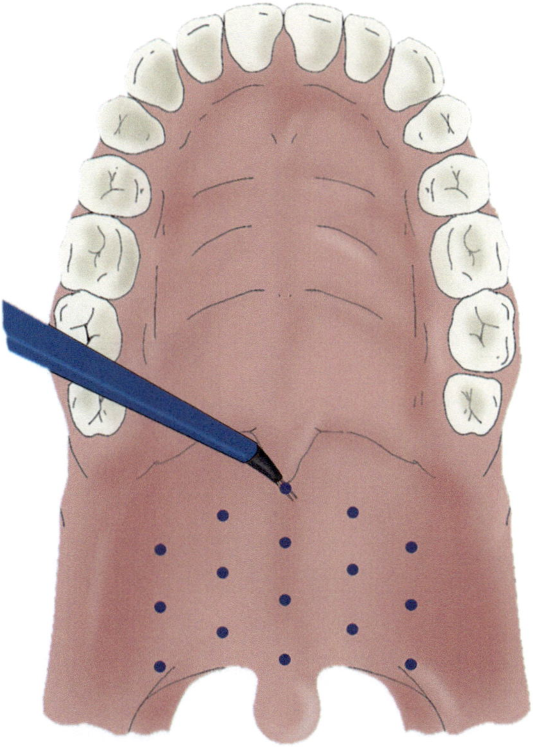

Fig. 4.11 First entry point in midline, just distal to hard and soft palate junction

4.2.4.2 Postoperative Care

- Warn patients some pain and throat discomfort is expected. Analgesia such as paracetamol, arcoxia, as well as lozenges such as Difflam lozenges/gargle should be prescribed and patient can be advised to take soft cool diet.
- Avoid spicy or acidic food for 2–3 weeks.
- Edema of the soft palate can cause globus sensation, temporary difficulties swallowing, and minor speech disturbances, which typically lasts 2 weeks or so. Edema of the soft palate can also cause snoring to be worse during the initial 2 weeks before it becomes better.
- Warn patient that snoring may be more pronounced in the first few days following procedure
- Healing should be complete by 2–3 weeks
- Assess results in 8–12 weeks; consider repeat procedure if necessary.

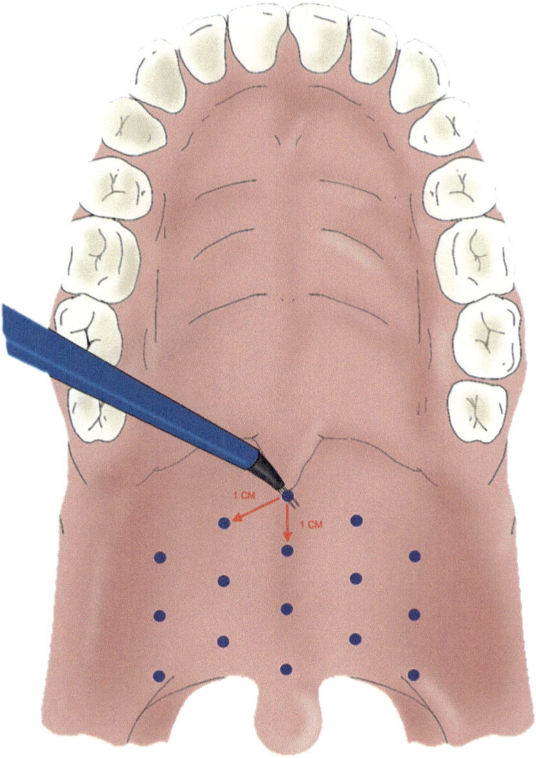

Fig. 4.12 Entry points for RF palate

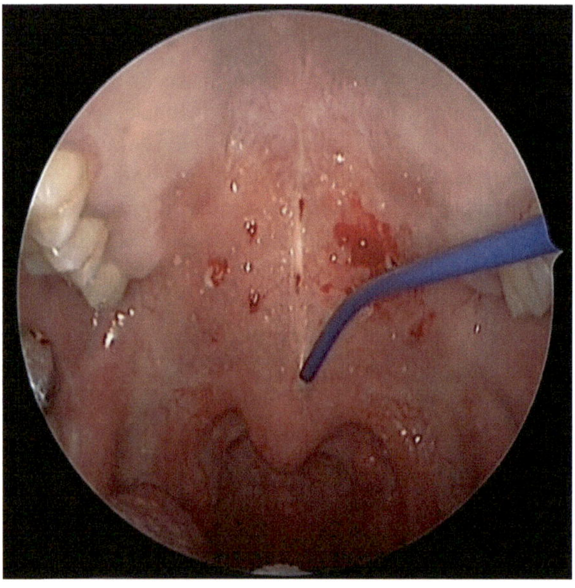

Fig. 4.13 RF to base of uvula

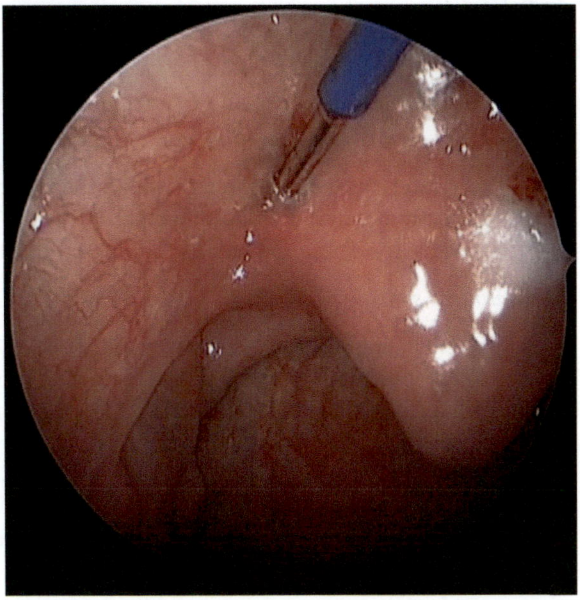

Fig. 4.14 RF to tonsillar pillar

Complications [19, 23]

Complications associated with radiofrequency ablation of soft palate are as follows:

1. *Pain*
   (a) During first to second week after operation, it is common for patients to experience mild to moderate throat discomfort or pain, which can be easily controlled with pain killers.
2. *Bleeding*
   (a) Blood-stained saliva is to be expected for first 3–5 days. Very rarely, excessive bleeding can occur and immediate hospital consultation should be sought.
3. *Edema of soft palate*
   (a) Swelling of the soft palate can occur and cause globus sensation, temporary swallowing difficulties, and minor speech disturbances. Snoring may potentially be worse initially before it improves.
4. *Infection*
   (a) Infection at the surgical wound site can occur, but this is rare.

5. *Palate ulcer*
   (a) After the procedure, soft palate ulcers may occur. These are usually self-limiting.
6. *Fistula or abnormal connection with nasal cavity*
   (a) Very rarely, if there is through and through puncture of the radiofrequency probe from anterior to posterior palate, fistula can form between oral and nasal cavity. These can be self-limiting or may require further repair.
7. *Continued snoring*
   (a) Patients should be warned that radiofrequency ablation of palate aims to reduce loudness and frequency of disruptive snoring. However, it is not possible to guarantee complete resolution of snoring. Some patients will continue to snore to some extent after surgery.
8. *Scarring*
   (a) Scarring can happen following surgery, and scar thickening can sometimes give patients potential globus sensation.
9. Transient velopharyngeal insufficiency
   (a) Patient may experience temporary reflux of food or water from oral cavity into the nose. This usually resolves with time.

Alternatives
- CPAP
- Dental appliance
- Positional therapy
- Weight loss
- Myofunctional therapy
- More invasive palatal surgery like an uvulopalatopharyngoplasty

4.2.5 Conclusion

Radiofrequency ablation of the soft palate is a useful procedure for selected patients. It offers a *safe, effective, and repeatable* solution for patients with palatal snoring or mild obstructive sleep apnea. It is particularly valuable in patients seeking minimally invasive interventions. While not suitable for all patients, proper selection, technique, and postoperative care can yield high patient satisfaction and symptom relief. It should be considered as one of the many tools *of sleep surgeons*, especially in the era of personalized sleep medicine.

4.3 Uvulopalatal Flap

Song Tar Toh and Liang Chye Goh

4.3.1 Introduction

The uvulopalatal flap (UPF) is a muscle-preserving, reversible palatal-shortening, and advancement procedure developed to treat retropalatal obstruction in primary snoring and mild–moderate obstructive sleep apnea (OSA). Conceptually, UPF advances and "tucks" the redundant distal soft palate (including the uvula) onto the oral (oropharyngeal) surface of the soft palate, achieving functional shortening while maintaining palatal muscular continuity—thereby mitigating the risk of velopharyngeal insufficiency (VPI) that complicated earlier resective operations such as traditional uvulopalatopharyngoplasty (UPPP) [24].

Historically, Powell and colleagues introduced the UPF in 1996 as a conservative modification to UPPP specifically aimed at lowering VPI risk without sacrificing anatomic efficacy. In their prospective comparison, UPF improved snoring at least as well as UPPP and, notably, showed no early VPI despite producing equivalent postoperative palatal shortening—supporting the mechanistic value of tissue repositioning over resection [3]. Subsequent reconstructive literature also established the UPF as a versatile flap for soft-palate repairs after oncologic oropharyngeal surgery, indicating its reliability, simplicity, and favorable functional profile [24].

From a pathophysiologic standpoint, UPF targets the most common site of upper airway collapse—the retropalatal segment—by reducing palatal redundancy and tethering the uvula/velum anteriorly, which can decrease inspiratory flow limitation and snoring intensity. Patient selection is crucial: ideal candidates have DISE-demonstrated retropalatal collapse with an elongated/bulky uvula and soft palate, relatively preserved lateral wall tone, and disease limited to the palate or as part of a planned multilevel strategy. Preservation of palatal musculature is central to maintaining speech and swallowing function, and the reversibility of the flap is appealing for patients and surgeons seeking nondestructive options [25].

Evidence for efficacy spans observational cohorts and a randomized comparative trial. In a prospective clinical trial with long-term follow-up (mean $\approx$ 54 months), Neruntarat reported marked short-term improvements in AHI ($\approx$46 $\rightarrow$ 13 events/h) with sustained though attenuated benefit at long term ($\approx$19 events/h); about half of patients met long-term success criteria, and serious complications were not observed—highlighting both durability for some and relapse risk for others [25]. In an RCT of patients with mild–moderate OSA and retropalatal obstruction, UPF and anterior palatoplasty achieved comparable 6-month outcomes (surgical success $\approx$83% in both; AHI reductions to ~8 to 9 events/h), with lower early postoperative pain in the palatoplasty arm—useful when counseling on morbidity profiles across palatal options [26].

When contextualized against legacy palatal surgery, UPF's tissue-sparing philosophy is clinically relevant. Classic long-term series of UPPP demonstrate waning response over time, reinforcing the need for procedures that preserve function and allow iterative, multilevel planning [27]. Contemporary reviews of palatal surgery likewise position UPF among conservative techniques that can be combined (e.g., with lateral wall or tongue-base procedures) to address multilevel disease while maintaining a favorable balance between efficacy and adverse effects [28]. In addition, the advent of minimally invasive palatal implants offers another treatment option for selected patients with snoring and mild OSA, broadening the spectrum of palatal interventions beyond resective surgery [29].

In summary, UPF is a pragmatic, patient-centric palatal operation that (1) improves retropalatal airway patency by anteriorly advancing the uvula/velum, (2) preserves palatal muscle and function to minimize VPI and nasopharyngeal regurgitation, (3) performs competitively with other contemporary palatal procedures for appropriately selected mild–moderate OSA, and (4) remains reversible and compatible with staged multilevel strategies. The accumulating evidence base—including prospective long-term data and randomized comparisons—supports UPF as a key option in the modern palette of palatal surgeries for snoring and OSA [3, 25–29].

4.3.2 Principles

- The uvulopalatal flap works by *advancing the uvula and redundant distal soft palate* forward, tucking it onto the oropharyngeal side of the palate.
- A *diamond-shaped mucosal and submucosal excision* facilitates this fold and allows for secure soft tissue repositioning.
- The muscular continuity of the palate is preserved, minimizing functional disruption.
- The procedure is *reversible*, which makes it ideal for patients who prefer nondestructive surgical options.

4.3.3 Indications

The uvulopalatal flap is suitable for patients with:

- *Primary snoring* without significant apneas
- *Mild to moderate OSA* with retropalatal collapse identified on DISE
- An *elongated or bulky uvula and soft palate* contributing to airway obstruction
- Preference for *minimally invasive or reversible techniques*
- Contraindications to or dissatisfaction with previous resective palatal surgery (e.g., UPPP)

4.3.4 Contraindications

- *Severe OSA* requiring multilevel or lateral pharyngeal wall procedures
- Presence of *palatal hypotonia*, neuromuscular disease, or preexisting VPI
- Prior *extensive palatal surgery* resulting in fibrosis or scarring
- Anatomical factors such as *short soft palate* where folding would result in overshortening

4.3.4.1 Surgical Technique

1. *Patient Preparation and Exposure*
   - The patient is placed in the *supine position* with standard sterile draping.
   - A *Boyle–Davis mouth gag* is inserted and suspended to provide exposure of the oropharynx and soft palate.
2. *Identification of the Palatal Dimple*
   - The *uvula is gently grasped* with forceps, and *tension is applied anteriorly and upward.*
   - This maneuver reveals the *palatal dimple*, a key anatomical marker indicating the safe extent of shortening.

     Tip: Shortening the soft palate *beyond the dimple* increases the risk of *velopharyngeal insufficiency.*
3. *Creating the Mucosal Fold*
   - The uvula is *reflected upward (cephalad)* to create a *crease in the mucosa* at the junction of the uvula and posterior soft palate.
   - This crease will form the *new palatal edge* once the flap is completed.

     Tip: The ideal final position of the *uvular tip* should be *5–10 mm posterior to the hard–soft palate junction* for optimal function.
4. *Flap Design and Mucosal Excision (Figs. 4.15 and 4.16)*
   - A *diamond-shaped outline* is marked using diathermy:
     - The diamond includes the *entire mucosal surface of the uvula.*
     - A matching *reciprocal diamond-shaped defect* is created on the *oral surface of the soft palate.*
   - *Mucosa and submucosal tissue* within the diamond are dissected off the *underlying palatal musculature* to facilitate flap placement.
5. *Flap Inset and Closure (Fig. 4.17)*
   - The uvula is folded anteriorly and *sutured into the reciprocal defect* on the soft palate.

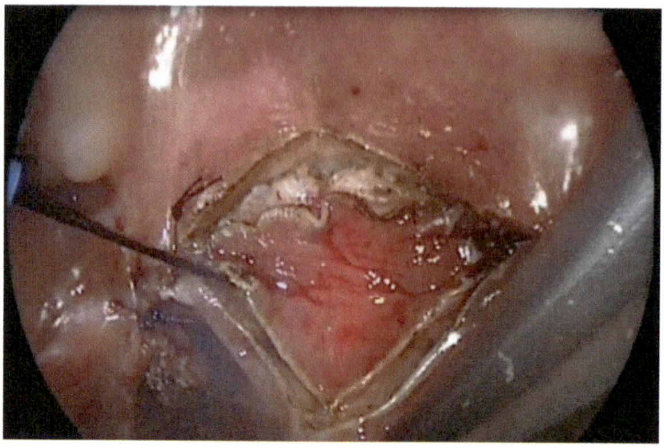

Fig. 4.15 After determination of the desired palatal position, the outline for a diamond-shaped flap is marked out with diathermy

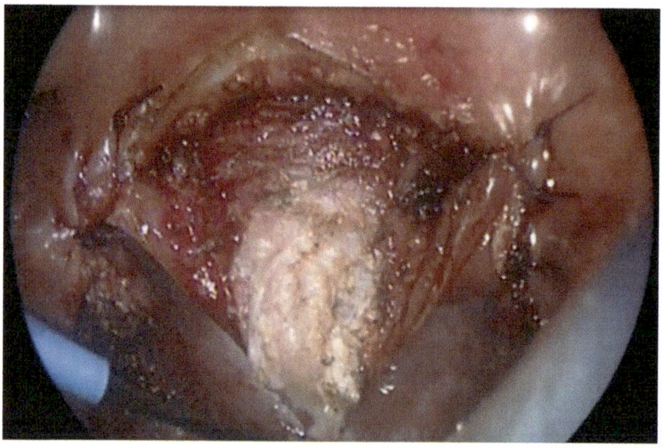

Fig. 4.16 Mucosal and submucosal tissue dissected off the underlying muscle layer

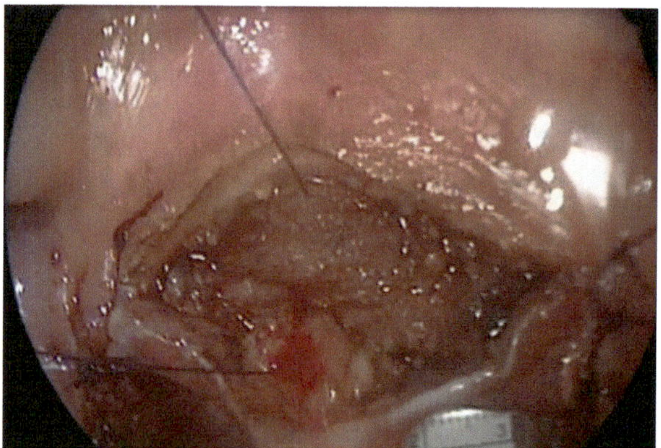

Fig. 4.17 Closure of muscular layer with tagging sutures

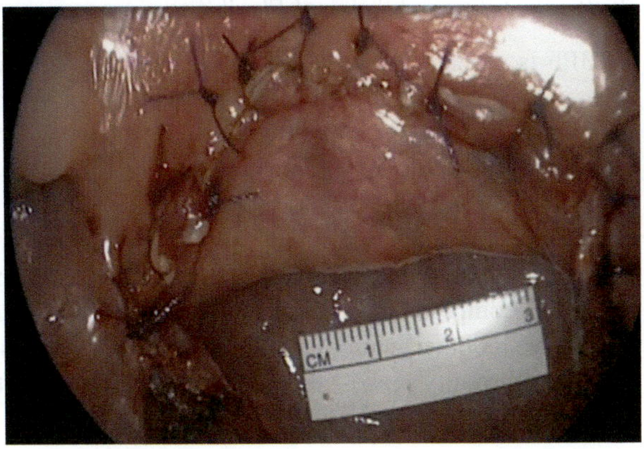

Fig. 4.18 Soft palate defect closed

- The *muscular layer is approximated* first using *tagging sutures* (e.g., 3–0 Vicryl).
- The *mucosal edges* are then closed meticulously using *absorbable sutures* (e.g., 4–0 or 5–0 Vicryl Rapide).
- Hemostasis is ensured throughout, and no packing is typically required (Fig. 4.18).

Postoperative Care

- Patients are advised to maintain a *soft or pureed diet* for 7–10 days to minimize mechanical disruption of the sutures.
- *Oral hygiene*, saline gargles, and analgesics are prescribed postoperatively.
- Most patients can resume *normal speech and swallowing* within 2 weeks.
- A follow-up evaluation should include both visual and functional assessment of the flap.

4.3.5 Advantages of the Uvulopalatal Flap

The uvulopalatal flap (UPF) offers several distinct advantages over traditional resective procedures such as uvulopalatopharyngoplasty (UPPP) and even some of the newer palatal techniques. These advantages lie primarily in its *muscle-preserving design, functional outcomes*, and *surgical versatility*.

1. *Muscle-Preserving and Functional Safety*

Unlike UPPP, which involves partial resection of the uvula and soft palate musculature, UPF repositions tissue rather than removing it. This preserves muscular integrity, thereby minimizing the risks of velopharyngeal insufficiency (VPI), nasopharyngeal regurgitation, and dysphonia [24, 25]. Postoperative speech and swallowing function are generally well maintained, even in long-term follow-up cohorts [3].

2. *Reversibility and Surgical Flexibility*

UPF is essentially a reconstructive "folding" procedure, making it potentially reversible. If required, the flap can be taken down and repositioned without the permanent tissue loss associated with resective palatal surgery [24]. This flexibility is particularly valuable in patients who may require staged or multilevel surgery.

3. *Reduced Morbidity*

Patients undergoing UPF typically report less postoperative pain and fewer complications compared to those receiving traditional UPPP [25, 26]. Early recovery is generally smoother, with faster return to normal diet, speech, and swallowing. The reduced morbidity makes it an attractive option for patients hesitant about aggressive surgical interventions.

4. *Shorter Operative Time and Low Bleeding Risk*

The UPF can be performed relatively quickly under local or general anesthesia. Since the procedure preserves musculature and involves minimal excision, intraoperative bleeding is reduced compared to resective techniques. This translates to shorter operating times and fewer perioperative complications [24].

5. *Compatibility with Multilevel Surgery*

Because the UPF is tissue-sparing, it can be easily integrated into multilevel surgical strategies (e.g., combined with tongue-base reduction or lateral pharyngeal wall procedures). This makes it a versatile tool in the surgeon's skill for comprehensive OSA management [27, 28].

4.3.6 Potential Complications

Although the uvulopalatal flap (UPF) is designed to minimize morbidity compared to traditional resective palatal procedures, complications can still occur. Fortunately, most are mild, transient, and manageable with conservative care.

1. *Early Postoperative Morbidity*
   - *Odynophagia and throat discomfort*: Transient pharyngeal pain is common in the first postoperative week but is generally milder than after uvulopalatopharyngoplasty (UPPP) [24, 25].
   - *Edema and mucosal irritation*: Local swelling may contribute to mild dysphagia or globus sensation but typically resolves within days.
2. *Bleeding*
   - *Intraoperative bleeding* is uncommon due to limited resection of palatal tissue and preserved muscular integrity.

- *Postoperative bleeding* may occur from suture dehiscence or vessel injury but is generally minor and self-limited [24].

3. *Flap-Related Issues*
   - *Suture dehiscence or flap mispositioning* can occur, particularly if patients resume a solid diet prematurely or have poor wound care compliance. This may lead to partial flap failure, asymmetry, or persistent snoring [3].
   - *Infection* is rare but possible, usually presenting as localized erythema or discharge; oral antibiotics and saline gargles are usually sufficient.
4. *Functional Disturbances*
   - *Velopharyngeal insufficiency (VPI)* and *nasopharyngeal regurgitation* are very uncommon compared to UPPP, owing to muscle preservation [24, 25]. When they do occur, they are usually transient and resolve with tissue remodeling.
   - *Speech changes* are minimal; however, rare cases of hypernasality may be observed in patients with excessive palatal shortening.
5. *Residual or Recurrent Symptoms*
   - *Persistent snoring* or *residual OSA* may occur if patient selection is suboptimal (e.g., lateral wall collapse, multilevel obstruction not addressed).
   - *Relapse over time* has been reported in long-term follow-up, with some patients experiencing recurrence of OSA symptoms after several years [3].
6. *Rare Complications*
   - *Excessive scarring or fibrosis*, though rare, may lead to palatal stiffness and reduced compliance.
   - *Exaggerated shortening* of the palate may cause mild nasal regurgitation in exceptional cases.

4.3.7 Conclusion

The uvulopalatal flap provides a reliable and patient-centered approach to managing *retropalatal obstruction*, especially in individuals with *mild disease or anatomical soft palate redundancy*. Its *muscle-preserving* and *reversible* nature makes it an attractive alternative to more invasive procedures. Careful attention to surgical landmarks and patient selection is essential to achieving optimal results with minimal complications.

4.4 Relocation Pharyngoplasty

Song Tar Toh and Liang Chye Goh

4.4.1 Introduction

Obstructive sleep apnea (OSA) is a highly prevalent disorder characterized by recurrent upper airway collapse during sleep, leading to intermittent hypoxemia, sympathetic activation, and fragmented sleep. Beyond daytime sleepiness and impaired quality of life, untreated OSA contributes to systemic hypertension, arrhythmias, metabolic dysfunction, and increased cardiovascular morbidity and mortality [30–32]. Although continuous positive airway pressure (CPAP) remains the gold standard, long-term adherence is suboptimal, often due to discomfort, inconvenience, or intolerance [33, 34]. This gap has intensified interest in effective, anatomy-directed surgical therapies.

Among surgical targets, the retropalatal segment is frequently implicated in OSA pathogenesis. Drug-induced sleep endoscopy (DISE) and imaging consistently identify the soft palate and lateral pharyngeal walls as sites of collapse, often with circumferential narrowing [35, 36]. Traditional uvulopalatopharyngoplasty (UPPP), while historically common, is associated with variable efficacy and significant morbidity, including velopharyngeal insufficiency, dysphagia, and altered speech resonance [28]. Consequently, newer procedures emphasize functional reconstruction and vector realignment over resection.

Relocation pharyngoplasty (RP), first described by Li and colleagues in 2009, represents one such evolution [9]. Rather than excising tissue, RP repositions the palatopharyngeus muscle laterally and superiorly, effectively "splinting" the lateral pharyngeal wall to expand and stabilize the retropalatal airway. This muscle-preserving technique seeks to address both concentric and transverse collapse while maintaining physiologic palatal function. By redirecting muscular vectors instead of removing structures, RP minimizes the risk of velopharyngeal insufficiency and promotes faster recovery [37].

Multiple clinical studies, including prospective cohorts, have validated the efficacy of RP, demonstrating significant reductions in Apnea–Hypopnea Index (AHI), improvements in Epworth Sleepiness Scale (ESS) scores, and favorable subjective outcomes [37–39]. Furthermore, RP is often integrated into multilevel surgical strategies with tongue-base, nasal, or skeletal procedures, guided by DISE phenotyping [40, 41]. Compared with expansion sphincter pharyngoplasty (ESP) and barbed reposition techniques, RP is distinguished by its emphasis on anatomic preservation, predictable vector modification, and reproducible outcomes when applied to appropriate phenotypes [42].

As surgical management of OSA continues to move toward individualized, phenotype-driven therapy, RP is useful for patients with dominant retropalatal or lateral pharyngeal wall collapse who are intolerant of CPAP. Its emergence highlights a broader shift in sleep surgery: from resectional, one-size-fits-all procedures toward precise, reconstructive, and function-sparing approaches.

4.4.2 Principles

- The goal of relocation pharyngoplasty is to *laterally reposition the palatopharyngeus muscle* and *secure it to the superior pharyngeal constrictor*, effectively *pulling the lateral pharyngeal wall outward.*
- This creates a *stable and expanded oropharyngeal airway*, particularly in the retropalatal region.
- The procedure preserves *neurovascular integrity*, avoids unnecessary resection of pharyngeal musculature, and aims to reduce tissue collapse during negative inspiratory pressure.

4.4.3 Indications

Relocation pharyngoplasty is typically indicated for:

- *Moderate to severe OSA* with retropalatal obstruction
- *Nonresponders to CPAP therapy*
- *Low lying soft palate*
- Multilevel obstruction requiring a *palatal-level component*

4.4.4 Contraindications

- Soft palate shortening or defects that preclude muscle manipulation
- Significant scarring or fibrosis from previous palatal surgeries
- Neuromuscular weakness involving the pharyngeal musculature
- Velopharyngeal insufficiency or cleft palate history

4.4.5 Surgical Technique

1. *Patient Positioning and Exposure*
    - The patient is placed in the *supine position* under general anesthesia.
    - A *Boyle–Davis mouth gag* or equivalent is inserted to allow full oropharyngeal exposure.

- *Tonsillectomy* is performed if not already completed to facilitate muscle access.

2. *Triangular Incision and Tissue Removal (Figs. 4.19 and 4.20)*

   - Mucosa and *submucosal adipose tissue* in this triangular area are removed, exposing the *palatopharyngeus* and *superior constrictor*

3. *Mobilization and Rotation of the Palatopharyngeus (Fig. 4.21)*

   - The *palatopharyngeus muscle* is grasped near the uvula, then rotated *cephalad and laterally* to reach the *C point* on the posterior soft palate (Fig. 4.22)

4. *Lateral Fixation with Constrictor Muscle (Fig. 4.22, 4.23)*

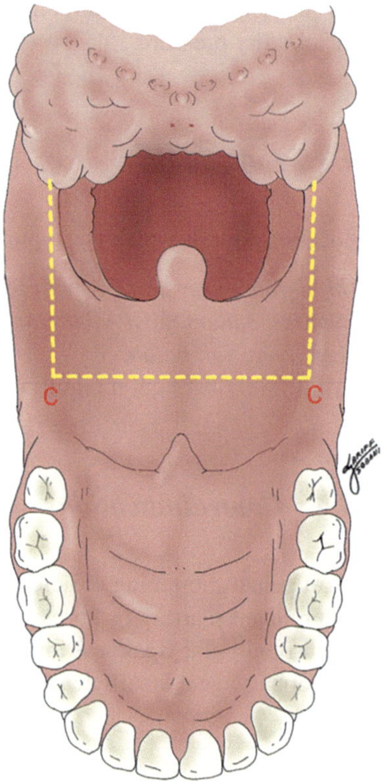

Fig. 4.19 C point represents the mid-occlusal plane

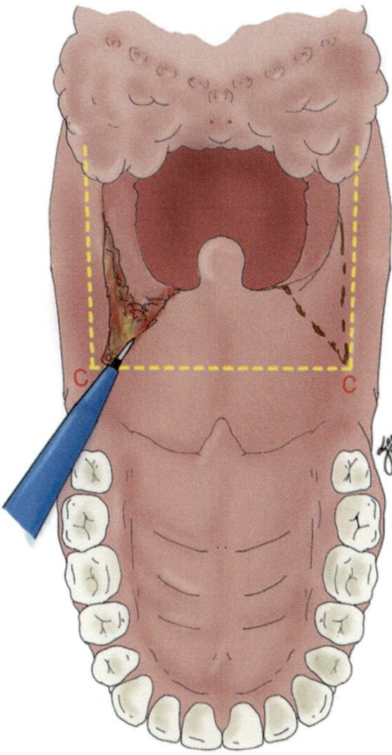

Fig. 4.20 Triangular cuts created at the upper pole of the Tonsillar Fossa. A *triangular incision* is made from the *upper pole of the tonsillar fossa* to the *mid-occlusal plane* (Fig. 7a)

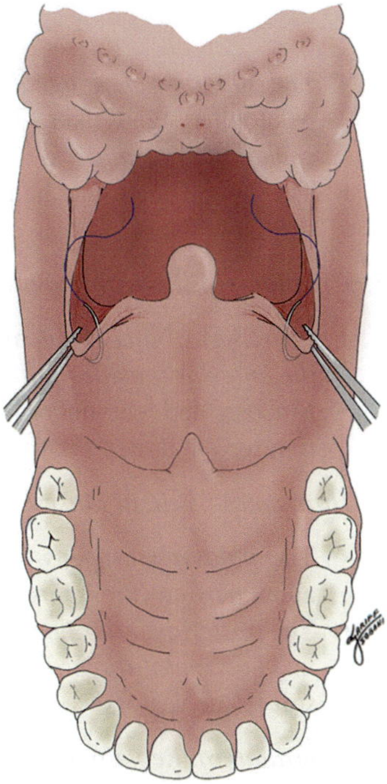

Fig. 4.21 Absorbable sutures used to suture apex of the supratonsillar cut to the palatopharyngeus using mattress sutures

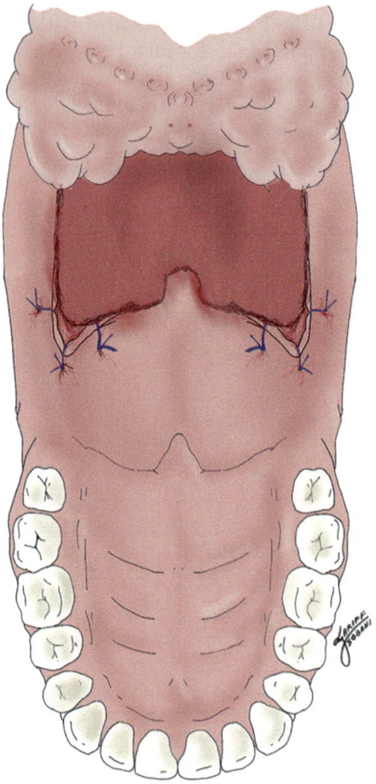

Fig. 4.22 Expected suture placement after completion of suturing procedure

- The *superior pharyngeal constrictor* is identified and approximated to the palatopharyngeus using *3–0 Vicryl* in a *mattress suture pattern*, directed from *cephalad to caudal*.
- This lateral anchoring helps maintain *airway expansion* and prevents posteromedial collapse.

5. *Creation of Elliptical Mucosal Flap* (*Fig. 4.23*)

   - An *elliptical incision* is made from the *uvular base* to the *inferior margin of the anterior tonsillar pillar*, with the *C point* forming the apex.
   - Mucosa and submucosa within this ellipse are carefully dissected and removed to *flatten the soft palate* and eliminate redundant tissue.

6. *Horizontal–Vertical Muscle Approximation*

   - The *palatopharyngeus muscle* is divided from the *superior constrictor* to allow *tension-free redirection*.
   - The *posterior pillar flap* is then sutured to the *palatoglossus muscle*, oriented in a *horizontal-to-vertical plane*, allowing dynamic yet stable realignment of soft tissue vectors.

7. *Contralateral Repetition*

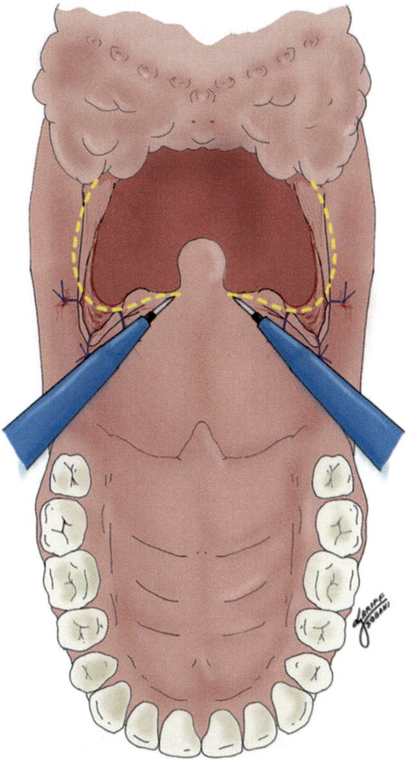

Fig. 4.23 Elliptical incision made to connect the base of uvula and the inferior margin of the anterior pillar while avoiding jagged edges

- The entire process is then *repeated on the contralateral side* with identical steps and careful tension balancing to ensure symmetry and airway patency.

8. *Uvula Trimming (Fig. 4.24)*

   - The *distal nonmuscular portion of the uvula* is resected (Fig. 4.25), completing the reconstruction and reducing potential vibratory tissue contributing to snoring.

4.4.5.1 Postoperative Care

- Patients should be advised a *soft diet* for 7–10 days to avoid mechanical disruption of the suture lines.
- Adequate *oral hygiene* with saline gargles and prescribed *analgesics* should be maintained.
- *Mild odynophagia* and globus sensation may occur initially and typically resolve within 1–2 weeks.
- Endoscopic review may be performed in the clinic after 2–3 weeks to assess healing and airway patency.

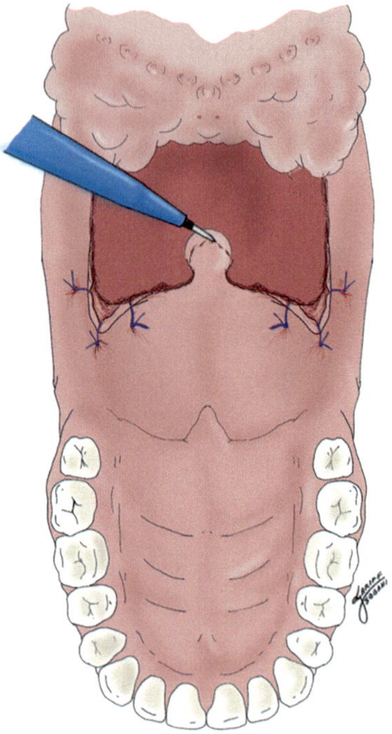

Fig. 4.24 Uvula trimming made to the nonmuscular portion of the uvula if uvula is visibly elongated

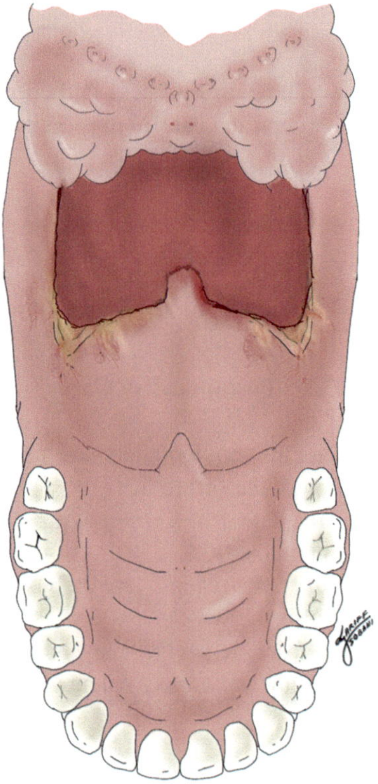

Fig. 4.25 Expected end results once sutures have absorbed

4.4.5.2 Advantages of Relocation Pharyngoplasty

- Effective for *lateral pharyngeal wall collapse*, especially in moderate to severe OSA
- Preserves *muscular and neurovascular structures*
- Does not require permanent implants or foreign material
- Can be tailored to *individual anatomy and airway vector*
- Excellent adjunct to *multilevel sleep surgery* protocols

4.4.6 Potential Complications and Mitigation Strategies

1. Hemorrhage
   Risk:
   - Intraoperative or postoperative bleeding is the most common early complication after palatal surgery.
   - Source typically includes tonsillar/parapharyngeal vessels, palatopharyngeus branches, or superior constrictor.

   Mitigation:
   - Perform meticulous dissection with bipolar or cold instrumentation.
   - Adequate hemostasis before closure; avoid excessive cautery that can compromise muscle viability.
   - Postoperatively: blood pressure control, avoidance of NSAIDs in high-risk patients, clear patient instructions to report delayed bleeding.
2. Airway Compromise and Edema
   Risk:
   - Edema of the soft palate or lateral pharyngeal wall may transiently narrow the airway; rare cases of significant obstruction are reported.
   - Exacerbated in severe OSA patients with baseline critical airway.

   Mitigation:
   - Administer perioperative corticosteroids to reduce edema.
   - Admit high-risk patients to monitored settings with continuous oximetry (HDU/ICU for severe OSA, BMI >40, or multilevel surgery).
   - Early application of CPAP/BiPAP at lower titration when safe.
3. Velopharyngeal Insufficiency (VPI) and Speech Changes
   Risk:
   - Altered palatal dynamics may cause hypernasality, nasal regurgitation, or difficulty with certain consonants.
   - More common in aggressive resectional procedures (UPPP), but can occur if sutures are misapplied or vectors are overtightened in RP.

Mitigation:

- Preserve uvular mucosa whenever possible.
- Avoid over-rotation or excessive lateralization of the palatopharyngeus.
- Symmetric bilateral technique reduces risk of asymmetric palatal closure.
- Most VPI is transient; persistent cases may require speech therapy or revision surgery.

4. Dysphagia and Globus Sensation

   Risk:

- Short-term difficulty swallowing solids/liquids is relatively common due to muscular reorientation and edema.
- Rarely, scar tethering can lead to persistent dysphagia.

Mitigation:

- Gentle handling of the palatopharyngeus and minimal mucosal excision.
- Postoperative soft diet and hydration.
- Early speech/swallowing therapy if symptoms persist beyond 6–8 weeks.

5. Pain and Neuropathic Sequelae

   Risk:

- Significant odynophagia is expected postoperatively, especially when combined with tonsillectomy.
- Rare reports of glossopharyngeal neuralgia-like symptoms if nerve fibers are injured.

Mitigation:

- Employ multimodal, opioid-sparing analgesia.
- Adequate hydration and topical agents (e.g., saline rinses, topical anesthetic sprays) can improve comfort.
- Avoid deep cautery in the parapharyngeal space to reduce nerve injury risk.

6. Taste Disturbance

   Risk:

- Temporary dysgeusia reported in some RP and ESP series due to manipulation of the glossopharyngeal nerve endings in the tonsillar fossa.

Mitigation:

- Careful dissection along avascular planes.
- Inform patients preoperatively that changes are usually mild and self-limiting.

7. Scarring and Asymmetry

   Risk:

- Excessive fibrosis or asymmetric suturing may narrow one side of the oropharynx, leading to persistent snoring or sensation of asymmetry.

Mitigation:

- Use balanced, bilateral suturing with equal tension.
- Avoid overtightening, which predisposes to scar contracture.
- Consider postoperative nasal/oral saline irrigation to reduce crusting and fibrosis.

8. Residual or Recurrent OSA
   Risk:

- RP specifically addresses retropalatal and lateral wall collapse; residual disease persists if tongue-base, epiglottis, or skeletal restriction is uncorrected.

Mitigation:

- Preoperative DISE to phenotype obstruction sites.
- Plan multilevel surgery where indicated (e.g., tongue-base reduction, nasal surgery).
- Reassess with PSG 8–12 weeks post-op and integrate adjunctive therapies (CPAP, oral appliances) if residual AHI remains high.

4.4.7 Conclusion

Relocation pharyngoplasty is a useful yet anatomically respectful technique for treating *retropalatal airway collapse* in patients with obstructive sleep apnea. By *mobilizing and securing the palatopharyngeus muscle*, the lateral pharyngeal wall is expanded, improving airway stability during sleep. When performed with attention to anatomical vectors and tissue tension, this technique provides excellent outcomes with minimal risk.

4.5 Barbed Repositioning Palatopharyngoplasty (BRP)

Liang Chye Goh and Claudio Vicini

4.5.1 Introduction

Barbed repositioning palatopharyngoplasty (BRP) is a mucosa-sparing, *lateral-wall-oriented* palatal reconstruction that leverages bidirectional barbed sutures to *re-tension, lateralize, and stiffen* the velopharyngeal soft tissues without wide tissue resection. Conceptually, BRP was designed to counter the now well-recognized role of *oropharyngeal lateral wall collapse* in the pathophysiology of adult obstructive sleep apnea (OSA). By creating multiple distributed points of fixation from the pterygomandibular raphe/hamulus region to the soft palate and palatopharyngeus,

BRP widens the retropalatal cross-sectional area and resists inspiratory medialization while *preserving palatal length and function* [43].

The lateral pharyngeal wall has long been implicated as a dominant collapse substrate in OSA; phenotyping tools such as *drug-induced sleep endoscopy (DISE)* codified this observation (e.g., VOTE classification) [35] and accelerated a shift from resective uvulopalatopharyngoplasty (UPPP) toward *vector-modifying* procedures that specifically stabilize the lateral wall. BRP emerged within this shift, complementing DISE-guided multilevel planning and offering an anatomic, physiology-preserving alternative to wide palatal excision.

Technically, BRP achieves its effect through *knotless* barbed sutures (e.g., V-Loc/Stratafix) that translate surgeon-set tension into durable tissue repositioning along the soft palate and posterior pillar. This provides (1) *distributed load sharing* (many micro-anchors rather than a few knots), (2) *precise vector control* (lateralization and slight cranial elevation of the palatopharyngeus), and (3) reduced operative time and manipulation which are factors that may lower bleeding and edema risk compared with traditional palatal resections. These features align with contemporary goals of maintaining velopharyngeal competence while *stiffening the inlet* against negative inspiratory pressure [35, 43, 44].

Evidence Base The index pilot from Vicini et al. established *feasibility, safety, and teachability* of BRP, catalyzing widespread adoption. Subsequent prospective cohorts and comparative series including studies against expansion sphincter pharyngoplasty—have shown *clinically meaningful AHI reduction*, high surgical success, and low complication rates when patients are selected for retropalatal/lateral-wall collapse on DISE [43, 45, 46]. Long-term series document sustained subjective benefits (e.g., Palate Postoperative Problem Score), while meta-analyses synthesize multicenter experience and support BRP as an effective palatal strategy within multilevel surgery [43, 46, 47].

Technique Family and Evolution BRP sits within a broader *barbed pharyngoplasty* family (barbed anterior; barbed suspension; barbed expansion sphincter), each modulating vectors to address specific collapse patterns [47, 48]. This taxonomy shows that barbed sutures are not "one technique" but a toolkit to tailor *lateral-wall stabilization* to DISE phenotypes [44] which is an approach supported by narrative and systematic reviews and by emerging randomized and learning-curve data.

Clinical Role In practice, BRP is most valuable for patients with *retropalatal concentric or lateral collapse* who are CPAP-intolerant and are undergoing *multilevel* correction (e.g., tongue-base/epiglottic procedures, nasal optimization).

Contemporary comparative studies suggest BRP achieves success rates comparable to other advanced palatal reconstructions while maintaining a *muscle-preserving*, profile; selection should therefore be *phenotype-driven* rather than procedure-driven [49–51].

4.5.1.1 Indications

Barbed repositioning palatopharyngoplasty (BRP) is indicated in patients with obstructive sleep apnea (OSA) where *retropalatal collapse* is a predominant component of airway obstruction. It is particularly suited for those with concentric or lateral pharyngeal wall collapse, which may not respond adequately to conventional uvulopalatopharyngoplasty (UPPP). Specific indications are as follows.

1. *Obstructive Sleep Apnea (OSA) Patients*
   - Patients who have moderate to severe OSA (AHI >15) with intolerance or noncompliance to CPAP therapy
   - Patients who have undergone drug-induced sleep endoscopy (DISE) demonstrating:
   - Patients who have *redundant soft palate and posterior pillar laxity/low lying soft palate* contributing to obstruction
2. *Failed Previous Palatal Surgery*
   - Patients with persistent or recurrent OSA symptoms after traditional UPPP or other palatal procedures where palatal scarring and tissue tethering need to be addressed with improved vector control
3. *Multilevel Surgery Candidates*
   - As part of *multilevel sleep surgery*, particularly when combined with tongue-base procedures, epiglottoplasty, or nasal surgery
   - As an adjunct to *hypoglossal nerve stimulation* in cases with persistent retropalatal obstruction
4. *Favorable Anatomic Features*
   - Adequate tonsillar fossa exposure
   - No significant velopharyngeal incompetence
   - Soft palate length suitable for redirection and barbed suspension

4.5.1.2 Patient Preparation and Positioning

- The procedure is performed under general anesthesia with orotracheal intubation.
- The patient is placed in the *supine position*, with neck slightly extended.
- A *Boyle–Davis mouth gag* or equivalent is inserted to provide optimal exposure of the oropharynx.
- Antibiotic prophylaxis is administered per institutional protocol.
- Hemostasis throughout the procedure is critical and typically achieved with bipolar cautery.

4.5.2 Surgical Steps

1. Bilateral Tonsillectomy
   - Begin with complete removal of the tonsils using cold dissection or bipolar diathermy, taking care to avoid injury to the superior constrictor and parapharyngeal structures.
   - Ensure meticulous hemostasis at this stage, as visibility during the following steps is critical.
2. *Creation of Triangular Incision*
   - A *triangular mucosal incision* is made beginning at the *upper pole of the tonsillar fossa*, extending inferomedially toward the *mid-occlusal plane*.
   - Both *mucosa and underlying adipose tissue* are removed to expose the *palatopharyngeus muscle*.
3. *Dissection and Partial Transection of the Palatopharyngeus*
   - The *palatopharyngeus muscle* is carefully dissected away from the *posterior pillar mucosa*.
   - A *partial inferior transection* of the palatopharyngeus muscle is performed to allow adequate mobilization for anterior and lateral repositioning.

4.5.2.1 Suturing Technique Using Barbed Suture

- A *Stratafix™ 2–0 or V-Loc™ 2–0 barbed suture (dual needle, unidirectional)* is used for muscle suspension and repositioning.
- The suture is applied without the need for knot tying, relying on barbed tension and anchoring (Fig. 4.26).

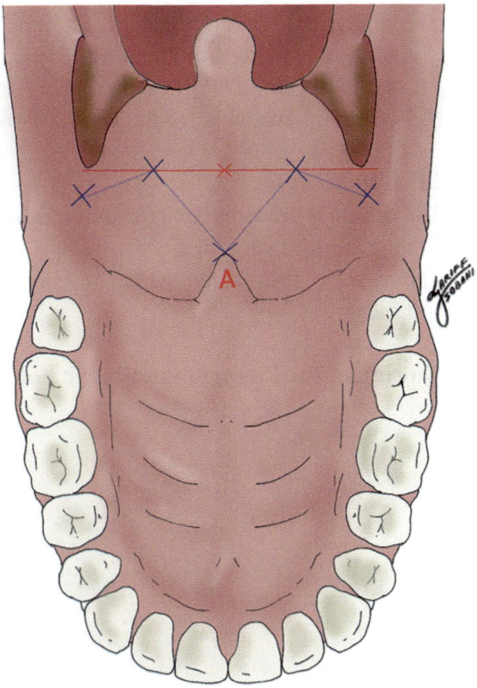

Fig. 4.26 Surgeon's view depicting sites of entry of barbed sutures. Point A, B, and C. Red X depicting midway point between uvula base and transition point

Initiation of the Suture (Midline—Point A)

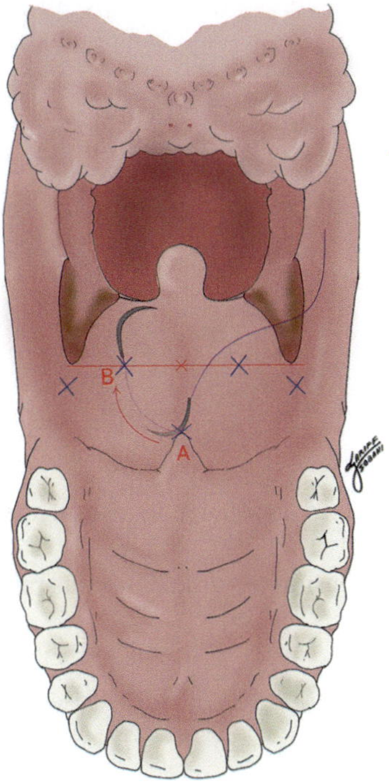

- The first needle is introduced at the junction between the hard and soft palate (Point A), traversing from anterior to posterior soft palate.
- The suture is *pulled halfway through* the soft palate, leaving the other half of the barbed suture available for the *contralateral side*.

Guiding to Point B

- The needle is guided to exit the *anteroinferior surface of the soft palate* (Point B) from posterior to anterior.
- The same needle is *reinserted at Point B*, traversing back into the posterior soft palate.

Anchoring at the Pterygomandibular Fold (Point C)

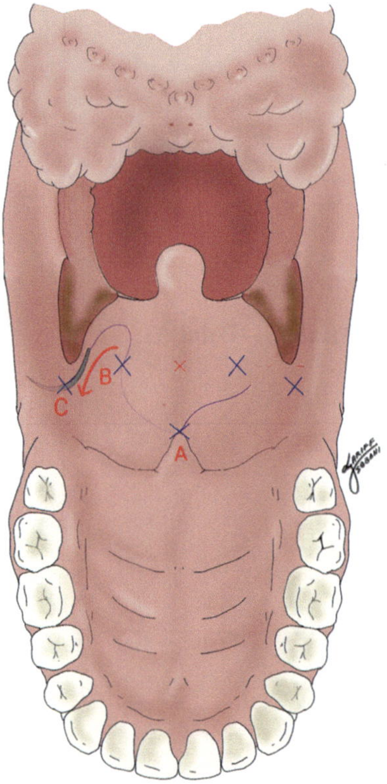

- The needle is now directed anteriorly to exit at the pterygomandibular raphe (Point C).
- This establishes lateral tension toward the fibrous raphe.

Reentry to Tonsillar Fossa (Point D)

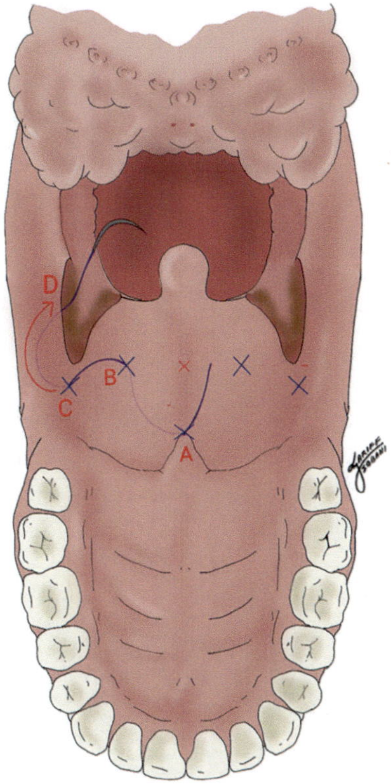

- The needle is reinserted at the raphe (Point C), traveling posteriorly to exit at the *tonsillar fossa (Point D)*.

Suspension of Palatopharyngeus (Point E)

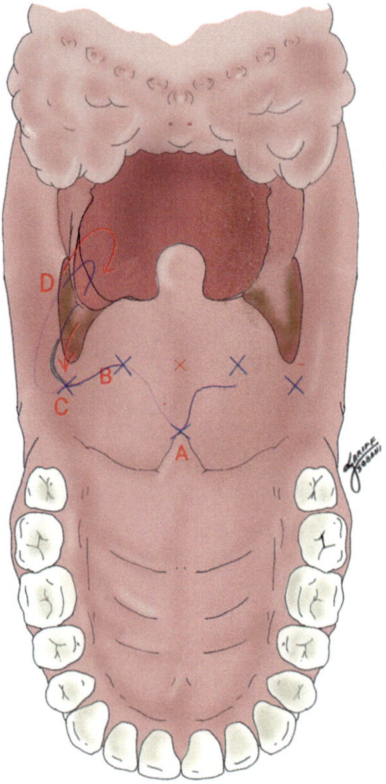

- The suture is now used to *hitch the partially transected palatopharyngeus muscle* (Point E) in a superior and lateral vector.
- The suture is directed anteriorly again to exit once more at the *pterygomandibular raphe*, securing the muscle in its new position.

Repeat on Contralateral Side

- The *same technique* is performed on the *contralateral side* using the other needle and remaining half-length of barbed suture.
- Ensure symmetrical muscle positioning and tension.

Final Steps

- *Excess suture* is trimmed as no knot tying is required due to the locking mechanism of the barbs.
- *Free mucosal edges* of the posterior pillar and tonsillar fossa are re-approximated using *4–0 Vicryl Rapide* or equivalent absorbable suture.

4.5.2.2 Postoperative Considerations

1. *Immediate Postoperative Period*
   - *Airway monitoring:* Patients should be observed closely in the recovery unit for early signs of airway compromise, particularly due to edema or bleeding.
   - *Analgesia:* Pain is usually moderate, localized to the oropharynx, and managed with a combination of paracetamol and NSAIDs. Short courses of opioids may be required in selected cases.
   - *Diet:* Clear fluids are initiated once the patient is fully awake, with advancement to soft, cool foods as tolerated. Avoidance of hot, spicy, or coarse foods in the first week reduces discomfort and risk of trauma to the surgical site.
   - *Hemostasis:* Minor oozing is common but typically self-limiting. Any significant bleeding requires prompt intervention.
2. *Early Postoperative Care (First 1–2 Weeks)*
   - *Oral hygiene:* Gentle mouth rinsing with antiseptic or saline solutions reduces bacterial load and aids mucosal healing. Vigorous gargling should be avoided.
   - *Suture care:* Barbed sutures are absorbable and require no removal. Patients should be reassured that mild foreign-body sensation or transient asymmetry is expected during healing.
   - *Activity restriction:* Patients should avoid strenuous physical activity, heavy lifting, or phonatory strain (e.g., excessive shouting) for at least 2 weeks.
   - *Follow-up visits:* Early endoscopic inspection ensures that suture placement remains intact, there is no dehiscence, and healing progresses as expected.
3. *Late Postoperative Care*
   - *Diet advancement:* A return to normal diet is usually possible by 2–3 weeks, depending on mucosal healing and patient comfort.
   - *Monitoring for complications:* Rare late issues include palatal tethering, velopharyngeal insufficiency, suture extrusion, or persistent pain. These should be addressed promptly if identified.
   - *Functional outcomes:* Snoring reduction, improved airway stability, and patient-reported sleep quality should be reassessed at 6–8 weeks, often supplemented by repeat sleep testing.

4.5.2.3 Advantages of BRP Technique [35, 43, 44]

- Minimally invasive tissue handling
- Knotless, time-saving suture technique
- Preservation of palatal muscle function and structure
- Enhanced lateral wall stabilization
- Reduced operative time and bleeding

4.5.2.4 Complications [35, 43–46]

Early Complications

- *Bleeding and hemorrhage:* Intraoperative bleeding is uncommon but may occur due to injury of tonsillar or palatal vessels. Postoperative secondary hemorrhage, though rare, requires prompt intervention.
- *Edema and airway compromise:* Palatal or pharyngeal swelling may transiently narrow the airway, necessitating close observation in the immediate postoperative period.
- *Pain and dysphagia:* Moderate throat pain and difficulty swallowing are common in the first week but usually manageable with analgesics and dietary modification.
- *Infection:* Superficial wound infection or localized abscess formation is infrequent but possible.
- *Foreign-body sensation:* Some patients may initially perceive the barbed suture as a foreign body, though this typically subsides as healing progresses.

Late Complications

- *Suture extrusion or palpability:* Although uncommon, barbed sutures may extrude or become palpable in the lateral pharyngeal wall, occasionally requiring removal or revision.
- *Velopharyngeal insufficiency:* Rare, but excessive tension or improper suture placement may lead to nasal regurgitation, altered speech resonance, or velopharyngeal dysfunction.
- *Palatal tethering or asymmetry:* Overtightening of sutures can create tethering of the palate or lateral wall asymmetry, potentially affecting swallowing or speech.
- *Persistent or recurrent obstruction:* In some cases, residual pharyngeal collapse may persist or recur, requiring adjunctive or revision procedures.
- *Chronic discomfort or sensory changes:* Rarely, patients report ongoing throat discomfort, numbness, or altered mucosal sensitivity.

4.5.3 Conclusion

Barbed repositioning palatopharyngoplasty (BRP) is an innovative, efficient, and anatomically respectful surgical technique in the management of retropalatal obstruction in OSA patients. Its knotless approach and dynamic palatal repositioning offer excellent control over airway architecture with reduced morbidity. Mastery of the stepwise suturing technique is critical for ensuring consistent outcomes and patient safety.

4.6 Transpalatal Advancement Pharyngoplasty

Stephen Shih-Teng Kao and Stuart Grayson Mackay

4.6.1 Introduction

Upper airway pathology in obstructive sleep apnea commonly involves the palate, often in combination with other subsites. Since its inception in 1981, the uvulopalatopharyngoplasty (UPPP) and its various modifications has been the workhorse in the surgical management of obstructive sleep apnea [52, 53]. Patients with a narrow retropalatal space and long, vertically orientated soft palate may have poorer outcomes following UPPP alone [54]. This led to the development of the transpalatal advancement (TPA) pharyngoplasty first described in 1993 by Woodson and Toohill [54].

Conceptually, TPA is analogous to an "internal" maxillary component of a maxillomandibular advancement without alteration of dentofacial skeleton [55]. TPA advances the soft palate anteriorly, anchoring to the robust hard palate, without soft tissue resection [54, 56]. This results in a significantly increased retropalatal space, beyond what is achievable with a UPPP-alone [56]. This technique facilitates multilevel airway surgery when combined with modified-UPPP and tongue procedures as a simultaneous or staged procedure.

TPA has steadily evolved to improve surgical outcomes and reduce complication rates. The initial description by Woodson et al. involved removing the 1–2 cm of posterior hard palate with advancement of the soft palate anteriorly into the defect [54]. In 2005, Woodson and Robinson published an alteration to the technique where a bony island attached to the soft palate aponeurosis was retained and both advanced in continuity [57]. The advancement of this bony and soft unit allowed for a more robust bone-to-bone apposition with intent to reduce oronasal fistula formation [57]. Variations in the palatal incision have been described in the literature, with modifications developed to reduce wound breakdown and fistula formation, without compromising access.

Woodson originally described the "gothic arch" incision and modified this by shortening the arch and adding an anterior limb to improve palatal access [55]. Shine and Lewis developed the "propeller" incision demonstrating reduction in oronasal fistula rates [58]. A follow-up study by Chan et al. employing both "gothic arch" and "propeller" incisions in different patients found similar results [59]. Fundamentally, these mucosal incision modifications aim to preserve the perfusion of the mucosal flap from the greater palatine neurovascular bundle, which originates posteriorly from the greater palatine foramina.

Surgery is central to contemporary management of adult OSA treatment [52]. It becomes particularly important in patients with moderate or severe OSA who are intolerant or failed PAP therapy. The ability of a surgeon to recognize patients with appropriate anatomic phenotypes for TPA is fundamental.

4.6.2 Principles

The goals of transpalatal advancement pharyngoplasty are to advance the soft palate anteriorly and improve the caliber of the retropalatal space without soft tissue excision. This expansion, particularly in the anteroposterior plane, is larger than what is achievable with a modified UPPP alone.

TPA converts an unfavorable vertically orientated palate into a more favorable intermediate or oblique position [56, 60]. The shorted soft palate stiffens leading to reduced pharyngeal collapse [55].

4.6.3 Indications

- Moderate to severe obstructive apnea with PAP failure or intolerance
- Ideal candidate
  - Long vertical soft palate
  - Broad hard palate >20 mm wide
  - Retropalatal AP collapse
- Other
  - Lateral and complete concentric collapse have less predictable results
  - Narrower palates may have higher rates of oronasal fistula [59]

4.6.4 Contraindications

- Absolute
  - Cleft palate, submucous cleft
  - Velopharyngeal insufficiency
  - Unreasonable patient expectations
- Relative
  - Craniofacial anomalies
  - Large torus palatini (requires removal prior or during TPA)

- Maxillomandibular advancement surgery is a consideration (compromise/alteration vascular supply)
- Prior radiation, heavy smoker, T2DM, osteoporosis (risk of poor wound healing)
- Prior "resective" palate surgery (increased risk of VPI and swallowing dysfunction)

4.6.5 Surgical Technique

1. *Patient Positioning and Exposure*
    - The surgery is performed under general anesthesia with the airway established via a nasal tracheal tube.
    - The patient is placed in the Rose position with a shoulder roll.
    - Perioperative antibiotics, dexamethasone 8 mg, and tranexamic acid 1 g.
    - Oropharyngeal exposure with Boyle–Davis gag or Dingman mouth retractor.
    - Modified-UPPP and tongue procedures are performed at this stage (if multilevel airway surgery is planned).
2. *Mucosal Incisions*
    - Infiltration with lignocaine 2% with adrenaline 1:80,000 to the hard palate mucoperiosteum at the planned incision sites and greater palate foramen to assist with hemostasis and hydro-dissection.
    - Mark the greater palatine foramen bilaterally to identify path of the greater palatine neurovascular bundle.
    - Irrespective of incision type, care must be taken when marking incision to remain medial to the greater palatine neurovascular bundle to improve perfusion of the mucosal flap and reduce risk of postoperative wound dehiscence and breakdown.
    - Mucoperiosteal incisions are made with a needle tip diathermy down to bone.
    - Mucosal incision variations
        - "Gothic arch" is employed for a broad and wide palate.
        - "Propeller" is employed for a narrow palate.
    - Gothic arch incision (Fig. 4.27a)
        - Apex of the arch is 2–3 cm from the alveolus (ease of mucosal closure).
        - Posterolateral limbs are medial to the greater palatine foramen, then flare out laterally toward pterygoid hamulus.
    - Propellor incision (Fig. 4.27b)
        - Centered at level of greater palatine foramen, approximately 5 mm anterior to the hard and soft palate junction. Approximately 120° between limbs.

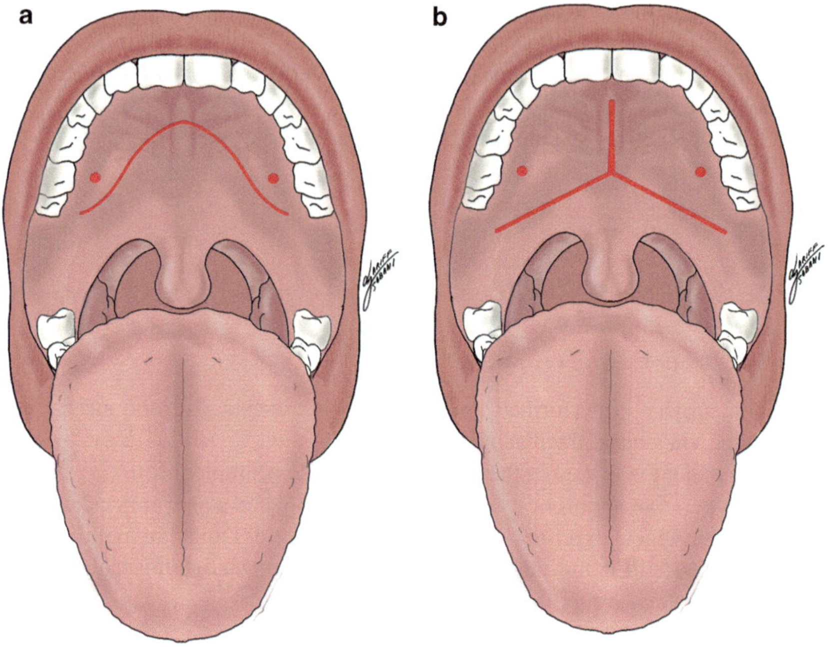

Fig. 4.27 Palatal incisions. The greater palatine foramina are marked with red dots. (**a**) "Gothic arch" incision with anterior limit 20 mm from alveolus. (**b**) "Propeller" incision with trifurcation 5 mm anterior to hard and soft palate junction

  - Extend anterior limb to 2–3 cm from alveolus.
  - Posterolateral limbs are medial to the greater palatine foramen extending to the pterygoid hamulus.

3. *Flap Elevation and Tendonolysis*

   - The mucoperiosteal flap is elevated carefully exposing hard palate and proximal soft palate aponeurosis.
   - The flap is elevated posteriorly and superficial to the soft palate aponeurosis until the "silvery" color of the tensor veli palatini (TVP) tendon is identified.
   - For the "propeller" incision, stay sutures are placed through the apex of the triangular flaps as retraction to improve surgical access (Fig. 4.28a).
   - The TVP tendon is divided laterally with a needle point diathermy or blade to identify the intact levator veli palatini muscle beneath.
   - This maneuver allows for improved mobility of the central soft palate.

4. *Osteotomy*

   - Perform box osteotomy approximately 7–10 mm (AP) × 20 mm (lateral) in size with the posterior segment *attached* to the soft palate aponeurosis (Fig. 4.29a).
     - This is ideally performed with a Piezosurgery® device with the microsaw attachment for improved mucosal preservation on the nasal surface.

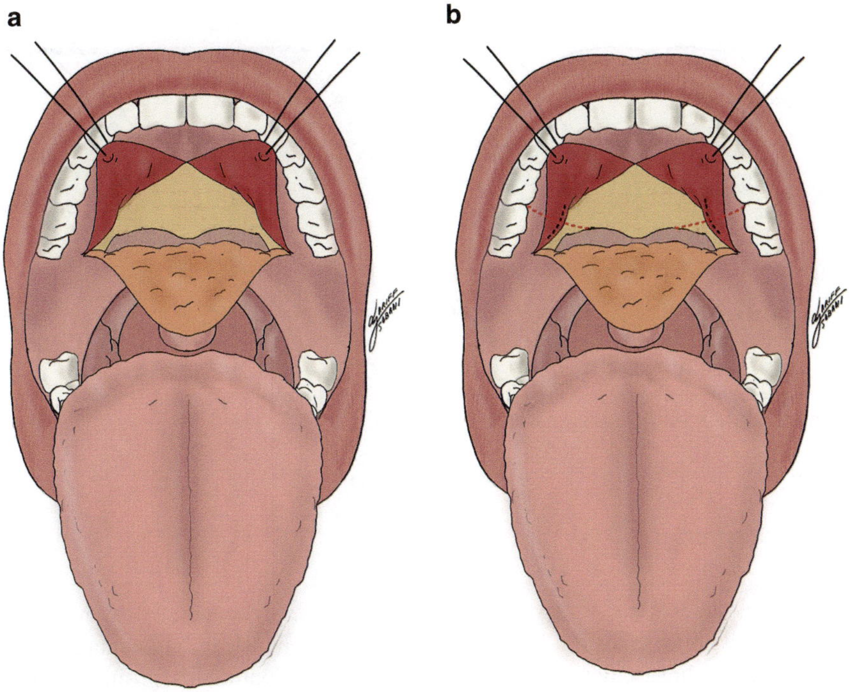

Fig. 4.28 Flap elevation and tendonolysis. (**a**) Mucoperiosteal flaps are elevated to expose the underlying hard palate and soft palate aponeurosis and retracted with stay sutures. (**b**) Tensor veli palatini (red line) tendon is exposed and divided as demonstrated by the black lines

  - Alternatively, an otology drill with a 1.5 mm diamond bur can be used.
- Once the bony island is freed anteriorly and laterally, the island is elevated, and mayo scissors are used to divide the vomer attachment.
  - Care is taken to not tear the soft palate mucosa and aponeurotic attachment when instrumenting the bony island.
  - Bleeding is typically from the nasal mucosa, which can be controlled with bipolar cautery.
- Kerrison rongeur 2–3 mm is used to remove 8–15 mm of the hard palate anterior to the bony island.
- The edges of the hard palate anterior to the bony island can be smoothed with the Piezosurgery® device with the osteoplasty circular scalpel smoother or previously mentioned drill.
  - This improves apposition between the bony island and the anterior hard palate.
- Nasal mucosa over the hard palate anteriorly is elevated with curved Obwegeser periosteal elevator.
  - This step reduces risk of entering the nasal cavity mucosa during the hole drilling stage.

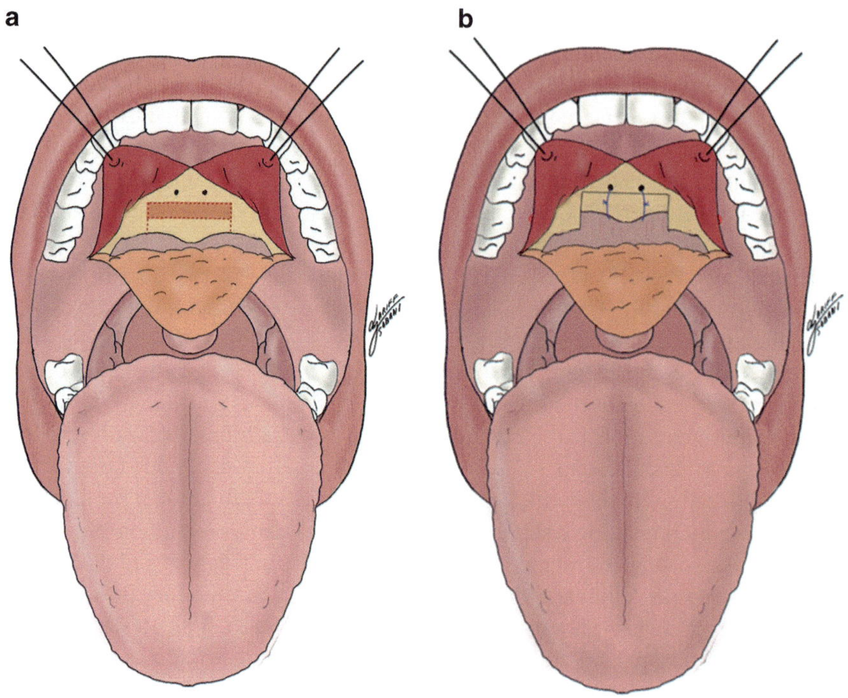

Fig. 4.29 Osteotomy and advancement. (**a**) The box osteotomy is performed ensuring posterior attachment to the soft palate aponeurosis is maintained. 5–15 mm of bone is removed anterior to the bony island (red box). Drill holes are placed through the hard palate anterior to section of removed hard palate. (**b**) Sutures are placed on the medial and lateral aspects of the soft palate aponeurosis to assist in robust anterior advancement

- Two holes are drilled through the hard palate 10 mm anterior to the proposed point of attachment of the bony island, with either the Piezosurgery® device with the micro-perforation sharp cylinder insert or the 1.5 mm diamond otology drill.
  - Ensure adequate bone stock between holes and free edge to prevent fracture during advancement.

5. *Advancement*

- A 0 Vicryl on a 5/8th circle tapered needle is used for advancement, as the curvature of the needle is required for improved mobility.
- The suture is passed in reverse through the drill hole, then regrasped where the sharp end is passed medially through the soft tissue aponeurosis around bony island and clipped (Fig. 4.29b).
- A second suture is passed through the same drill hole, with the same technique as before, and passed laterally through the flaps of aponeurotic soft tissues and clipped.
  - Ensure the sutures remain submucosal, taking care not to breach the mucosa of the flaps.

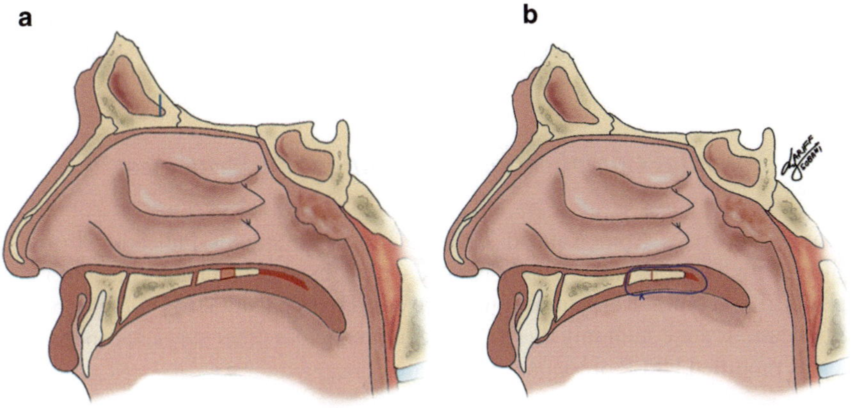

Fig. 4.30 Palatal advancement. (**a**) Sagittal view section of bone removed (red box) anterior to bony island. (**b**) Sagittal view depicting the anterior advancement of the soft palate with the corresponding bony island. The soft palate reconfigured from a vertical into a more favourable oblique orientation

- The same is performed on the contralateral size.
- The medial bony island sutures are tied and secured sequentially ensuring adequate bony apposition (Fig. 4.30).
- The lateral aponeurotic soft tissue sutures are tied to further advance the soft palate.
- Bone patte or bone graft collected from the drilling or Kerrison punch may be applied to osteotomy and drill holes to improve bony healing.

6. *Closure*

- The palatal incisions are closed with 2–0 undyed Vicryl on a 5/8th tapered needle.
- Gothic arch incisions should be closed in a posterior to anterior direction.
- Propeller incisions are closed in a lateral to medial direction with the apex closed last.
- Excess mucosa and fat can be trimmed after complete closure to prevent a palpable thickening.
- This must be performed after closure to prevent excessive mucosal removal resulting in exposed palatal bone, leading to breakdown or fistula formation.
- The patient is extubated sitting at >30° at the completion of the surgery.

4.6.6 Postoperative Management

- Patients should be monitored in a high dependency unit with continuous oximetry and positioned with their head elevated to >30°.
- Initiate oral intake once awake and encourage swallowing.
- Intravenous steroids for 48 h postoperatively.

- Regular analgesia with a combination of opioid and non-opioid analgesics (selective COX2 inhibitor nonsteroidal anti-inflammatory drugs, acetaminophen).

4.6.7 Potential Complications and Mitigation Strategies

Complication rates from isolated TPA are low, with studies indicating the vast majority are transient and typically resolve with conservative management [55, 59, 61]. The most common complication reported is oronasal fistula [61]. Other reported complications are commonly due to TPA combined with other surgical procedures, such as modified UPPP or tongue surgeries.

1. Oronasal Fistula

   - Oronasal fistulae formation occurs between 2% and 16% of patients within 4 weeks following surgery [55, 58, 59].
   - Invariably preceded by wound dehiscence or breakdown, presenting as nasal regurgitation of food or liquids or hypernasal speech.
   - Majority of oronasal fistulae close with conservative management with the use of a dental obturator plate or re-suture under local anaesthethsia [55, 59].

   Mitigation:

   - Avoid disruption of greater palatine vessels
   - Careful elevation of palate mucoperiosteum
   - Postoperative antibiotics to reduce bony island infection
   - No dentures until wounds heal
   - "Propeller" incision for high arched palates

2. Hemorrhage

   - Postoperative bleeding is uncommon from isolated TPA [55, 61, 62].
   - Hemorrhage is more commonly from the other components of multilevel airway surgery, such as tonsillectomy and modified UPPP, which can occur within 14 days following surgery.

   Mitigation:

   - Careful intraoperative hemostasis
   - Return patient to a normotensive state at the end of the case to ensure no active bleeding
   - Encourage early oral intake with regular hydration
   - Avoid non-selective COX nonsteroidal anti-inflammatory drugs and anticoagulants pre- and post-operatively
   - Smoking cessation prior to surgery [63]

3. Dysphagia, Globus Pharyngeus, Velopharyngeal Insufficiency

   - Swallowing difficulties was commonly seen in the early postoperative period secondary to pain and repositioning of soft tissue musculature [57].

- Permanent VPI is very rare.
- The pain and dysphagia are typically secondary to the tonsillectomy, pharyngeal, and tongue surgeries more so than the TPA component.

  Mitigation:

- Soft tissue edema can be managed with 1–2 doses of steroids
- Majority of VPI is transient and resolves with time
- Speech therapy and swallowing exercises are encouraged when incision sites have healed

4. Pain and Neuropathic Sequelae

   - Pain and odynophagia are expected postoperatively.
   - The pain is typically from the tonsillectomy or pharyngeal or tongue surgeries, and not the osteotomies of TPA.

     Mitigation:

   - Encouraging early oral intake postoperatively
   - Regular multimodal analgesia
   - Avoid disruption of greater palatine neurovascular bundle

5. Recurrent or Residual OSA

   - TPA is effective in enlarging the retropalatal space; however, it has unpredictable outcomes in complete concentric collapse or isolated lateral wall collapse.
   - Unsatisfactory outcomes can be secondary to unidentified multilevel disease.
   - Patient selection is vital with assessment of all components of the upper airway, including retropalatal, oropharyngeal, and retrolingual segments.

     Mitigation:

   - Judicious patient selection with optimal anatomical phenotype
   - Combine TPA with multilevel airway surgery to address pathologic segments of the airway
   - Weight loss and maintenance postoperatively

4.6.8 Surgical Outcomes

Isolated TPA was found to reduce Apnea–Hypopnea Index (AHI) with improvements in lowest oxygen saturation (LSAT) indices [61]. These results may correlate with increased retropalatal space, particularly in the AP plane [54]. Woodson and Robinson compared TPA with UPPP and found increased improvement of AHI in the TPA group. They concluded that TPA may have increased benefit to UPPP alone in patient with Friedman stage 3 [57]. More often, TPA is performed as a component of multilevel airway surgery; studies have indicated improvements across AHI, LSAT indices, and Epworth Sleepiness and Snoring Severity scales [59, 64]. Multilevel airway surgery demonstrated comparable mean disease alleviation when compared with PAP therapy [65].

4.6.9 Conclusion

Transpalatal advancement (TPA) pharyngoplasty is an effective surgical technique when used in conjunction with multilevel airway surgery in the management of moderate to severe OSA. By advancing and anchoring the soft palate to the robust hard palate bone, the retropalatal space enlarges and palate stiffens. This in turn increases upper airway caliber and reduces collapsibility, improving OSA.

References

1. Ikematsu A, Yaku Y, Niho M. The Ikematsu system for the diagnosis of snoring: a review of 39 years of clinical studies. In: Sleep apnea and rhonchopathy: 3rd world congress. Tokyo: S. Karger AG; 1991.
2. Fujita S, Conway W, Zorick F, Roth T. Surgical correction of anatomic abnormalities in obstructive sleep apnea syndrome: Uvulopalatopharyngoplasty. Otolaryngol Head Neck Surg [Internet]. 1981 [cited 2025 Oct 12];89(6):923–34. Available from: https://doi.org/10.1177/019459988108900609
3. Powell N, Riley R, Guilleminault C, Troell R. A reversible uvulopalatal flap for snoring and sleep apnea syndrome. Sleep. 1996;19(7):593–9.
4. Fairbanks DNF. Operative techniques of uvulopalatopharyngoplasty. Ear Nose Throat J. 1999;78(11)
5. Cahali MB. Lateral pharyngoplasty: a new treatment for obstructive sleep apnea hypopnea syndrome. Laryngoscope. 2003;113(11)
6. Friedman M, Ibrahim HZ, Vidyasagar R, Pomeranz J, Joseph NJ. Z-palatoplasty (ZPP): a technique for patients without tonsils. Otolaryngol Head Neck Surg. 2004;131(1)
7. Han D, Ye J, Lin Z, Wang J, Wang J, Zhang Y. Revised uvulopalatopharyngoplasty with uvula preservation and its clinical study. ORL. 2005;67(4)
8. Pang KP, Woodson BT. Expansion sphincter pharyngoplasty: a new technique for the treatment of obstructive sleep apnea. Otolaryngol Head Neck Surg. 2007;137(1)
9. Li HY, Lee LA. Relocation pharyngoplasty for obstructive sleep apnea. Laryngoscope. 2009;119(12)
10. Li HY, Tsai MS, Lee LA, Hsin LJ, Lee YC, Lin WN, et al. Palatal hybrid surgery for obstructive sleep apnea-state-of-the-art annotation of uvulopalatopharyngoplasty. Biomed J. 2023;46(3)
11. Mantovani M, Minetti A, Torretta S, Pincherle A, Tassone G, Pignataro L. The velo-uvulo-pharyngeal lift or "roman blinds" technique for treatment of snoring: a preliminary report. Acta Otorhinolaryngol Ital. 2012;32(1)
12. Mantovani M, Minetti A, Torretta S, Pincherle A, Tassone G, Pignataro L. The "Barbed Roman Blinds" technique: a step forward. Acta Otorhinolaryngol Ital. 2013 Apr;33(2):128.
13. Vicini C, Faedi F, Iannella G. Barbed reposition pharyngoplasty (BRP). In: Barbed pharyngoplasty and sleep disordered breathing. Cham: Springer; 2022.

14. MacKay SG, Carney AS, Woods C, Antic N, McEvoy RD, Chia M, et al. Modified uvulopalatopharyngoplasty and coblation channeling of the tongue for obstructive sleep apnea: a multicentre Australian trial. J Clin Sleep Med. 2013;9(2)
15. Friedman M, Salapatas AM, Bonzelaar LB. Updated Friedman staging system for obstructive sleep apnea. Adv Otorhinolaryngol. 2017;80:41–8.
16. Sundman J, Nerfeldt P, Fehrm J, Bring J, Browaldh N, Friberg D. Effectiveness of tonsillectomy vs modified Uvulopalatopharyngoplasty in patients with tonsillar hypertrophy and obstructive sleep apnea: the TEAMUP randomized clinical trial. JAMA Otolaryngol Head Neck Surg. 2022;148(12)
17. Chiu FH, Chen CY, Lee JC, Hsu YS. Effect of modified uvulopalatopharyngoplasty without tonsillectomy on obstructive sleep apnea: polysomnographic outcome and correlation with drug-induced sleep endoscopy. Nat Sci Sleep. 2021;13:11.
18. Vutukuri R, Kitagawa N, Fukino K, Tubbs RS, Iwanaga J. The pterygomandibular raphe: a comprehensive review. Anat Cell Biol. 2024;57(1)
19. Powell NB, Riley RW, Troell RJ, Li K, Blumen MB, Guilleminault C. Radiofrequency volumetric tissue reduction of the palate in subjects with sleep-disordered breathing. Chest. 1998;113(5):1163–74.
20. Stuck BA, Sauter A, Hörmann K, Verse T, Maurer JT. Radiofrequency surgery of the soft palate in the treatment of snoring. A placebo-controlled trial. Sleep. 2005;28(7):847–50. https://doi.org/10.1093/sleep/28.7.847.
21. Randerath WJ, Verbraecken J, Andreas S, et al. Non-CPAP therapies in obstructive sleep apnoea. Eur Respir J. 2011;37(5):1000–28.
22. Bäck LJ, Liukko T, Rantanen I, Peltola JS, Partinen M, Ylikoski J, Mäkitie AA. Radiofrequency surgery of the soft palate in the treatment of mild obstructive sleep apnea is not effective as a single-stage procedure: a randomized single-blinded placebo-controlled trial. Laryngoscope. 2009;119(8):1621–7.
23. Hofmann T, Schwantzer G, Reckenzaun E, Koch H, Wolf G. Radiofrequency tissue volume reduction of the soft palate and UPPP in the treatment of snoring. Eur Arch Otorhinolaryngol. 2006;263(2):164–70.
24. Gillespie MB, Eisele DW. The uvulopalatal flap for reconstruction of the soft palate. Laryngoscope. 2000;110(4):612–5.
25. Neruntarat C. Uvulopalatal flap for obstructive sleep apnea: short-term and long-term results. Laryngoscope. 2011;121(3):683–7.
26. Haytoğlu S, Arıkan OK, Muluk NB, Tuhanioğlu B, Çörtük M. Comparison of anterior palatoplasty and uvulopalatal flap placement for treating mild and moderate obstructive sleep apnea. Ear Nose Throat J. 2018;97(3):E12–8.
27. Boot H, van Wegen R, Poublon RML, Bogaard JM, Schmitz PI. Long-term results of uvulopalatopharyngoplasty for obstructive sleep apnea syndrome. Laryngoscope. 2000;110(3):469–75.
28. Sher AE, Schechtman KB, Piccirillo JF. The efficacy of surgical modifications of the upper airway in adults with obstructive sleep apnea syndrome. Sleep. 1996;19(2):156–77.
29. Friedman M, Schalch P, Lin HC, Kakodkar KA, Joseph NJ, Mazloom N. Palatal implants for the treatment of snoring and obstructive sleep apnea/hypopnea syndrome. Otolaryngol Head Neck Surg. 2008;138(2):209–16.
30. Young T, Peppard PE, Gottlieb DJ. Epidemiology of obstructive sleep apnea: a population health perspective. Am J Respir Crit Care Med. 2002;165(9):1217–39.
31. Punjabi NM. The epidemiology of adult obstructive sleep apnea. Proc Am Thorac Soc. 2008;5(2):136–43.
32. Marin JM, Carrizo SJ, Vicente E, Agustí AG. Long-term cardiovascular outcomes in men with obstructive sleep apnoea-hypopnoea with or without treatment with CPAP: an observational study. Lancet. 2005;365(9464):1046–53.
33. Weaver TE, Grunstein RR. Adherence to continuous positive airway pressure therapy: the challenge to effective treatment. Proc Am Thorac Soc. 2008;5(2):173–8.

34. Rotenberg BW, Murariu D, Pang KP. Trends in CPAP adherence over twenty years of data collection: a flattened curve. J Otolaryngol Head Neck Surg. 2016;45(1):43.
35. Kezirian EJ, Hohenhorst W, de Vries N. Drug-induced sleep endoscopy: the VOTE classification. Eur Arch Otorhinolaryngol. 2011;268(8):1233–6.
36. Vanderveken OM, Maurer JT, Hohenhorst W, et al. Evaluation of drug-induced sleep endoscopy as a patient selection tool for implanted upper airway stimulation for obstructive sleep apnea. J Clin Sleep Med. 2013;9(5):433–8.
37. Li HY, Cheng WN, Chuang LP, et al. Positional dependency and surgical success of relocation pharyngoplasty among patients with severe obstructive sleep apnea. Otolaryngol Head Neck Surg. 2013;149(3):506–12.
38. Oh H, Kim HG, Pyo S, et al. The clinical efficacy of relocation pharyngoplasty to improve retropalatal circumferential narrowing in obstructive sleep apnea patients. Sci Rep. 2020;10(1):2101. PMID: 32034229.
39. Koutsourelakis I, Safiruddin F, Ravesloot MJ, de Vries N. Surgery for obstructive sleep apnea: sleep endoscopy determinants of outcome. Laryngoscope. 2012;122(12):2587–91.
40. Green KK, Kent DT, D'Agostino MA, et al. Drug-induced sleep endoscopy and surgical outcomes: a multicenter cohort study. Laryngoscope. 2019;129(3):761–70.
41. Gottlieb DJ, Punjabi NM. Diagnosis and management of obstructive sleep apnea: a review. JAMAs. 2020;323(14):1389–400.
42. Pang KP, Pang EB, Win MTM, Terris DJ. Expansion sphincter pharyngoplasty for the treatment of OSA: a systematic review and meta-analysis. Eur Arch Otorhinolaryngol. 2016;273(9):2329–33. PMID: 26541714.
43. Vicini C, Hendawy E, Campanini A, et al. Barbed reposition pharyngoplasty (BRP) for OSAHS: a feasibility, safety, efficacy and teachability pilot study. Eur Arch Otorhinolaryngol. 2015;272(10):3065–70.
44. Barbieri M, Murru FM, Pascu M, et al. Barbed suspension pharyngoplasty for treatment of lateral pharyngeal wall collapse in OSA. Eur Arch Otorhinolaryngol. 2019;276(9):2627–32.
45. Iannella G, Vallicelli B, Magliulo G, et al. Long-term subjective outcomes of barbed reposition pharyngoplasty for obstructive sleep apnea syndrome treatment. Int J Environ Res Public Health. 2020;17(5):1542.
46. Saenwandee P, Neruntarat C, Saengthong P, et al. Barbed pharyngoplasty for obstructive sleep apnea: a meta-analysis. Am J Otolaryngol. 2022;43(2):103306.
47. Salamanca F, Costantini F, Mantovani M, et al. Barbed anterior pharyngoplasty: an evolution of anterior palatoplasty. Acta Otorhinolaryngol Ital. 2014;34(6):434–8.
48. Moffa A, Iannella G, Ralli M, et al. Different barbed pharyngoplasty techniques for retropalatal collapse: a systematic review. Sleep Breath. 2020;24(3):1115–27.
49. Vicini C, Cammaroto G, Stilli A, et al. Effectiveness of barbed repositioning pharyngoplasty for OSA: randomized clinical trial protocol and preliminary data. Eur Arch Otorhinolaryngol. 2020;277(9):2619–26.
50. Leone F, Raggi A, Novara C, et al. Barbed pharyngoplasty for OSA: the surgical learning curve. Sleep Breath. 2022;26(4):1869–74.
51. Emara TA, Eliwa AR, Aldesouky OM, et al. Anterolateral advancement pharyngoplasty versus barbed repositioning pharyngoplasty for obstructive sleep apnea with lateral wall collapse: a comparative study. Int Arch Otorhinolaryngol. 2024;28:e489–98.
52. MacKay SG, Lewis R, McEvoy D, Joosten S, Holt NR. Surgical management of obstructive sleep apnoea: a position statement of the Australasian Sleep Association*. Respirology. 2020;25(12):1292–308. https://doi.org/10.1111/resp.13967.
53. MacKay SG, Chan L. Surgical approaches to obstructive sleep apnea. Sleep Med Clin. 2016;11(3):331–41. https://doi.org/10.1016/j.jsmc.2016.04.003.
54. Woodson BT, Toohill RJ. Transpalatal advancement pharyngoplasty for obstructive sleep apnea. Laryngoscope. 1993;103(3):269–76. https://doi.org/10.1288/00005537-199303000-00006.
55. Woodson BT. Transpalatal advancement pharyngoplasty. Oper Tech Otolaryngol Head Neck Surg. 2007;18(1):11–6. https://doi.org/10.1016/j.otot.2007.02.001.

56. Woodson BT. Changes in airway characteristics after transpalatal advancement pharyngoplasty compared to uvulopalatopharyngoplasty (UPPP). Sleep. 1996;19(suppl_10):S291–3. https://doi.org/10.1093/sleep/19.suppl_10.S291.
57. Woodson BT, Robinson S, Lim HJ. Transpalatal advancement pharyngoplasty outcomes compared with uvulopalatopharygoplasty. Otolaryngol Head Neck Surg. 2005;133(2):211–7. https://doi.org/10.1016/j.otohns.2005.03.061.
58. Shine NP, Lewis RH. The "Propeller" incision for transpalatal advancement pharyngoplasty: a new approach to reduce post-operative oronasal fistulae. Auris Nasus Larynx. 2008;35(3):397–400. https://doi.org/10.1016/j.anl.2007.09.001.
59. Chan L, Kitpornchai L, Mackay S. Causative factors for complications in transpalatal advancement. Ann Otol Rhinol Laryngol. 2020;129(1):18–22. https://doi.org/10.1177/0003489419867969.
60. Woodson BT. A method to describe the pharyngeal airway. Laryngoscope. 2015;125(5):1233–8. https://doi.org/10.1002/lary.24972.
61. Volner K, Dunn B, Chang ET, et al. Transpalatal advancement pharyngoplasty for obstructive sleep apnea: a systematic review and meta-analysis. Eur Arch Otorhinolaryngol. 2017;274(3):1197–203. https://doi.org/10.1007/s00405-016-4121-3.
62. Shine NP, Lewis RH. Transpalatal advancement pharyngoplasty for obstructive sleep apnea syndrome: results and analysis of failures. Arch Otolaryngol Head Neck Surg. 2009;135(5):434–8. https://doi.org/10.1001/archoto.2009.45.
63. Demars SM, Harsha WJ, Crawford JV. The effects of smoking on the rate of postoperative hemorrhage after tonsillectomy and uvulopalatopharyngoplasty. Arch Otolaryngol Head Neck Surg. 2008;134(8):811. https://doi.org/10.1001/archotol.134.8.811.
64. Stewart S, Huang J, Mohorikar A, Jones A, Holmes S, MacKay SG. AHI outcomes are superior after upper airway reconstructive surgery in adult CPAP failure patients. Otolaryngol Head Neck Surg. 2016;154(3):553–7. https://doi.org/10.1177/0194599815621729.
65. Every JD, Mackay SG, Sideris AW, Do TQ, Jones A, Weaver EM. Mean disease alleviation between surgery and continuous positive airway pressure in matched adults with obstructive sleep apnea. Sleep. 2023;46(9):zsad176. https://doi.org/10.1093/sleep/zsad176.

Chapter 5
Tongue Base and Hypopharyngeal Surgery for Obstructive Sleep Apnea

Liang Chye Goh, Song Tar Toh, Srinivas Kishore, Moideen Sanu, Ahmad Kusyairi Khalid, Mohd Zulkiflee Abu Bakar, and Claudio Vicini

5.1 Coblation Channeling Ablation of the Tongue

Liang Chye Goh and Song Tar Toh

5.1.1 Introduction

Coblation channeling ablation of the tongue is a minimally invasive surgical technique designed to reduce tongue volume and improve retrolingual airway patency in patients with *obstructive sleep apnea (OSA)*. By creating linear thermal ablation

L. C. Goh (✉) · M. Z. Abu Bakar
Department of Otorhinolaryngology, Faculty of Medicine, Universiti Malaya, Kuala Lumpur, Malaysia
e-mail: juliusglc@um.edu.my; abzulkiflee@um.edu.my

S. T. Toh
Department of Otorhinolaryngology-Head & Neck Surgery, Singapore General Hospital, Singapore, Singapore
e-mail: toh.song.tar@singhealth.com.sg

S. Kishore
AIG Hospitals, Gachibowli, Hyderabad, India

M. Sanu
Centre for Advanced Care in ENT, Head and Neck Oncology, Muvattupuzha, India

A. K. Khalid
KPJ Healthcare University, Nilai, Negeri Sembilan, Malaysia
e-mail: ahmad.kusyairi@kpju.edu.my

C. Vicini
Department of Head-Neck Surgery, Otolaryngology, Head-Neck and Oral Surgery Unit, Morgagni Pierantoni Hospital, Azienda USL Della Romagna, Forlì, Italy
e-mail: claudio@claudiovicini.com

L. C. Goh, S. T. Toh (eds.), *Sleep Surgery in a Nutshell*,
https://doi.org/10.1007/978-981-95-9749-9_5

channels within the intrinsic musculature of the tongue—primarily targeting the tongue base—the procedure stiffens and scars the tissue, limiting its collapse during sleep [1–3].

This technique is particularly useful in *multilevel sleep surgery* protocols, especially in patients with significant *tongue-base collapse* identified on drug-induced sleep endoscopy (DISE) [3]. Coblation or radiofrequency energy delivers controlled tissue ablation with minimal collateral damage, preserving critical surrounding structures.

Coblation channeling of the tongue (CCT)—also termed coblation tongue-base reduction or coblation endoscopic lingual lightening—treats *retrolingual collapse* by creating submucosal ablation tracts (channels) inside the tongue base, thereby *reducing tissue bulk* and *stiffening the lamina* with minimal surface trauma. The plasma-mediated ablation operates at lower temperatures than electrocautery, aiming to limit collateral thermal injury while allowing controlled volumetric reduction.

Patients most likely to benefit exhibit *drug-induced sleep endoscopy (DISE)-confirmed tongue-base collapse* (VOTE "T" level), often with small tonsils and Friedman tongue position III, where palatal surgery alone underperforms. In meta-analytic syntheses, coblation-based tongue procedures show *clinically meaningful improvement* in Apnea–Hypopnea Index (AHI), sleepiness, and oxygenation, with *success rates* that compare favorably to radiofrequency ablation (RFA) of the tongue base [1, 3–6].

5.1.2 Principles [6]

- The goal is to *reduce the volume and collapsibility of the tongue base* via multiple, strategically placed submucosal ablation channels.
- This is achieved using *thermal tissue coagulation* with *coblation* (low-temperature radiofrequency energy in a saline medium) or *bipolar RF technology*.
- Over time, healing and fibrosis result in *stiffening of the tongue tissue*, reducing dynamic collapse during sleep.

5.1.3 Procedure Steps

5.1.3.1 Anesthesia and Preparation

- General anesthesia with oral endotracheal intubation is employed. The endotracheal tube is pushed to the contralateral retromolar trigon.
- The patient is positioned supine with standard draping.
- Perioperative medications:
  - Antibiotics and Analgesics
  - Steroid (e.g., Dexamethasone 8 mg IV at induction)
- Head is placed extended using a shoulder roll.

5.1.3.2 Intraoral Exposure

- A Doyen retractor or appropriate mouth gag is positioned to expose the oral cavity.
- A silk 1-0 anchoring stitch is placed through the anterior dorsum of the tongue to provide gentle outward traction during the procedure (Fig. 5.1a) or a wet gauze then a Duval artery forceps.

5.1.3.3 Marking Channeling Points (Fig. 5.1)

Using a surgical marker pen, ablation points are marked:

- The *posterior-most point* is located at or just anterior to the *foramen caecum* at the midline dorsum.
- *Subsequent points* are marked *1 cm anterior* to each previous point (Fig. 5.1b).
- The *number of points* depends on tongue size and exposure. The *posterior limit* is determined by the surgeon's ability to visualize and insert the wand safely.
- The *anterior limit* should not exceed the area corresponding to the *base of the frenulum*, in order to avoid through-and-through lesions.
- Pull the tongue gently to the side. Do not retract it forcefully as this may distort the location of lingual arteries, making them more prone to injury).

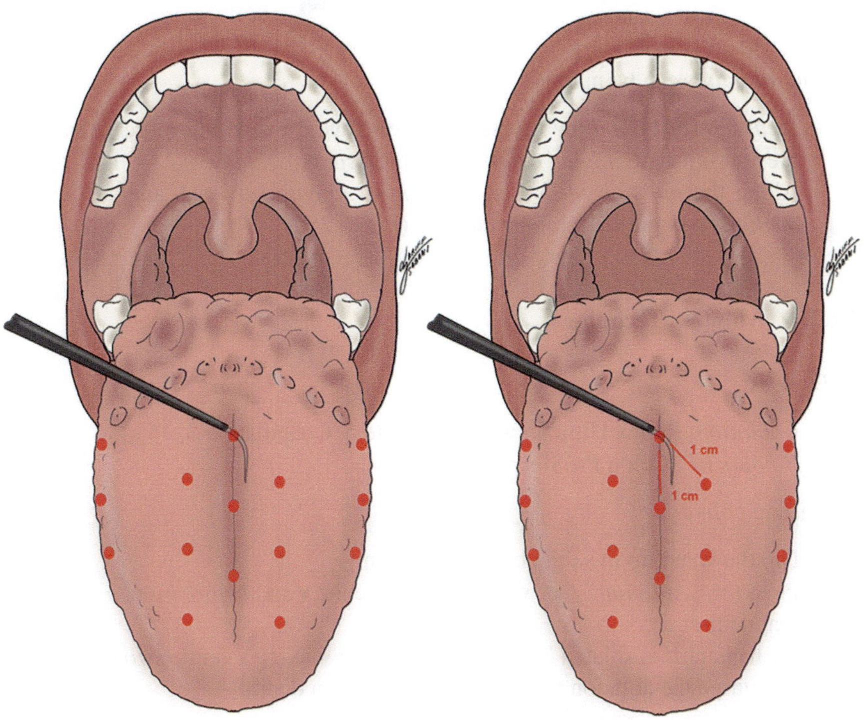

Fig. 5.1 Area of coblation is marked and coblated 1 cm apart as seen above

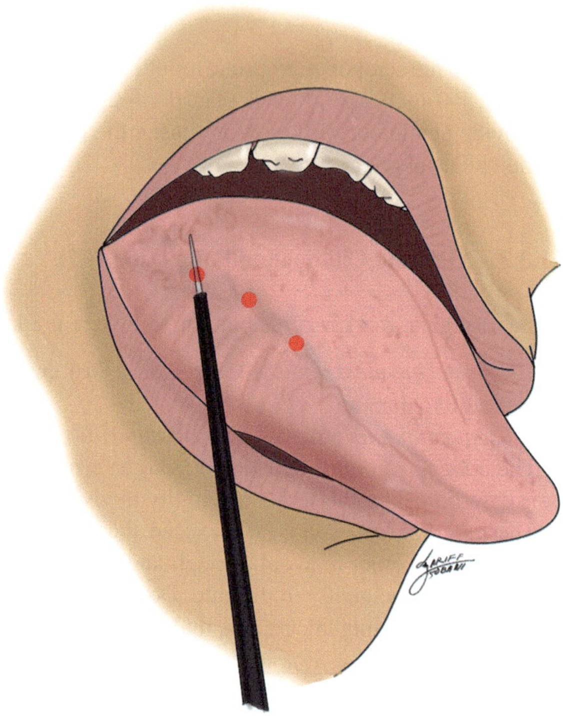

Fig. 5.2 Coblation made at the lateral surface of the tongue at the squamo-mucosal junction

- *Lateral points* can be marked
  - *1 cm lateral to midline* (dorsal surface)—avoid extending more laterally to prevent injury to *lingual arteries* and the *hypoglossal nerve*.
  - Along the *junction of dorsal and ventral tongue surfaces*, angled *postero-medially* toward the foramen caecum (Fig. 5.2).

5.1.3.4 Ablation Technique

- *Devices*:
  - *Coblation*: Reflex Ultra 55 wand (Coblate 5, Coagulation 3, 15 s)
  - *Bipolar RF*: Celon ProSleep Plus (6–8 W)
- If using *coblation*:
  - Dip the wand tip in saline before insertion.
  - Press the *"Ablation" foot switch* to activate the wand *before insertion* into the tongue tissue.
  - Each channel is ablated for approximately *15 s*, using a gentle *swirling motion* to enlarge the ablation path and ensure uniform depth.
- Avoid excessive force to prevent mechanical trauma. Ensure that the *metallic active tip* is fully embedded in the tongue muscle before ablation.

5.1.3.5 Hemostasis

- As the wand is being withdrawn, the *"Coagulation" setting* may be activated briefly to seal the mucosal entry point and limit bleeding.
- Any remaining bleeding is controlled with *gentle pressure* using *moist gauze*.
- The *retraction stitch* and *mouth gag* are removed at the conclusion of the procedure.

5.1.3.6 Postoperative Care

- *High-dependency observation* for airway monitoring should be considered in patients with moderate to severe OSA. Consider a nasopharyngeal airway sized 4.0–5.5 mm ID while monitoring.
- *Antibiotics*: Continue oral antibiotics or equivalent for *7 days*.
- *Steroids*: IV Dexamethasone 4 mg *twice daily for 3 doses* to reduce edema.
- *Analgesia*: Paracetamol or NSAIDs for *5–7 days*, with escalation if required.
- *Throat gargles* or *lozenges* may be prescribed based on surgeon preference.
- *Diet*: Soft diet for the first few days. Patients should be advised to maintain good oral hygiene.
- *Follow-up*: Review at *1 week* to assess for signs of infection, wound healing, and airway adequacy. Follow-up visits should assess for persistent dysphagia, taste disturbance, or residual tongue-base obstruction. Rare complications such as fibrosis or altered speech mechanics should be identified early.
- *Functional outcomes:* Symptom improvement in snoring, daytime sleepiness, and airway patency should be reassessed after 6–8 weeks, often supplemented by repeat sleep testing in selected cases.
- *Adjunctive care:* In patients with multilevel obstruction, coblation may be part of a staged or combined surgical plan.

5.1.4 Clinical Considerations

- Patients typically report *mild discomfort*, with significant improvement in symptoms over 1 week.
- *Minimal intraoral scarring* and preservation of tongue function are expected when ablation is done properly.
- This procedure is particularly effective when combined with *palatal or lateral wall surgery* as part of a *multilevel OSA management strategy*.

5.1.5 Complications

5.1.5.1 Early Complications

- *Pain and dysphagia:* Mild to moderate throat pain and discomfort during swallowing are common in the first postoperative week but usually resolve with conservative management.
- *Edema and airway compromise:* Localized swelling at the tongue base may transiently narrow the airway. Patients with severe OSA or comorbidities should be monitored closely in the immediate postoperative period.
- *Bleeding:* Intraoperative bleeding is rare due to the coagulative effect of coblation. Delayed hemorrhage is uncommon but can be serious if a lingual vessel is involved.
- *Ulceration or mucosal injury:* Surface burns or ulcerations may occur if energy delivery extends beyond the submucosal layer, potentially leading to pain and delayed healing.
- *Infection:* Although rare, submucosal infection or abscess formation can occur and should be treated promptly with antibiotics and drainage if needed.

5.1.5.2 Late Complications (Table 5.1)

- *Fibrosis and scar formation:* Excessive scarring may alter tongue-base mobility, though the controlled nature of coblation usually minimizes this risk.
- *Persistent dysphagia or dysarthria:* Rare but possible, particularly if fibrotic changes involve deeper tongue musculature.
- *Altered sensation:* Numbness, paresthesia, or taste disturbance may result from inadvertent injury to lingual nerve branches, although this is uncommon.
- *Insufficient response or residual obstruction:* Some patients may experience limited improvement, especially if collapse is multilevel. Repeat procedures or adjunctive surgeries may be required.
- *Airway stiffness:* In rare cases, excessive stiffening may alter normal tongue dynamics and impact swallowing or speech.

Table 5.1 Comparison of coblation vs. bipolar RF in tongue channeling ablation

Parameter	Coblation (e.g., Reflex Ultra 55)	Bipolar RF (e.g., Celon ProSleep Plus)
Energy delivery	Radiofrequency energy in saline medium (plasma field formation)	Direct bipolar radiofrequency current between two electrode poles
Operating temperature	~40–70 °C (low-temperature ablation)	~85–90 °C (higher thermal range)
Tissue effect	Controlled *volumetric ablation* with minimal lateral thermal injury	*Coagulative necrosis* leading to fibrosis
Lesion characteristics	Cleaner, well-defined, with *less char or carbonization*	Slightly more *eschar and stiffness* around channel margins

(continued)

Table 5.1 (continued)

Swelling/edema	Generally *less post-op edema*	Moderate edema may occur due to higher heat
Visual feedback	Requires *saline immersion* and real-time tactile feedback	Direct contact with tissue, easier to use *"dry"*
Wand tip design	Longer and thinner; needs activation *prior to entry*	Shorter tip; can be used in tighter fields
Ease of use	Slightly *steeper learning curve*; saline contact important	*More forgiving* in confined surgical fields
Pain profile (post-op)	Generally *less painful*	Mild to moderate discomfort in first 3–5 days
Device cost	Typically *higher*	Relatively *lower*
Best used when	Precision and minimal collateral damage are priorities	Rapid and effective fibrosis in large tongue-base volume

5.2 Endoscopic Coblation-Assisted Tongue-Base Resection

Srinivas Kishore

5.2.1 *Introduction*

Retrolingual obstruction—arising from the bulk, compliance, and collapse dynamics of the tongue base—represents a central pathophysiological mechanism in many adults with obstructive sleep apnea (OSA). In particular, lingual tonsillar hypertrophy and posterior tongue enlargement narrow the retroglossal airway, making it especially vulnerable during sleep. Under normal wakeful conditions, tonic activity of the genioglossus muscle counteracts posterior displacement of the tongue. However, as neuromuscular tone diminishes during sleep, the posterior tongue readily encroaches into the airway lumen. This collapse is further amplified by negative intraluminal pressure generated during inspiration, which accentuates medialization, elongation, and dynamic narrowing of the retroglossal segment [7, 8].

Traditional surgical approaches to this region, such as midline glossectomymidline glossectomy or lingual tonsillectomy [18] were often associated with significant morbidity due to wide resections and risk of bleeding, dysphagia, or prolonged recovery [7–9]. In contrast, the advent of endoscopic coblation has provided a safer and more targeted alternative. Coblation employs plasma-mediated, low-temperature ablation to create submucosal channels within the tongue base. This technique achieves a dual effect: debulking excess tissue while also inducing controlled fibrotic stiffening of the remaining musculature. By reducing tongue-base volume and enhancing laminar rigidity, coblation decreases retroglossal collapsibility and improves airway patency, while limiting surface thermal damage and postoperative discomfort [2].

Modern practice emphasizes careful patient selection to maximize therapeutic benefit. Phenotype-guided strategies are now standard, with drug-induced sleep endoscopy (DISE) serving as a critical diagnostic adjunct. Using the widely adopted

VOTE classification system—Velum, Oropharyngeal lateral walls/tonsils, Tongue base, and Epiglottis—surgeons can determine whether tongue-base collapse is the primary site (T-dominant), part of a multilevel obstruction (codominant), or a secondary contributor. This information is vital in tailoring treatment, as isolated tongue procedures may suffice for T-dominant collapse, whereas multilevel interventions are often required in more complex patterns [10].

Retrolingual obstruction remains a pivotal target in OSA surgery. Endoscopic coblation, guided by careful phenotyping and DISE assessment, represents a minimally invasive yet effective strategy that balances efficacy with safety. It embodies the broader evolution of sleep surgery toward precision-based, anatomy-specific interventions designed to optimize patient outcomes [11, 12].

5.2.2 *Indications and Selection*

Coblation tongue-base procedures are considered in adults with symptomatic OSA or socially disruptive snoring when *retrolingual collapse* on DISE materially contributes to disease burden. Typical *high-yield* candidates include:

- Friedman tongue position III with relatively small tonsils;
- *Lingual tonsillar hypertrophy*;
- Persistent OSA after palatal surgery or adenotonsillectomy; and
- Patients pursuing multilevel correction in whom the tongue is a rate-limiting site. In mixed phenotypes, nasal resistance (septum, turbinates, valve) should be optimized to reduce ventilatory load and to facilitate positive airway pressure (PAP) as adjunct or fallback therapy.

Preoperative baseline should capture *polysomnography* (or standardized HSAT) with AHI/ODI and sleep architecture, *Epworth Sleepiness Scale* (ESS), disease-specific quality-of-life metrics, such as the Functional Outcomes of Sleep Questionnaire (*FOSQ*) *score*. In borderline anatomy, DISE can be augmented with a jaw-thrust maneuver to estimate likely benefit from mandibular advancement versus tongue surgery.

Because retrolingual disease rarely exists in isolation, coblation is often combined with *lateralizing palatal surgery* (e.g., ESP/BRP) when *O-level (Oropharyngeal)* lateral-wall behavior is present, and with *epiglottic* procedures when DISE shows trapdoor or book-type epiglottic collapse. Nasal surgery (septum, turbinates, valve) is frequently additive—improving nasal breathing, reducing PAP pressures, and stabilizing postoperative airflow.

5.2.2.1 Advantages

- *Hemostasis-friendly*: Minimal or no intraoperative bleeding.
- *Clear visual field*: Simultaneous irrigation and suction maintain excellent visibility.

- *Efficient bleeding control*: Coagulation is easily achieved with integrated irrigation and suction.
- *Enhanced safety*: Electrical current enables detection of nerve or muscle stimulation.
- *Non-compressive exposure*: Provides wide access to the tongue base without mechanical compression.

5.2.2.2 Disadvantages

- *Cost considerations*: Use of disposable coblation wands increases procedural cost.
- *Learning curve*: Requires prior experience, preferably through coblation adenotonsillectomy training.

5.2.3 Preoperative Setup

- *Device settings:*
  - Ablation (yellow pedal): Level 9
  - Coagulation (blue pedal): Levels 3–4
  - Irrigation: Normal saline elevated ~1 m above the surgical bed to ensure adequate gravity-assisted flow
  - Suction: Maximal strength to prevent clogging of the coblator tip
- *Endoscopy:*
  - Equipment identical to that used in endoscopic sinus surgery

5.2.4 Patient Positioning and Preparation

- *Anesthesia*: Nasotracheal intubation
- *Draping*: As per standard tonsillectomy protocol
- *Patient position*: Supine with head in a neutral position
- *Surgeon position*: Same orientation as for endoscopic sinus surgery

5.2.5 Surgical Field Exposure

- *Mouth opening*: Secured using a Denhardt mouth retractor (right-side engagement)

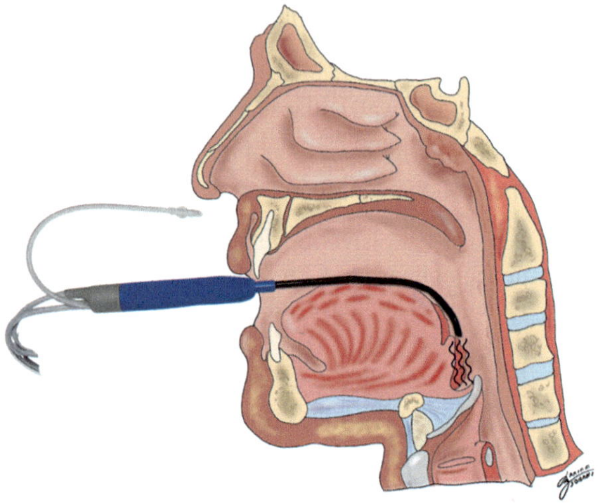

Fig. 5.3 Bent coblator wand to approach the lingual tonsils

- *Tongue traction* (three-point method):
  - One midline suture (3-0 Vicryl) anterior to the foramen cecum
  - Two paramidline sutures (3-0 Vicryl), 1.5 cm lateral to midline on each side
- *Uvula management*:
  - Tag and lift using a nasal or oral approach, or
  - Retract upward with a malleable retractor to protect the soft palate
- *Visualization*: Achieved with a 30° or 70° rigid endoscope

5.2.6 Technique: Tongue-Base Ablation (Figs. 5.3, 5.4 and 5.5)

- *Starting point*: Posterior to the circumvallate papillae
- *Anterior tongue base:*
  - Begin with one side to gauge safe depth
  - Proceed to the opposite side
  - Ablate lingual tonsils
- *Depth considerations:*
  - Neurovascular structures lie =1.5 cm deep from mucosal surface and =1.5 cm lateral from the midline
  - Optional: Use Doppler to delineate lingual arteries
- *Posterior tongue base*: Ablate in similar fashion
- *Closure*: No suturing required

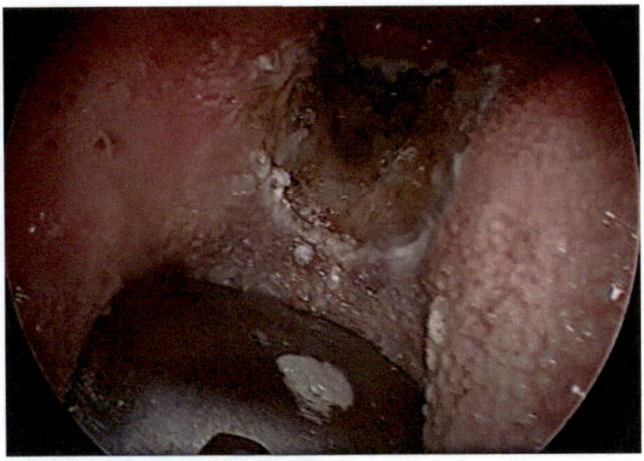

Fig. 5.4 Gag suspended and coblation started posterior to circumvallate papillae toward vallecula

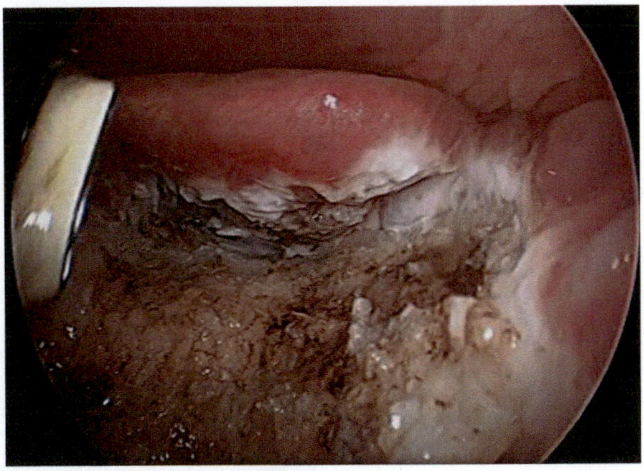

Fig. 5.5 Inferior limit of coblation

5.2.7 Practical Tips on Coblator Use (Figs. 5.6 and 5.7)

- Coblation depth: Typically 1–2 mm per pass
- Technique:
  - Use gentle contact with tissue
  - Avoid plunging or burying the tip
  - Maintain constant motion and suction to reduce clogging
  - Periodically clean the tip for optimal performance

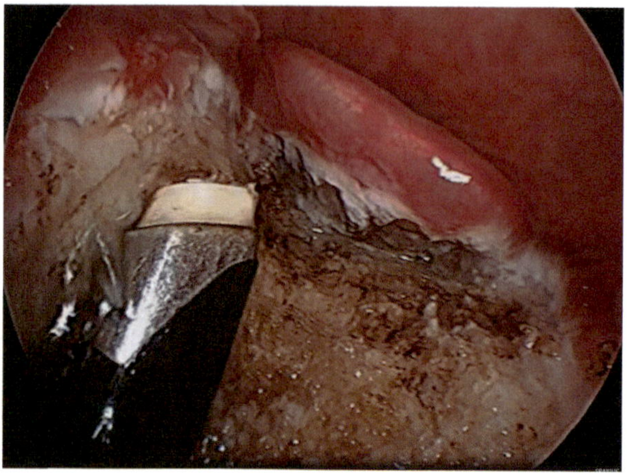

Fig. 5.6 Coblation of lingual tonsil

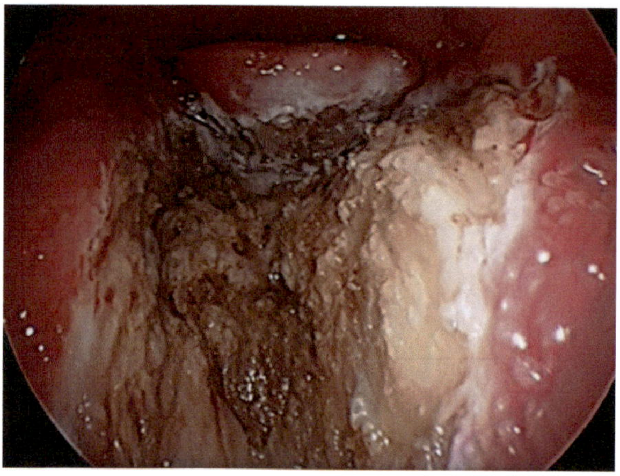

Fig. 5.7 Post-coblation

5.2.8 Postoperative Care

5.2.8.1 Immediate Care

- *ICU monitoring:* Patients are best managed in a high-dependency or intensive care setting overnight, where airway patency, hemodynamics, and oxygenation can be closely monitored. Sedation is maintained to minimize agitation, with planned *extubation the following morning* once airway stability and protective reflexes are assured.

5.2.8.2 Diet

- *Soft diet initiation:* Patients may begin a *soft diet by lunch on the first postoperative day*, provided there is no significant airway swelling or bleeding.
- *Duration:* A *soft diet is continued for 14 days*, minimizing trauma to the operative site and reducing the risk of secondary bleeding.

5.2.8.3 Medications

- *Analgesia:* Scheduled *analgesics for 10 days* help control postoperative pain, which can be significant due to tongue-base manipulation.
- *Antimicrobial rinses: Oral gargles with chlorhexidine* are prescribed for 7 days to maintain oral hygiene and reduce local microbial load.
- *Antibiotics:* A short course of *systemic antibiotics (3 days)* may be used prophylactically, though institutional protocols may vary.

5.2.8.4 Precautions

- *Activity restriction:* Patients should be advised to *avoid strenuous activity, heavy lifting, or vigorous exercise for 4 weeks*. This precaution is essential given the risk of *delayed postoperative hemorrhage*, with documented cases occurring as late as 3 weeks postoperatively.
- *Patient counseling:* Clear instructions regarding signs of bleeding (e.g., hemoptysis, blood-tinged saliva, or sudden oral bleeding) should be provided, and patients should be encouraged to seek immediate medical attention if these occur.

5.2.9 Safety, Complications, and Mitigation

Across adult and pediatric series, serious adverse events are *uncommon* when exposure, planes, and energy are controlled. Expected morbidities include *odynophagia* (several days), *tongue edema*, mild *dysphagia*, *transient taste alteration*, and small-volume *bleeding*. Airway compromise due to edema or hematoma is rare but preventable with midline/paramedian channeling, conservative lateral extent, perioperative steroids where appropriate, and prudent observation in high-risk patients (severe OSA, high BMI, extensive multilevel procedures). Neurologic complications (hypoglossal neurapraxia) are very uncommon with careful depth and lateral boundaries. Your postoperative precautions (soft diet, oral hygiene, avoidance of strenuous activity for several weeks) and the caution about *delayed hemorrhage* are appropriate and should remain highlighted for patient counseling.

5.3 Submucosal Minimally Invasive Lingual Excision (SMILE)

Srinivas Kishore and Moideen Sanu

Submucosal minimally invasive lingual excision (SMILE) is a *mucosa-sparing, submucosal debulking* of the tongue base performed through a small anterior midline incision, typically using coblation [13, 14]. By reducing retroglossal bulk while preserving the dorsal mucosa, it aims to lessen postoperative pain and dysphagia compared with open wedge resections, yet achieve greater volumetric change than needle-based radiofrequency. Early comparative work showed *higher success with SMILE than radiofrequency base-of-tongue (RFBOT)* (64.6% vs 41.7%) but with more complications [14]—an experience-dependent trade-off that many centers mitigate via strict midline tunneling, Doppler mapping, and disciplined hemostasis. Conventional tongue-base ablation procedures often damage the mucosa, resulting in significant postoperative pain and dysphagia.

The best candidates are *CPAP-intolerant* adults whose DISE demonstrates *dominant tongue-base collapse* (VOTE "T" component, often AP or concentric) with or without lingual tonsillar hypertrophy. DISE—standardized by the *VOTE* system—improves site-specific selection and planning for tongue-base procedures and multilevel strategies [10]. Concomitant epiglottic collapse may require adjunctive procedures (e.g., epiglottopexy) to avoid persistent obstruction.

Cadaveric and radiologic work consistently supports a *midline, submucosal "safe zone"* posterior to the foramen caecum: major neurovascular structures (hypoglossal/lingual artery neurovascular bundle (HLNVB)) course *inferolateral* and are rarely encountered if the tunnel stays central and depth-controlled [15]. Notably, *lingual artery proximity increases with tongue protrusion*, reinforcing neutral positioning and the value of *intraoperative Doppler* before lateral extension [15, 16]. Practical rules of thumb derived from these studies: stay within *~7–10 mm of midline* near the vallecula, keep debulking relatively shallow in the most posterior third, and expand laterally only after confirming vessel location.

The dominant hazards are *bleeding (immediate/delayed), edema-related airway compromise, infection, and dysphagia/dysgeusia*. Risk reduction hinges on: (1) *strict midline tunneling* with shallow, incremental passes; (2) *neutral tongue positioning* and *Doppler mapping* prior to lateral/deeper work; (3) meticulous *irrigation–suction* to keep the coblation tip efficient; and (4) clear post-op instructions and surveillance for *delayed hemorrhage* (7–21 days), with a low threshold for return if sentinel bleeding occurs. The cadaveric/CTA studies underpinning the midline "safe zone" are particularly relevant for counseling and team drills (airway + hemostasis protocols) [22].

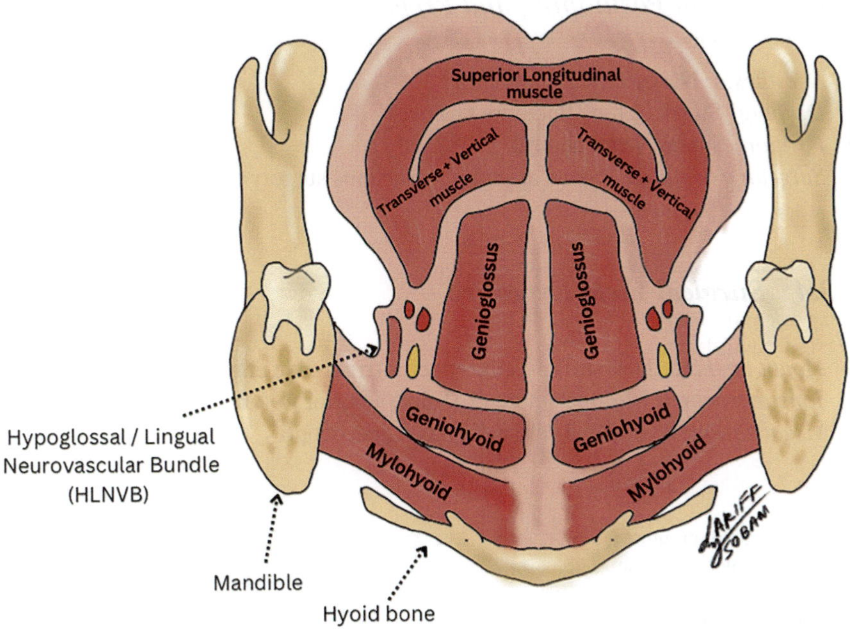

Fig. 5.8 Coronal section through the tongue showing location of lingual artery and nerve bundle approximately 1–2 cm lateral and 2.5 cm deep to foramen caecum. Adapted from Maturo and Mair [13]

5.3.1 Relevant Anatomy (Fig. 5.8)

- The *hypoglossal–lingual neurovascular bundle* [17] lies >1.5cm lateral to the midline at the level of the foramen cecum.
- Posterior to the foramen cecum, the *lingual artery and nerve* course more laterally, ~2.5 cm from midline.
- The *hypoglossal nerve* runs more inferior and lateral compared to the lingual artery.

5.3.2 Preoperative Setup

- *Device settings*
  - Ablation (yellow pedal): Level 9
  - Coagulation (blue pedal): Level 3–4
  - Irrigation: Normal saline, ~1 m above surgical bed for gravity flow
  - Suction: Maximal, to avoid coblator tip clogging
- *Endoscopy*
  - Standard endoscopic sinus surgery equipment

5.3.3 Patient Positioning and Preparation

- *Anesthesia:* Nasotracheal intubation
- *Draping:* Standard tonsillectomy protocol
- *Position:* Supine, head neutral
- *Surgeon orientation:* Same as endoscopic sinus surgery

5.3.4 Surgical Field Exposure

- *Mouth opening:* Denhardt mouth retractor (right-side engagement)
- *Tongue traction:* Midline suture (2-0 silk) anterior to foramen cecum (Fig. 5.9)
- *Visualization:* 0° or 30° 4 mm rigid nasal endoscope.

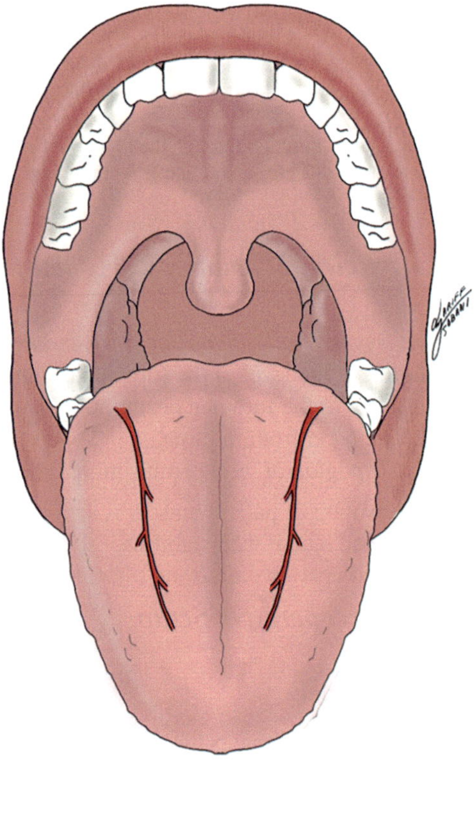

Fig. 5.9 Retraction suture through the anterior tongue and the course of the lingual artery marked with help of Doppler. Adapted from Maturo and Mair [13]

5.3.5 Technique: Tongue-Base Ablation

- *Infiltration*: Inject 2 mL of 1% lidocaine with 1:100,000 adrenaline, 2 cm posterior to tongue tip.
- *Incision:*
  - Make a midline incision with EVac 70 T&A Plasma Wand Coblator, 2 cm posterior to tongue tip (Fig. 5.10).
  - Create a *submucosal tunnel* (2 cm diameter: 1 cm lateral to foramen on each side) in an anteroposteroinferior direction (Fig. 5.11).
  - Use nondominant finger to palpate coblator tip externally (Fig. 5.12).
  - Endoscope may be inserted into the cavity to follow the coblator tip for *direct visualization.*
- *Depth considerations:*
  - Neurovascular structures lie =1.5 cm deep and = 1.5 cm lateral. Staying midline avoids injury.
  - Optional: Intraoral Doppler to map lingual arteries.
- *Extent of resection:*
  - Extend excision up to vallecula.
  - At completion, a *midline depression* posterior to circumvallate papilla should be palpable.
  - Resection volume: ~20 cm^3 (approximately 30-50% of total adult tongue base volume) (Fig. 5.13).
- *Closure*: Leave anterior incision open.

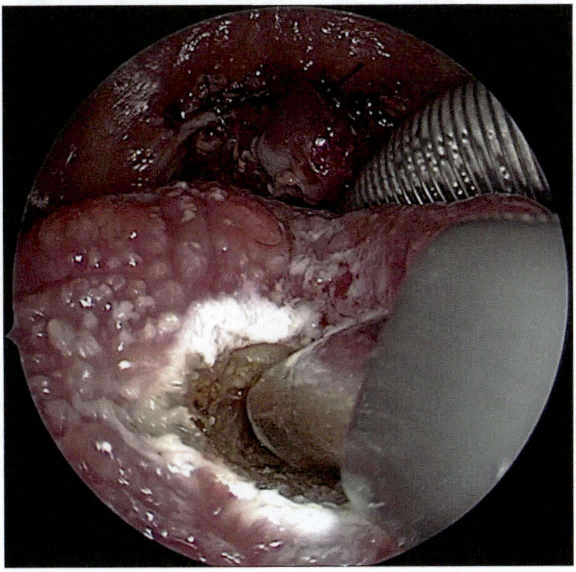

Fig. 5.10 Creating the incision with the coblator wand

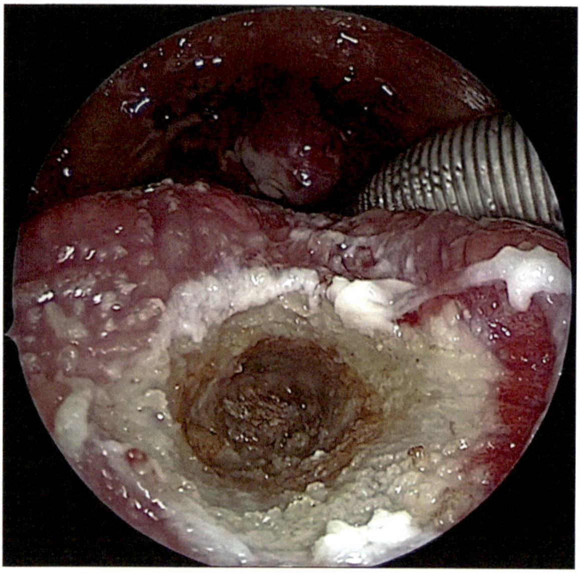

Fig. 5.11 The submucosal tunnel getting created

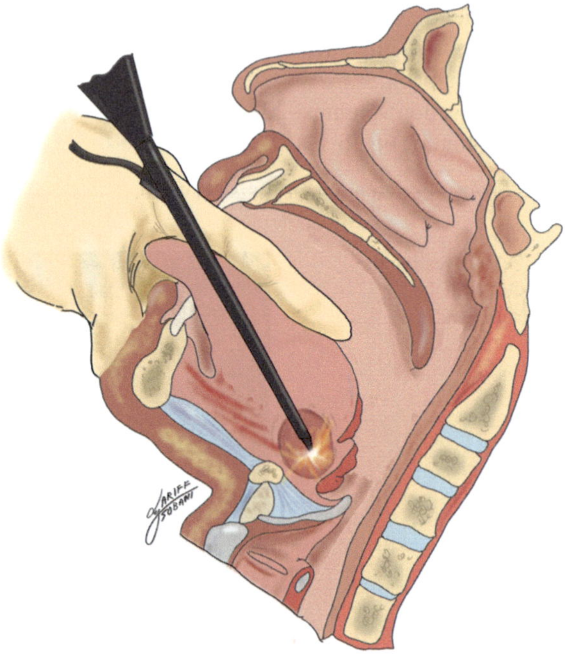

Fig. 5.12 Sagittal view of the tongue showing position of coblation wand and the nondominant hand. Adapted from Maturo SC et al.

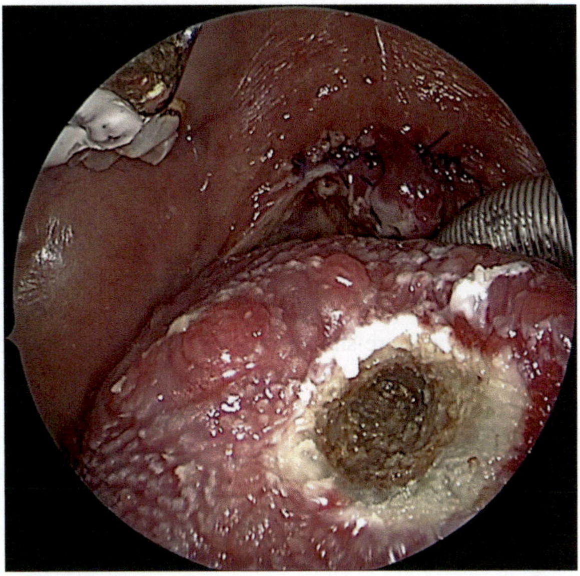

Fig. 5.13 The final picture of the cavity created

5.3.6 Practical Tips on Coblator Use

- Depth: 1–2 mm per pass
- Gentle, gliding contact—avoid plunging
- Maintain constant suction and motion to prevent clogging
- Regularly clean tip for efficiency

5.3.7 Postoperative Care [19, 20]

- *Immediate*
  - *Airway monitoring:* Patients should be closely observed in the recovery unit for signs of airway obstruction due to lingual edema or bleeding. Those with severe OSA or comorbidities often benefit from overnight monitoring.
  - *Hemostasis:* Although intraoperative bleeding is usually well controlled, the tongue's vascularity warrants vigilance for early or delayed hemorrhage.
  - *Pain control:* Moderate throat pain and swallowing discomfort are expected. Analgesia typically includes paracetamol or NSAIDs; opioids are reserved for breakthrough pain.
  - *Diet:*
  - IV steroids (Dexamethasone × 3 doses), analgesics, antibiotics

- *Diet*
  - Patients should begin with clear fluids once fully alert, advancing to soft, cool foods to reduce irritation and minimize discomfort.
  - Analgesics × 5 days
  - Chlorhexidine oral gargle × 7 days
  - Antibiotics × 7 days
  - Follow-up: Day 7, 14, 28
- *Precautions*
  - Strenuous physical exertion, heavy lifting, or activities that increase intrathoracic pressure should be avoided to reduce bleeding risk: × 4 weeks (risk of delayed hemorrhage, reported up to 3 weeks post-op)

5.3.8 Complications

5.3.8.1 Hemorrhage (Intra-op, Early, Delayed)

- *Mechanisms*: Injury to lingual artery branches or submucosal venous plexus; extension off midline; deep tunneling near the vallecula where vessels lie closer to the surface (especially with tongue protrusion). Cadaveric/CTA work supports a midline "safe zone" posterior to the foramen cecum; protrusion brings the lingual artery closer to the surface.
- *Mitigation*: Strict midline tunnel; neutral tongue position; intra-op Doppler mapping before any lateral/deeper work; incremental passes with continuous irrigation–suction; coagulation on low settings; post-op steroid/ice protocols and explicit delayed-bleed counseling.

5.3.8.2 Airway Edema and Obstruction

- *Mechanisms*: Submucosal tissue trauma, fluid shifts, and inflammatory response.
- *Mitigation*: Dexamethasone; head-up positioning; cool humidified O_2; low threshold for overnight monitored setting (HDU/ICU) in severe OSA, high BMI, or difficult airway; avoid tongue protrusion splints that could shift tissue in the first 48–72 h. (Risk framed by broader transoral airway surgery data.)

5.3.8.3 Dysphagia, Odynophagia, and Altered Swallowing Biomechanics [19]

- *Mechanisms*: Temporary edema, mucosal sensory changes, and reduced tongue-base bulk altering bolus propulsion.
- *Mitigation*: Graduated diet; analgesia; early swallow hygiene instructions; consider SLP input for high-risk phenotypes.

5.3.8.4 Taste Disturbance (Dysgeusia) and Oral Sensory Changes [21]

- *Mechanisms*: Thermal/edematous effects on dorsal mucosa and taste buds; traction effects; less commonly neuropraxia.
- *Mitigation*: Mucosa-sparing technique (core advantage of SMILE), midline tunneling, gentle retraction, and avoidance of lateral extension that increases nerve/vessel exposure.

5.3.8.5 Nerve Injury (Lingual Nerve, Hypoglossal Nerve)

- *Mechanisms*: The lingual nerve runs laterally in the oral tongue; hypoglossal trunk/branches are inferolateral; both are well away from midline in neutral position, forming the anatomical basis for the "safe corridor."
- *Mitigation*: Centerline tunnel, depth control by external palpation, neutral positioning, Doppler before lateral work.

5.3.8.6 Infection, Abscess, Hematoma

- *Profile*: Uncommon with mucosa-sparing tunnels and antiseptic mouthwash regimens; tongue-base hematoma/abscess is described after RF or open resections but remains infrequent with modern coblation.
- *Mitigation*: Peri-op oral hygiene, short course antibiotics (center-dependent), suction–irrigation to limit dead space, and early review if fever, trismus, or focal fluctuation.

5.3.8.7 Pain, Dysarthria, Scarring/Granulation

- *Profile*: Pain is expected but typically less than open wedge resections due to mucosa preservation; dysarthria is usually mild/transient compared with anterior oral-tongue resections. General glossectomy data emphasize speech/swallow trade-offs with larger resections—useful for counseling on extent-related risks.
- *Mitigation*: Multimodal analgesia; limit resection volume to planned endpoints; saline rinses and early tongue mobility exercises.

5.3.8.8 Dental, Temporomandibular Joint, and Anesthesia-Related Events

- *Profile*: Dental trauma, lip commissure injury, or TMJ strain can occur with prolonged retraction; cardiopulmonary/anesthetic risks as per any airway surgery.
- *Mitigation*: Teeth guards, padding, time-limited mouth-gag intervals, and airway plans aligned with OSA physiology. (Inferred from TORS/transoral airway surgery care pathways.)

5.4 Robotic-Assisted Tongue-Base Reduction and Partial Epiglottidectomy

Liang Chye Goh, Ahmad Kusyairi Khalid, Song Tar Toh, Mohd Zulkiflee Abu Bakar, and Claudio Vicini

5.4.1 Principles

Obstructive sleep apnea (OSA) is a complex disorder characterized by recurrent upper airway collapse, leading to intermittent hypoxemia, sleep fragmentation, and heightened cardiovascular and metabolic risk [25]. Continuous positive airway pressure (CPAP) remains the gold standard therapy, yet its real-world adherence rates are suboptimal, driving the search for effective surgical alternatives. Historically, palate-focused resections such as uvulopalatopharyngoplasty (UPPP) dominated the surgical landscape but often failed to address multilevel obstruction, particularly at the tongue base and epiglottis. This limitation prompted development of minimally invasive tongue-base approaches, of which *transoral robotic surgery (TORS)* has become the most widely studied.

TORS uses the da Vinci® surgical platform to access the oropharynx, tongue base, and supraglottic structures with three-dimensional magnified vision, tremor filtration, and wristed instruments that permit precise dissection in confined spaces. Introduced to sleep surgery in the early 2010s, TORS enabled surgeons to resect lingual tonsillar hypertrophy, tongue-base tissue, and supraglottic obstructions that were previously challenging to address safely. Compared with open tongue-base reduction, TORS offers reduced morbidity, superior visualization of critical neurovascular structures, and improved patient recovery [23, 24].

The primary role of TORS in OSA is within *multilevel surgical strategies*, particularly for patients with tongue-base collapse identified on drug-induced sleep endoscopy (DISE). Meta-analyses confirm significant AHI reduction and improved Epworth Sleepiness Scale scores in appropriately selected patients [25]. Reported success rates are highest in carefully selected patients with moderate-to-severe OSA, high body mass index cutoffs (typically <35–40), and prominent tongue-base hypertrophy.

Complications including bleeding, airway edema, dysphagia, and taste disturbance are generally transient; structured perioperative protocols in high-volume centers have maintained a favorable safety profile. Enhanced recovery, meticulous hemostasis, staged multilevel planning, and selective postoperative monitoring have made TORS a safe option in high-volume centers. Ongoing refinements include hybrid TORS procedures, robotic-assisted epiglottoplasty, and combined use with hypoglossal nerve stimulation, broadening the range of patients who may benefit [26, 27].

Robotic-assisted transoral surgery provides three-dimensional magnification and wristed instrument articulation in a confined operative field, enabling resection of tongue-base and supraglottic tissue that is difficult to access safely through conventional approaches. This chapter describes the technique of *robotic tongue-base reduction* and *partial epiglottectomy* using the *Da Vinci Xi Surgical System*, primarily indicated for patients with *retrolingual and supraglottic collapse* as part of obstructive sleep apnea (OSA) management [23].

Key surgical objectives include:

- *Volumetric reduction* of hypertrophic *lingual tonsillar tissue* and *tongue-base musculature*.
- Partial resection of the *epiglottis* in cases of posterior prolapse or redundant tissue obstructing the laryngeal inlet.
- Utilization of robotic technology to enhance *three-dimensional visualization*, instrument articulation, and surgical access to the tongue base and supraglottic airway.

5.4.2 *Surgical Technique*

5.4.2.1 Patient Positioning and Preparation (Fig. 5.14)

- *Nasotracheal intubation* is performed to optimize transoral access.
- The patient is positioned in a *"sniffing the air"* posture with *no shoulder roll* to align the surgical axis.
- A *midline 0 silk retraction stitch* is placed on the anterior dorsum of the tongue to aid exposure.
- A *Crowe–Davis mouth gag* fitted with a *Davis–Meyer tongue blade* (with integrated suction ports) is inserted. The *shortest and widest blade* that allows adequate tongue-base exposure is selected.

5.4.2.2 Robotic Docking (Figs. 5.15, 5.16, and 5.17)

- The *da Vinci Xi system* is docked adjacent to the patient's bed.
- A *30° upward-facing endoscope* and two robotic arms are deployed, typically equipped with:
  - Maryland bipolar forceps
  - Spatulated monopolar cautery
- A *bedside assistant* stands at the head of the bed to provide countertraction, suctioning, and instrument exchange.

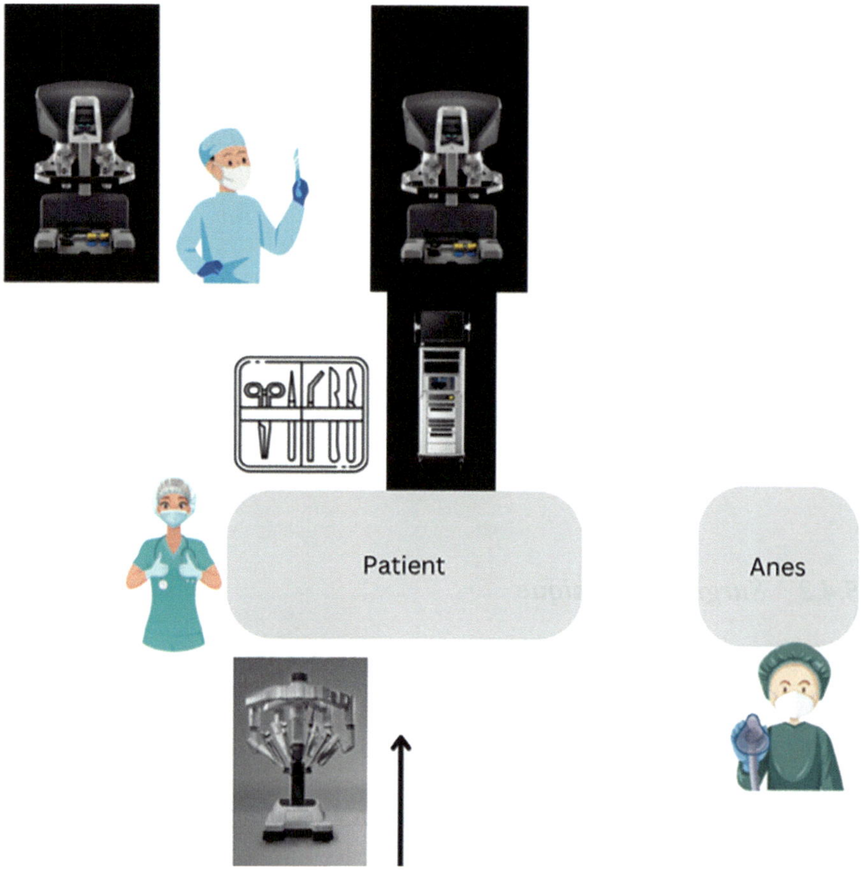

Fig. 5.14 Suggested DaVinci Xi Robot transoral tongue-base resection/partial epiglottidectomy operation theatre layout/setup

5.4.2.3 Robotic Tongue-Base Reduction

Initial Incision

- A *midline vertical incision* is made along the dorsum of the tongue base, starting from the *foramen caecum* and extending posteriorly to the *glossoepiglottic fold* (Fig. 5.18) [23, 24].
- The incision is deepened to the lymphomuscular junction, ensuring sufficient depth to allow complete retraction and dissection of the lingual tonsil (Figs. 5.18 and 5.19).

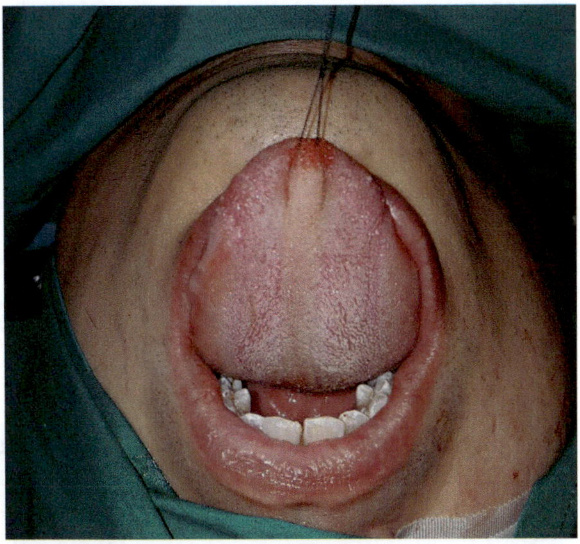

Fig. 5.15 Silk 1-0 is sutured at tongue dorsum and adjusted till the epiglottis is visible

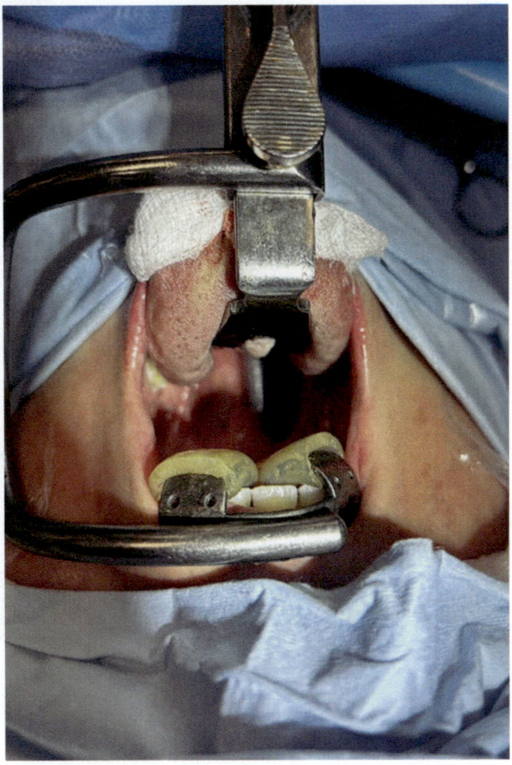

Fig. 5.16 Mouth gag placed and direct visualization made to identify the tip of epiglottis and lingual tonsils before commencement

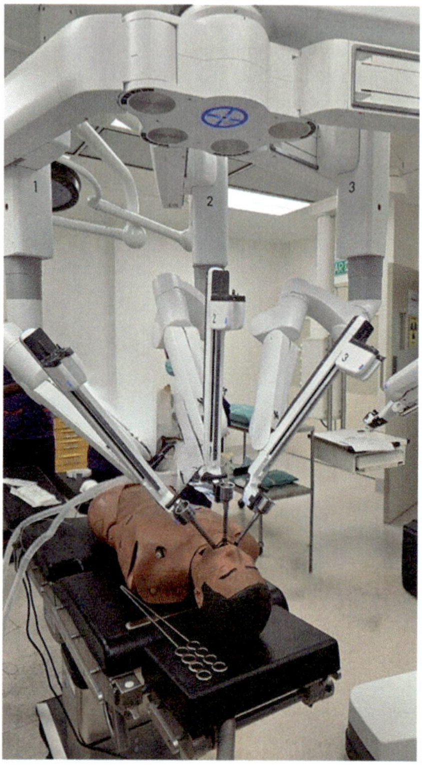

Fig. 5.17 Robot positioned into place with body approximately one foot length from patient's shoulder. Arms 1 and 3 to be used interchangeably with Maryland bipolar forceps and monopolar spatula. Arm 2 is reserved for the 8 mm 30° endoscopy

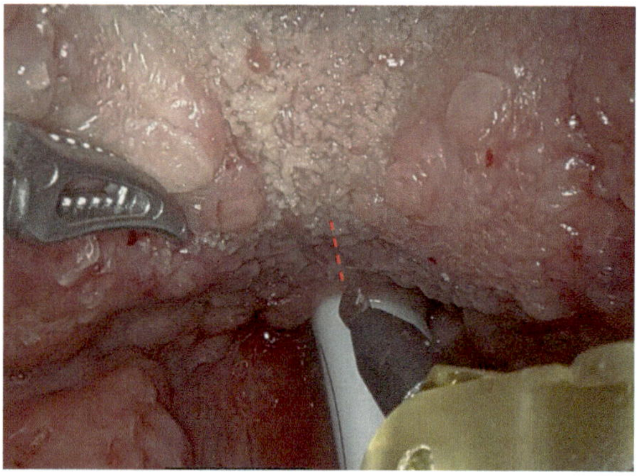

Fig. 5.18 Midline incision made starting from the foramen caecum to the edge of the lingual tonsil

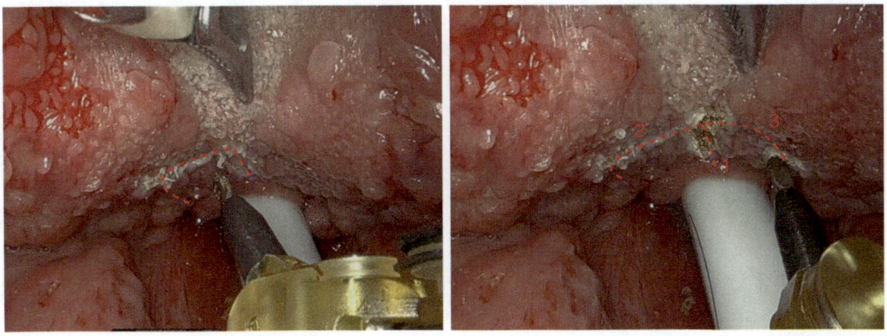

Fig. 5.19 Incision made at the midline (1) followed by left (2)- and right (3)-sided markings made to the paramedian area

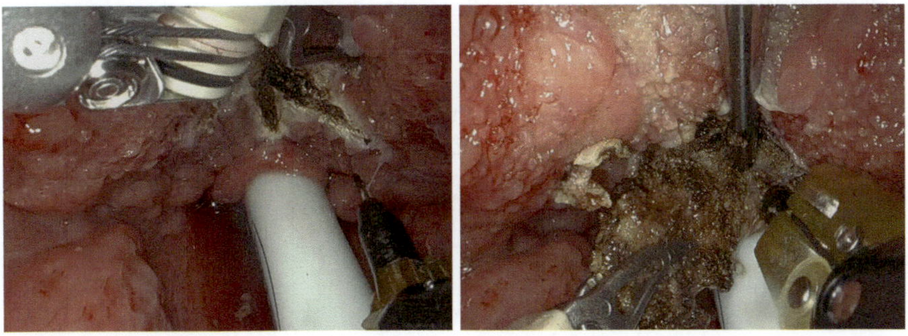

Fig. 5.20 Lingual tonsils carefully delineated to the vallecula region. Taking note to not remove too close to the tongue musculature

Right-Sided Resection (Fig. 5.20)

- The midline incision divides the tongue base into right and left halves.
- *Right lingual tonsil* resection begins by extending the incision laterally, posterior to the *sulcus terminalis*, toward the *glossotonsillar sulcus*.
- Tissue is removed in a *superior-to-inferior plane*, maintaining a plane between lymphoid and muscle layers.

Left-Sided Resection (Fig. 5.21)

- The same steps are repeated on the *left half* to complete bilateral lingual tonsillectomy and tongue-base debulking.

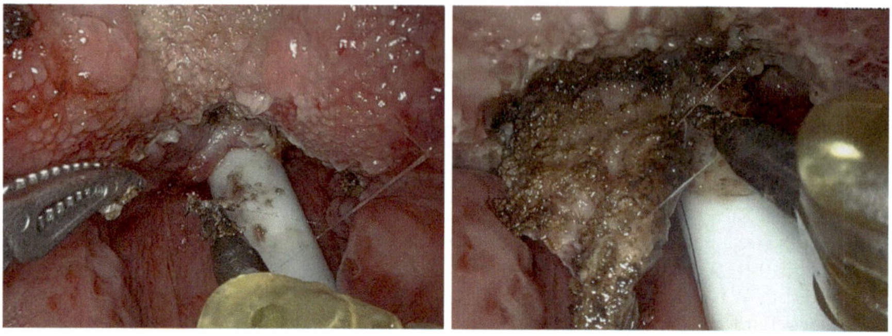

Fig. 5.21 Procedure repeated at the opposite side

5.4.2.4 Partial Epiglottidectomy (Fig. 5.22)

Midline Division

- The *epiglottis is split* vertically in the midline.
- The author recommends *limiting excision to the superior one-third* of the epiglottis to minimize aspiration risk.

Horizontal Transection

- A *horizontal incision* is then made connecting the midline split to the *lateral margins* of the epiglottis, completing partial resection of the obstructing portion.

5.4.3 Postoperative Management of Transoral Robotic Surgery (TORS) for OSA

5.4.3.1 Early Postoperative Management (First 24–72 h)

Monitoring and Setting

- Patients should be admitted to a *high-dependency unit (HDU)* or *ICU* for close airway observation, especially in cases involving:
  - Large-volume tongue-base reduction
  - Concurrent multilevel surgery (e.g., palatal or nasal)
  - High BMI (>35), severe OSA (AHI >30), or baseline hypoxia
- *Continuous pulse oximetry* and *capnography (if available)* are recommended
- A *nasopharyngeal airway* may be inserted to maintain patency in the first 24–48 h, especially if significant tongue-base edema is expected

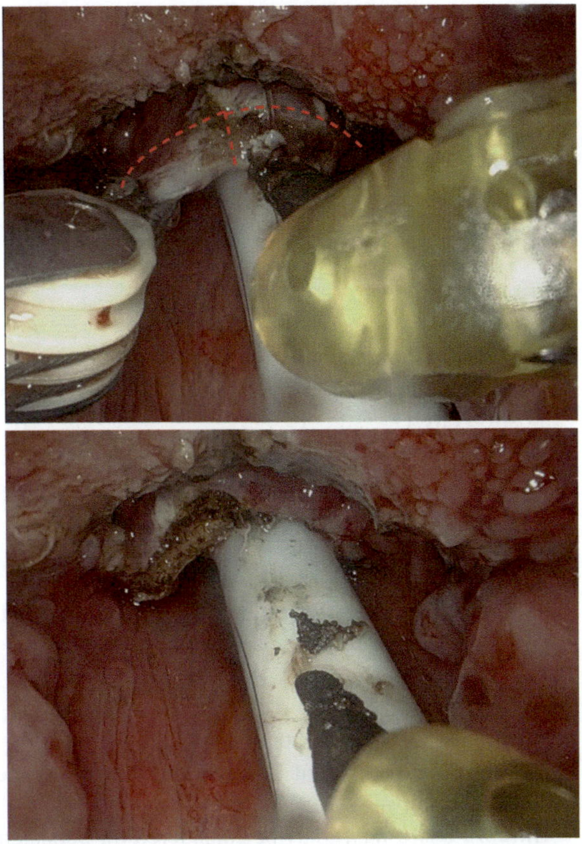

Fig. 5.22 Upper 1/3 of the epiglottis removed in the same manner

Airway and Bleeding Precautions

- Suction at bedside; avoid vigorous suctioning at tongue base to reduce bleeding
- Elevate head of bed to 30–45° to reduce edema
- Regular inspection for oropharyngeal bleeding; re-intervention may be needed if persistent oozing occurs
- Consider Nasopharyngeal airway (ID = 5.0–6.5 mm) for airway protection

Medication

- *Steroids:* IV dexamethasone (8 mg IV BD for 48 h) to reduce tongue-base edema
- *Antibiotics:* IV antibiotics, then transition to oral antibiotics for 5–7 days
- *Analgesia:*
  - Paracetamol + NSAIDs as first line

  - Opioids with caution (e.g., tramadol), ideally avoided due to risk of respiratory depression in OSA
  - Consider PCA (patient-controlled analgesia) if pain is moderate to severe, with monitoring
- *Proton pump inhibitors* (e.g., pantoprazole) may be added to reduce risk of reflux-induced irritation

Nutrition and Fluids

- NPO for first 6–12 h post-op
- Start with *sips of water* or cold clear fluids after airway deemed safe (usually by post-op day 1)
- Advance diet slowly to soft foods over 3–5 days
- *Nasogastric tube feeding* is rarely necessary unless patient has concurrent dysphagia or aspiration risk

5.4.3.2 Intermediate Postoperative Management (Day 3–Day 14)

Swallowing & Speech

- Most patients will tolerate oral intake by days 3–5
- Reassure patients about transient *odynophagia*, altered speech resonance, and thickened saliva
- *Swallow assessment* may be considered for persistent difficulty beyond day 7

Airway and Pain Management

- Monitor for *delayed bleeding*, especially around days 7–21 due to sloughing and surgical eschar.
- Continue *analgesia* on tapering schedule; most patients require paracetamol/ NSAIDs only beyond day 5
- Assess for *tongue-base edema* or signs of *airway compromise*—prolonged snoring or muffled voice may warrant in-clinic nasoendoscopy

Follow-up

- First follow-up at *1 week post-op* to assess wound healing, rule out infection, and review airway patency
- *AHI reassessment* is typically performed *at 3 months*, unless complications suggest earlier study is needed

- Counsel regarding *temporary dysgeusia*, mild tongue stiffness, or voice resonance changes—all of which typically improve over weeks

Activity and Recovery

- Recommend *voice rest* and avoidance of strenuous physical exertion during first 7 days
- Resume light activities after 1 week; full return to work typically by *2–3 weeks*
- Avoid CPAP or oral appliance therapy until reviewed by the surgical team unless indicated for severe desaturation

5.4.3.3 Optional Enhancements to Care

- Consider *perioperative use of corticosteroid-eluting dissolvable dressings* at tongue base (if available)
- *Digital oximetry monitoring* at home (Belun Ring, WatchPAT) may aid in early recognition of desaturation events
- *Multidisciplinary input* (e.g., ENT + sleep physician + dietitian) for complex cases

5.4.4 Complications and Management of Transoral Robotic Surgery (TORS)

Transoral robotic surgery, while effective in addressing tongue base and supraglottic obstruction, carries potential risks that require structured perioperative planning [25, 28].

- *Airway complications*

  Airway obstruction may occur due to *tongue-base edema, hematoma, or difficult reintubation*. Aspiration risk is heightened after partial epiglottectomy.

  Management: Admit high-risk patients (severe OSA, BMI >35, multilevel surgery) to HDU/ICU. Use *nasopharyngeal airway* for 24–48 h if edema is expected, administer IV steroids (e.g., dexamethasone), and maintain head-up positioning. Early recognition and readiness for reintubation are essential.
- *Hemorrhage*

  Both *intraoperative bleeding* and *delayed hemorrhage* (day 7–10 due to eschar sloughing) can occur.

  Management: Meticulous bipolar cautery or suture during surgery, bedside suction readiness, and urgent return to the operating room if persistent bleeding develops.

- *Swallowing and voice issues*

  Patients may develop *odynophagia, transient dysphagia, voice resonance changes, or aspiration.*

  Management: Limit epiglottic resection to the superior one-third. Advance diet slowly (fluids ? soft diet within 3–5 days). Perform swallow assessment if dysphagia persists beyond 7 days. Most voice and resonance changes resolve over weeks.
- *Sensory and motor sequelae*

  Dysgeusia, tongue stiffness, or numbness may result from traction or deep tissue involvement.

  Management: Reassure patients—these are usually temporary. Monitor at 1-week follow-up and provide dietary modifications if symptoms interfere with intake.
- *Systemic and medical risks*

  Respiratory depression from opioids, *infection*, and *reflux-related irritation* may complicate recovery.

  Management: Use multimodal analgesia (paracetamol + NSAIDs; avoid opioids where possible). Prescribe prophylactic antibiotics for 5–7 days. Add proton pump inhibitors to minimize reflux irritation.
- *Recovery and follow-up*

  Delayed complications may manifest as *bleeding or persistent airway symptoms.*

  Management: Review at 1 week for wound and airway assessment. Counsel patients on temporary taste disturbance or mild tongue changes. Reassess AHI at 3 months to confirm efficacy. Resume normal activities gradually, avoiding CPAP or oral appliances until cleared by the surgical team.

References

1. Hussain S, Hayat J, Chowdhury R, Ebrahim M, Alterki A, Bahgat A, Al-Sayed AA, Padhye V, Capasso R. Coblation versus radiofrequency for tongue base reduction in obstructive sleep apnea: a meta-analysis. OTO Open. 2025;9(1):e70076. PMID: 39835243.
2. Li HY, Lee LA, Kezirian EJ. Efficacy of coblation endoscopic lingual lightening in multilevel surgery for obstructive sleep apnea. JAMA Otolaryngol Head Neck Surg. 2016;142(5):438–43. PMID: 26987105.
3. MacKay SG, Carney AS, Woods C, Antic N, McEvoy RD, Chia M, Sands T, Jones A, Hobson J, Robinson S. Modified uvulopalatopharyngoplasty and coblation channeling of the tongue for obstructive sleep apnea: a multi-centre Australian trial. J Clin Sleep Med. 2013;9(2):117–24. PMID: 23372463.
4. Süslü AE, Katar O, Jafarov S, Özer S, Önerci M. Results of coblation midline glossectomy for obstructive sleep apnea. Auris Nasus Larynx. 2021;48(4):697–703. PMID: 33246747.
5. Wee JH, Tan K, Lee WH, Rhee CS, Kim JW. Evaluation of coblation lingual tonsil removal technique for obstructive sleep apnea in Asians: preliminary results of surgical morbidity and prognosticators. Eur Arch Otorhinolaryngol. 2015;272(9):2327–33. PMID: 25323152.

6. Zhang QF, Song W, She CP, Liu DL, Li DW, Zhang XR, Cheng C. Coblation-assisting uvulopalatopharyngoplasty combining coblation-channeling of the tongue for patients with severe OSAHS. Lin Chung Er Bi Yan Hou Tou Jing Wai Ke Za Zhi. 2012;26(3):114–7. Chinese. PMID: 22506427.
7. Duan X, Zhu M, Zhang C, Li M, Cai Y, Chen S, Zheng H. Modified coblation endoscopic lingual lightening in multilevel surgery for obstructive sleep apnea hypopnea syndrome: an open intervention study. Sleep Breath. 2024;28(2):647–56. PMID: 37843682.
8. Bahgat A, Bahgat Y, Alzahrani R, Montevecchi F, Cammaroto G, Vicini C. Transoral endoscopic coblation tongue base surgery in obstructive sleep apnea: resection versus ablation. ORL J Otorhinolaryngol Relat Spec. 2020;82(4):201–8. PMID: 32375151.
9. Chasens ER, Ratcliffe SJ, Weaver TE. Development of the FOSQ-10: a short version of the Functional Outcomes of Sleep Questionnaire. Sleep. 2009;32(7):915–9. PMID: 19639754; PMCID: PMC2706905.
10. Kezirian EJ, Hohenhorst W, de Vries N. Drug-induced sleep endoscopy: the VOTE classification. Eur Arch Otorhinolaryngol. 2011;268(8):1233–6. PMID: 21614467.
11. Babademez MA, Gul F, Sancak M, Kale H. Prospective randomized comparison of tongue base resection techniques: robotic vs coblation. Clin Otolaryngol. 2019;44(6):989–96. PMID: 31464082.
12. Ulualp SO. Outcomes of tongue base reduction and lingual tonsillectomy for residual pediatric obstructive sleep apnea after adenotonsillectomy. Int Arch Otorhinolaryngol 2019;23(4):e415–e421. PMID: 31649761.
13. Maturo SC, Mair EA. Submucosal minimally invasive lingual excision (SMILE): technique for tongue base reduction. Oper Tech Otolaryngol Head Neck Surg. 2007;18(1):29–32.
14. Friedman M, Soans R, Gurpinar B, Lin HC, Joseph N. Evaluation of submucosal minimally invasive lingual excision technique for treatment of obstructive sleep apnea/hypopnea syndrome. Otolaryngol Head Neck Surg. 2008;139(3):378–84. PMID: 18722216.
15. Guan J, Yin S, Yu D, et al. Anatomic characteristics and relationship of lingual artery and hypoglossal nerve with tongue base. Lin Chuang Er Bi Yan Hou Ke Za Zhi. 2005;19(3):108–11. Chinese. PMID: 15844608.
16. Ye J, Wang J, He L, Han D. Anatomic characteristics of lingual artery and midline glossectomy. Zhonghua Er Bi Yan Hou Ke Za Zhi. 2001;36(1):55–7. Chinese. PMID: 12761911.
17. Lauretano AM, Li KK, Caradonna DS, et al. Anatomic location of the tongue base neurovascular bundle. Laryngoscope. 1997;107(8):1057–9. PMID: 9261008.
18. Fujita S, Woodson BT, Clark JL, et al. Laser midline glossectomy as a treatment for obstructive sleep apnea. Laryngoscope. 1991;101(8):805–9. PMID: 1865726.
19. Lee JA, Byun YJ, Nguyen SA, Lentsch EJ, Gillespie MB. Transoral robotic surgery versus plasma ablation for tongue base reduction in obstructive sleep apnea: meta-analysis. Otolaryngol Head Neck Surg. 2020;162(6):839–52. PMID: 32204654.
20. Schar MS, Omari TI, Woods CM, Cock C, Doeltgen SH, Chai-Coetzer CL, Eckert DJ, Athanasiadis T, Ooi EH. Swallowing biomechanics before and following multi-level upper airway surgery for obstructive sleep apnea. J Clin Sleep Med. 2022;18(4):1167–76. PMID: 34913869; PMCID: PMC8974379.
21. Lin HC, Hwang MS, Liao CC, Friedman M. Taste disturbance following tongue base resection for OSA. Laryngoscope. 2016;126(4):1009–13. PMID: 26343916.
22. Ibrahim A, Kumar S, Patil AR, Aishwarya JG, Shah AS, Nair S. Radiological and cadaveric study of anatomical safe zone for transoral base of tongue surgery. J Robot Surg. 2021;15(5):711–6. PMID: 33108621.
23. Lin HS, Rowley JA, Badr MS, Folbe AJ, Yoo GH, Victor L, Mathog RH, Chen W. Transoral robotic surgery for treatment of obstructive sleep apnea-hypopnea syndrome. Laryngoscope. 2013;123(7):1811–6.
24. Vicini C, Dallan I, Canzi P, et al. Transoral robotic tongue base resection in obstructive sleep Apnea–hypopnoea syndrome: preliminary results. ORL J Otorhinolaryngol Relat Spec. 2010;72(1):22–7.

25. Miller SC, Nguyen SA, Ong AA, Gillespie MB. Transoral robotic base of tongue reduction for obstructive sleep apnea: a systematic review and meta-analysis. Laryngoscope. 2017;127(1):258–65.
26. Vicini C, Montevecchi F. Transoral robotic surgery for obstructive sleep apnea: past, present, and future. Sleep Med Clin. 2019;14(1):67–72.
27. Mouratidou S, Chaidas K. Transoral robotic surgery for patients with obstructive sleep apnea: a systematic literature review of current practices. Life (Basel). 2024;14(12):1700.
28. Hoff PT, D'Agostino MA, Thaler ER. Transoral robotic surgery in benign diseases including obstructive sleep apnea: safety and feasibility. Laryngoscope. 2015;125(5):1249–53.

Chapter 6
Hypoglossal Nerve Stimulation (HGNS) Implant

Liang Chye Goh, Song Tar Toh, and Clemens Heiser

6.1 Introduction

Hypoglossal nerve stimulation (HNS) is an implantable therapy for patients with moderate to severe obstructive sleep apnea (OSA) who are unable to tolerate or adhere to continuous positive airway pressure (CPAP) therapy. The treatment works by delivering electrical impulses to the hypoglossal nerve (cranial nerve XII), which activates the genioglossus muscle—the primary tongue protrusor. This action stabilizes the upper airway by pulling the tongue forward and stiffening it during inspiration, thereby preventing collapse of the pharyngeal airway during sleep.

Since its FDA approval in 2014, the Inspire® Upper Airway Stimulation (UAS) system has become the most widely adopted and studied HNS device. The Inspire system consists of an implantable pulse generator placed in the chest, a stimulation lead directed to the hypoglossal nerve in the neck, and a sensing lead placed between the intercostal muscles to detect the patient's breathing cycle. The newly developed Inspire V system introduces a significant technical advancement: it no longer requires a respiratory sensing lead placed between the ribs (in the intercostal space). Instead, the respiratory sensing function is now integrated directly into the

L. C. Goh (✉)
Department of Otorhinolaryngology, Faculty of Medicine, Universiti Malaya, Kuala Lumpur, Malaysia
e-mail: juliusglc@um.edu.my

S. T. Toh
Department of Otorhinolaryngology-Head & Neck Surgery, Singapore General Hospital, Singapore, Singapore
e-mail: song.tar@singhealth.com.sg

C. Heiser
ENT & Sleep Center Mangfall-Inn, Bad Aibling, Germany
e-mail: hno@heiser-online.com

L. C. Goh, S. T. Toh (eds.), *Sleep Surgery in a Nutshell*,
https://doi.org/10.1007/978-981-95-9749-9_6

implantable pulse generator (IPG). This integration simplifies the surgical procedure by eliminating the need for a second lead and reduces potential complications associated with the sensing component. The system delivers stimulation synchronized to inspiration, thereby targeting airway collapse only when needed. It is activated by the patient each night using a remote control. Clinical studies, such as the STAR trial and subsequent long-term follow-ups, have demonstrated significant reductions in Apnea–Hypopnea Index (AHI), improved oxygen saturation, and better quality of life in appropriately selected patients [1–4].

In recent years, additional systems have been developed, aiming to simplify implantation and improve patient comfort. The Genio® system by Nyxoah is one such alternative. Unlike Inspire, it is a battery-free, leadless system implanted under the chin in the submental space. It provides bilateral stimulation of the hypoglossal nerve and is activated nightly by an external patch worn on the skin. This design eliminates the need for chest incisions and respiratory sensing leads, making the implantation minimally invasive. Early clinical studies, including the BETTER SLEEP and BLAST OSA trials, have shown promising outcomes in patients with predominantly tongue base collapse and no complete concentric palatal collapse on drug-induced sleep endoscopy (DISE) [5].

Another emerging HNS option is the aura6000® system developed by LivaNova. This device includes an implantable pulse generator and a stimulation lead connected to the hypoglossal nerve but does not rely on a sensing lead for breath detection. Instead, the aura6000 delivers cyclic stimulation throughout the night, independent of the respiratory cycle. The system is turned on by the patient before sleep and delivers rhythmic stimulation in a preset pattern. Although it involves chest and neck implantation similar to Inspire, its simplified design may offer benefits in certain patient populations. Initial results from European cohorts and the ongoing OSPREY trial in the United States suggest that aura6000 may be a viable alternative, though further data are needed to establish its long-term efficacy [6].

Across all systems, careful patient selection remains critical. Candidates must typically have a moderate to severe AHI (generally 15–100 events per hour), a body mass index below 32–35 kg/m^2 (depending on guidelines), and an absence of complete concentric collapse of the soft palate on DISE (mandatory for Inspire®; not required for aura6000®, which carries no CCC contraindication in its FDA labeling). All currently available HNS therapies are intended for adults who are either intolerant of or unable to benefit from CPAP therapy [1, 7, 8, 9].

In summary, hypoglossal nerve stimulation represents a well-established and expanding therapeutic option for patients with OSA, particularly those who struggle with CPAP. While the Inspire system remains the most widely used and thoroughly studied device, newer systems such as Nyxoah's Genio and LivaNova's aura6000 are broadening the scope of this therapy with less invasive implantation methods and alternative stimulation strategies. As clinical experience and evidence grow, HNS is poised to play an increasingly central role in the personalized treatment of sleep apnea [5–7].

6.2 Principles (Fig. 6.1)

- *Targeted muscle activation*: HNS delivers electrical impulses to the hypoglossal nerve (cranial nerve XII), specifically activating the genioglossus muscle to protrude and stiffen the tongue, thereby maintaining upper airway patency during inspiration.
- *Breath-synchronized or cyclic stimulation*: Depending on the system, stimulation is either synchronized with the patient's breathing cycle (e.g., Inspire) or delivered in a preset rhythmic pattern (e.g., LivaNova aura6000), aiming to prevent airway collapse only when needed.
- *Implantable systems with varying complexity*: Devices range from multicomponent systems with implanted pulse generators and sensing leads (Inspire) to minimally invasive, leadless, and battery-free solutions (Nyxoah Genio), offering tailored options based on anatomical and clinical factors.
- *Strict patient selection based on anatomical and clinical criteria*: HNS is intended for patients with moderate to severe OSA who are CPAP-intolerant, have a body mass index within a defined range, and show no complete concentric palatal collapse on drug-induced sleep endoscopy (DISE) for the Inspire® system.

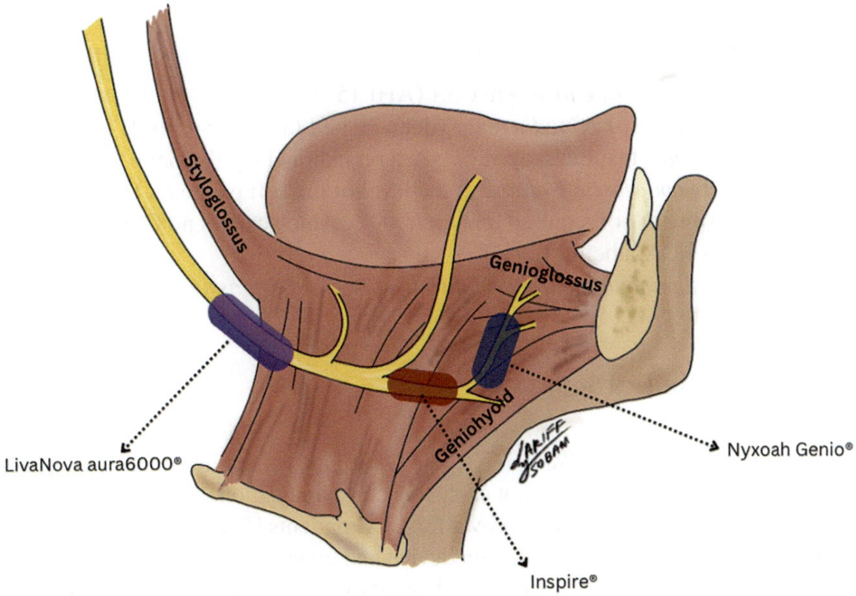

Fig. 6.1 Illustration showing the anatomical sites along the hypoglossal nerve where neurostimulation implants can be positioned

6.3 Commercially Available Systems

Several hypoglossal nerve stimulation (HGNS) systems have been developed globally; however, the *Inspire® Upper Airway Stimulation (UAS)* system (Inspire Medical Systems, Inc., Minnesota, USA) is currently *FDA-approved* and the most widely adopted device with long-term safety and efficacy data. This chapter focuses specifically on the Inspire® system, which has set the standard for HNS therapy.

Other investigational or regionally available systems include:

- *Genio® system* (Nyxoah, Belgium): A *bilateral stimulation device* with an external wearable activator, currently CE-marked, pre-market FDA approved in August 2025 and is undergoing expanded trials [5].
- *Aura6000®* (LivaNova, UK/Italy): An implantable device with an implantable pulse generator and stimulation lead surgically connected to the hypoglossal nerve. Which had recently received pre-market approval in March 2026 [6].

Despite promising innovations, these alternative systems are not yet FDA-approved and have limited global adoption. As such, the Inspire® system remains the *reference standard* for hypoglossal nerve stimulation in the management of obstructive sleep apnea [1–4].

6.4 Indications

HGNS is indicated in [1, 7, 8, 10]:

- Patients with *moderate to severe OSA* (AHI 15–100)
- *CPAP intolerance or nonadherence* (documented failure or refusal)
- *BMI = 32* kg/m^2 (Inspire; may vary based on national regulations)
- *No complete concentric collapse* at the level of the soft palate on DISE (mandatory for Inspire®; not required for aura6000®, which carries no CCC contraindication in its FDA labeling)
- *Absence of significant neuromuscular disease or hypoglossal nerve palsy*

6.5 Contraindications

- *Complete concentric collapse (CCC)* on DISE [1, 8]— applies to Inspire® [1, 8]; the aura6000® system does not carry this contraindication, and the Genio® system has received CE-mark approval for CCC patients [5, 6]
- *BMI > 32–35* kg/m^2 (depending on device and country approval) [1, 7]
- *Severe comorbidities*: uncontrolled cardiovascular disease, neuromuscular disorders
- Prior surgery or radiation affecting the *hypoglossal nerve anatomy* [8]
- Pregnancy, MRI incompatibility (depending on device model)

6.6 Device Components (Inspire® Implant) (Fig. 6.2)

1. *Stimulation electrode*
   - Placed around the *medial branch of the hypoglossal nerve* (primarily to stimulate genioglossus).
2. *Sensing lead*
   - Implanted in the *intercostal space* over the external/internal intercostal muscles.
   - Detects *inspiratory effort* and relays signal to the pulse generator.
3. *Pulse generator (IPG)*
   - Subcutaneous unit implanted in the *right upper chest.*
   - Controls timing and amplitude of nerve stimulation.
   - Activated by a *patient remote* prior to sleep.

6.7 Preoperative Preparation

- Informed consent obtained, including explanation of device components, function, and follow-up plan.
- DISE performed preoperatively to confirm *absence of complete concentric collapse (CCC)* — mandatory for Inspire®; not required for aura6000®.
- The right side of the neck and chest is preferred (to minimize heart interference), unless contraindicated.
- Prophylactic antibiotics administered.

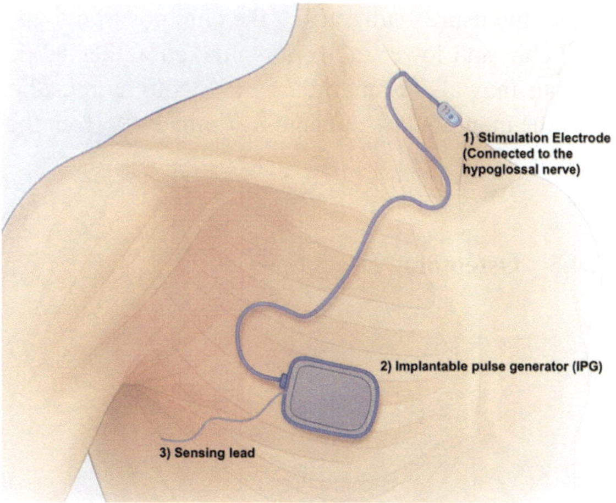

Fig. 6.2 Components of a hypoglossal nerve implant

6.8 Surgical Technique (Two-Incision Method)

It is typically performed under *general anesthesia*. Total operative time is 2–3 h (Fig. 6.3).

6.8.1 Patient Positioning and Electrode Placement

- Supine position with neck extended.
- Skin is prepped and draped from the *submental region to the right upper chest.*
- Two incisions will be made:
  - *Submandibular incision* (for hypoglossal nerve exposure)
  - *4th intercostal space incision* (for sensing lead)
- Nerve Integration Monitor (NIM) electrode monitor placed at the Tongue and floor of mouth.
  - Red lead placed at the lateral edge of the tongue
  - Blue lead placed at the floor of mouth opposite the canine tooth.
- Area is cleaned and draped in a sterile fashion

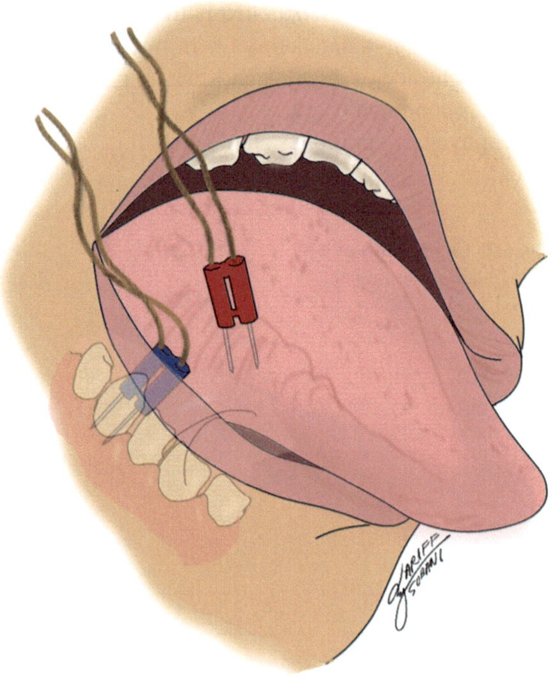

Fig. 6.3 NIM Electrode monitors placed within the oral cavity

6.8.2 *Hypoglossal Nerve Dissection*

Incision 1: Submandibular (4–5 cm) (Fig. 6.4)

- A horizontal incision is made 1–2 cm below the inferior border of the mandible.
- The *platysma* and *superficial cervical fascia* are dissected.
  - Identify and retract the *anterior belly of digastric* and *mylohyoid muscles* (Fig. 6.5).

- Digastric tendon identified and anchored inferiorly using Silk 1-0 sutures.
- Carefully isolate the *hypoglossal nerve* lateral to the hyoglossus and deep to the digastric.
- Careful manipulation of the hypoglossal nerve from the Ranine veins. Hemostasis is secured using Lahey's swab or low-powered bipolar diathermy while avoiding the hypoglossal nerve (Fig. 6.6).

- Using a nerve stimulator or NIM (nerve integrity monitor), differentiate *medial/ inclusion branches* (genioglossus-dominant) from lateral/exclusion ones that supply the tongue retractors.

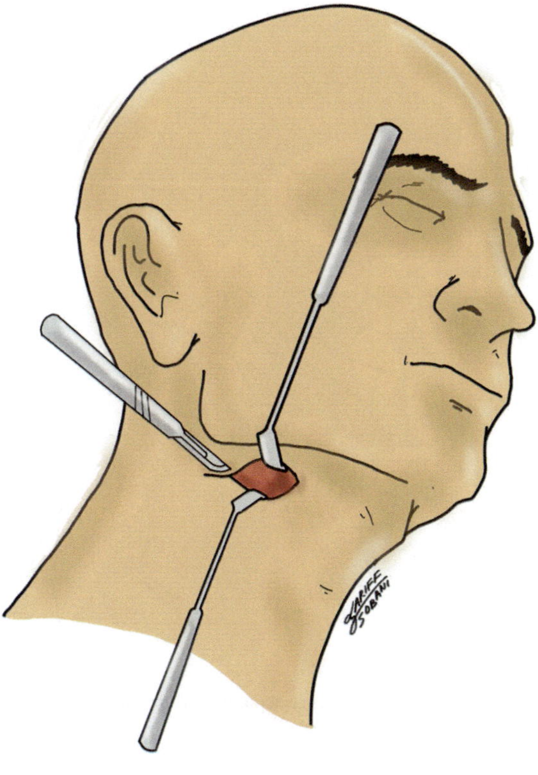

Fig. 6.4 4–5 cm horizontal marking placed 1 finger breath below the lower mandibular margin

Fig. 6.5 The digastric tendon is exposed and retracted downward to allow good visualization of the submandibular space and hypoglossal nerve

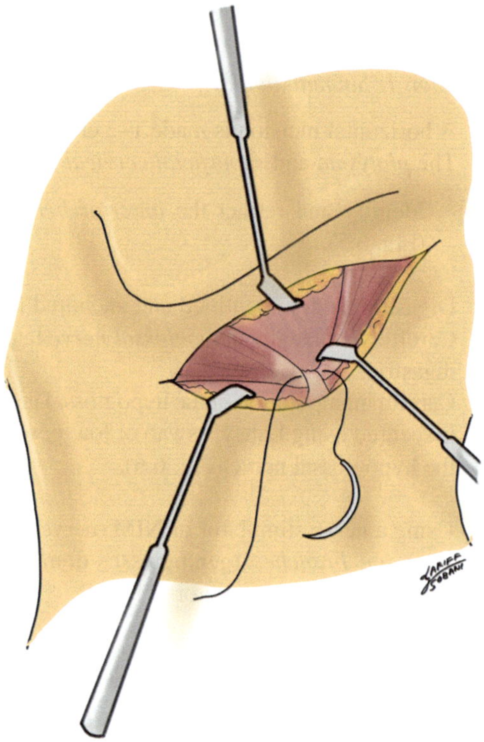

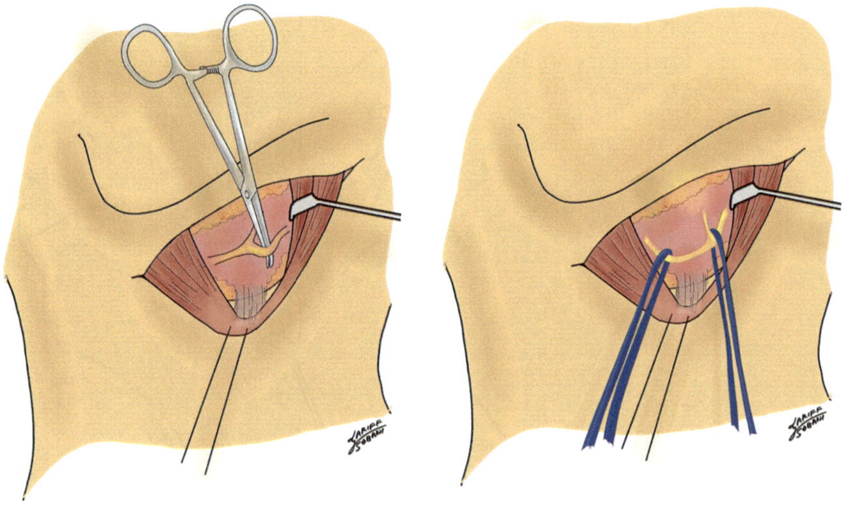

Fig. 6.6 Hypoglossal nerve separated from underlying fascia and exclusion branches. Vessel loop is used to elevate the nerve

- Once branch is free from exclusion branches, hook two vessel loops with 0.5–1 cm distance in between.
- The *medial branch* is dissected free from surrounding fascia and *encircled with the stimulation cuff electrode*.
  - Cuff should be placed without tension or kinking.
  - Ensure good contact and verify *tongue protrusion* with intraoperative stimulation (midline protrusion is ideal) (Fig. 6.7).

- Electrode is flushed with normal saline to clear debris before stimulation test is done.
- Electrode is carefully coiled within the submandibular space.
- Silk sutures from the digastric tendon is sutured on the anchor.
- The anchor is then sutured on the digastric tendon with *nonabsorbable sutures*.

6.8.3 Implantation of the Respiratory Sensing Lead

Incision 2: Right 4th intercostal space (~3 cm) (Fig. 6.8)

- A small oblique or horizontal incision is made in the *4th intercostal space*, anterior axillary line.

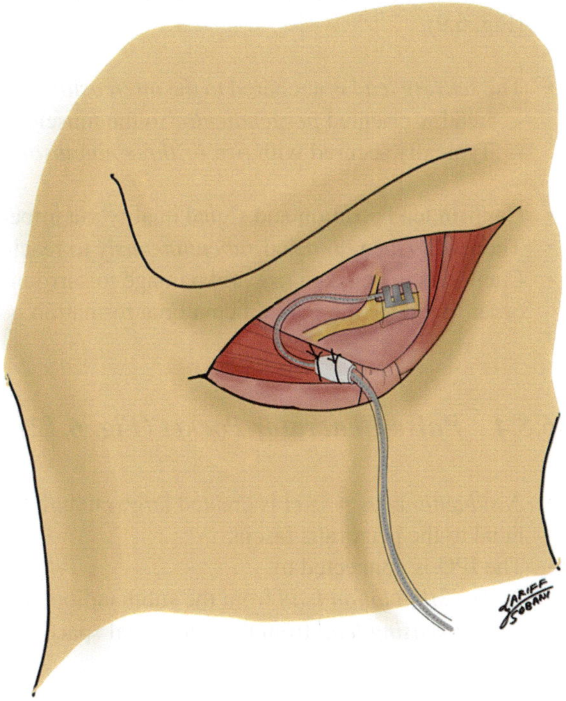

Fig. 6.7 Stimulating lead electrode cuff encircled around the hypoglossal nerve after NIM testing and exclusion of lateral branches. The husk is used to anchor onto the digastric tendon using absorbable sutures

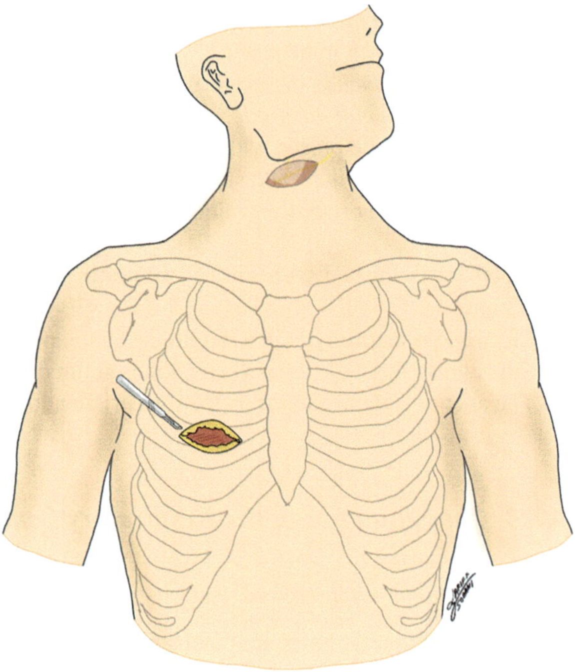

Fig. 6.8 Horizontal incision made at the right 4th intercostal space to implant the respiratory sensing lead

- The subcutaneous tissue is dissected to the *external intercostal muscle layer* (Fig. 6.9).

- The *sensing lead* is anchored *to the intercostal muscle*, avoiding pleural violation.
  - Lead is oriented *perpendicular* to the muscle fibers.
  - Typically secured with *two or three nonabsorbable sutures* (Fig. 6.10).

- Confirm lead position and signal quality via impedance testing/NIM probe.
- The lead is then tunneled *subcutaneously* to reach the pulse generator pocket.
- Caution is to be taken to avoid damage to surrounding tissue during tunneling in order to reduce the risk of hematoma formation postoperatively (Fig. 6.11).

6.8.4 Pulse Generator Pocket (Fig. 6.12)

- A *subcutaneous pocket* is created large enough to house the IPG, usually superficial to the pectoralis fascia.
- The IPG is connected to:
  - The *stimulation lead* from the submandibular incision
  - The *sensing lead* from the intercostal space

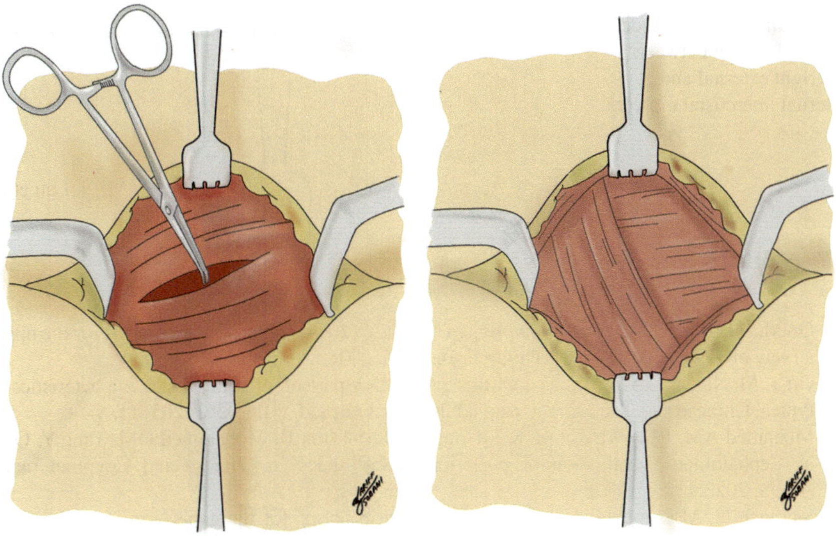

Fig. 6.9 Figure showing pectoralis muscle being incised (Left) and intercostal muscles being exposed (Right) at the 4th intercostal space

- After connection, an *impedance check* is performed on all channels to confirm functionality.

6.9 Intraoperative Testing

- With neuromuscular blockade avoided, the system is activated intraoperatively:
  - Confirm *tongue movement* with low-level stimulation (1–2 V)
  - Ideal movement is *symmetric tongue protrusion*
  - Lateral deviation may indicate stimulation of nontarget branches
- Adjust stimulation cuff position if required before final fixation.
- Leads are secured to prevent migration.

6.10 Closure and Device Programming

- Each incision is irrigated and closed in anatomical layers:
  - *Deep layers* with absorbable sutures (e.g., Vicryl 3-0)
  - *Skin* with monofilament absorbable suture or staples
- A *sterile dressing* is applied to each site.
- Final impedance and function checks are done before leaving the OR.

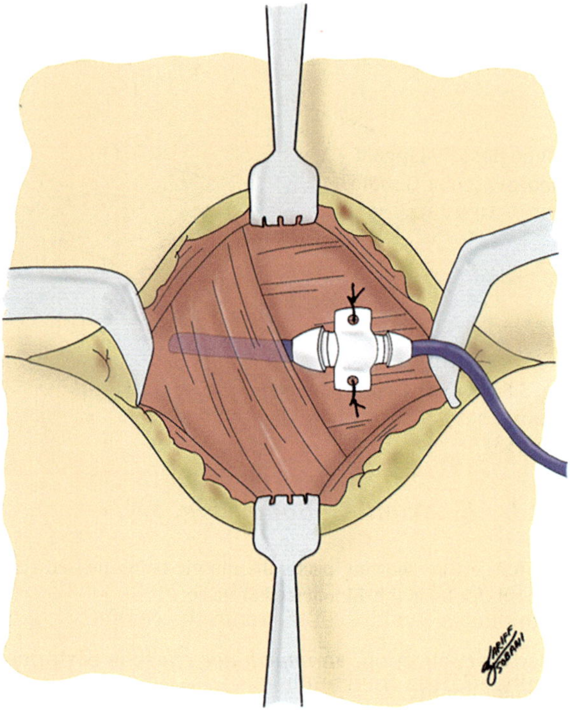

Fig. 6.10 Figure the tip of the sensing lead electrode being placed in between the right external and internal intercostal muscles

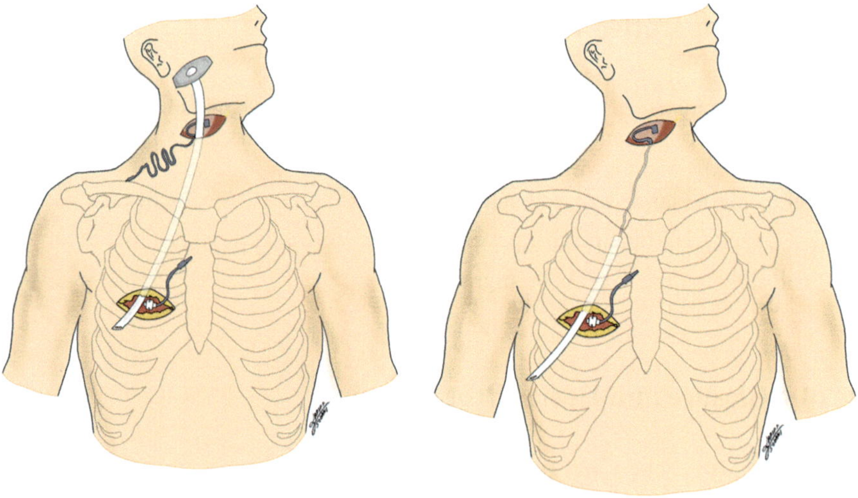

Fig. 6.11 An introducer is used to guide and tunnel the stimulating electrode from the right neck to the right chest

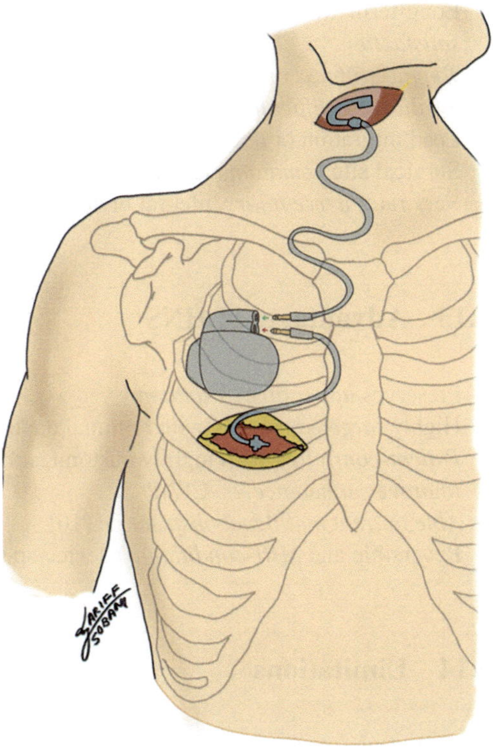

Fig. 6.12 The stimulating and sensing electrode is installed onto the IPG and is tested for response. The IPG is placed in a surgical pocket over the pectoralis fascia

- Device is left *OFF* until activation at 4–6 weeks.

6.11 Postoperative Management

- Most patients are discharged within 24 h.
- Analgesia, wound care instructions, and avoidance of shoulder strain are advised.
- *Device activation* occurs at ~4-6 weeks in clinic.
- *Titration polysomnography* is scheduled after initial activation to optimize therapeutic parameters.

6.12 Expected Outcomes

- Studies report *significant reductions in AHI* (average 68–80% decrease).
- *Daytime sleepiness* and *quality-of-life* scores (e.g., Epworth Sleepiness Scale, FOSQ) show substantial improvements.

- Long-term follow-up (5+ years) indicates *durable outcomes* and *high patient satisfaction.*
- *Tongue stiffness or discomfort* (usually transient)
- *Swallowing difficulty or tongue fasciculations*
- Lead migration or *device malfunction*
- Surgical site *hematoma* or *infection*
- Very rare: *nerve injury*, pleural breach, or device explantation

6.13 Advantages of HNS

- Preserves *upper airway anatomy*
- Highly *targeted therapy* with minimal daytime side effects
- *Patient-controlled* with nightly customization
- *Improves adherence* vs. CPAP
- *Able to treat multilevel obstruction* [10]
- Reversible and *MRI-conditional* (device-specific)

6.14 Limitations

- High *device cost*
- Requires *careful patient selection* [1, 7, 8]
- Contraindicated in complete concentric collapse (CCC), obesity, and certain anatomical variants
- Requires *long-term follow-up* and device maintenance [3, 4]

6.15 Complications

1. *Early wound issues: pain, swelling, hematoma/seroma (neck or IPG pocket)*

   Pain is among the most commonly reported adverse events in real-world databases; hematoma/seroma also appear regularly in reports.

   Management: limb/head elevation and ice; short NSAID/acetaminophen course; compressive dressing; *evacuate expanding hematomas*; resume anticoagulation cautiously once hemostasis assured.
2. *Infection/erosion (pocket or lead tract)*

   In large contemporary series, *1-year explant ~ 0.7%* and *revision ~ 1.5%*; infection is a leading reason for explantation.

   Management: Early superficial cellulitis -> oral antibiotics + wound care; *deep pocket infection/erosion ? culture-directed IV antibiotics and device explant*, with delayed reimplant after clearance.

3. *Stimulation-related or neural symptoms* (tongue stiffness/soreness, abrasions, dysarthria/dysphagia; rarely neuropraxia)

   Frequently reported but typically *transient*; database reviews list neuropraxia-type complaints among common adverse-event reports (selection-bias caveat).

   Management: Reassurance; topical/oral analgesia; *programming optimization* (lower amplitude/pulse width, ramp-up, adjust start delay); soft diet; speech/swallow therapy if persistent; consider imaging/device check if focal weakness.
4. *Respiratory-sensing lead complications* (older/current systems with intercostal/pleural-adjacent placement): *pneumothorax*, pleural effusion, intercostal pain

   A multi-institution database analysis found *pneumothorax ~ 2.4% on day of surgery*; pleural effusion ~0.6%.

   Management: Low threshold for *post-op CXR if dyspnea/pleuritic pain*; observe small, stable pneumothoraces; *tube thoracostomy* if large/symptomatic; technique refinement and site selection reduce risk.
5. *Lead/device issues* (migration/fracture; IPG malfunction; early battery or sensing-lead problems)

   Population-level data show *serious device-related events ~ 6% over 5 years* (mainly lead/device adjustments); within *1 year: explant ~ 0.7%, revision ~ 1.5%.*

   Management: Interrogate system; targeted reprogramming; imaging for suspected migration; *surgical revision/replacement* if malfunction persists.
6. *Stimulation intolerance/arousals/dry mouth*

   Management: Re-titrate parameters (amplitude, pulse width, duty cycle; extend start delay); add humidification; treat comorbid rhinitis/GERD; gradual acclimatization. Real-world registries report overall *low rates of device/procedure-related complications* when therapy is optimized.
7. *Perioperative serious adverse events (overall)*

   Pivotal trial data reported *<2% procedure-related serious adverse events at 12 months*; long-term cohort confirms *low serious event rates* with sustained benefit.

   Management: Standard perioperative risk mitigation and follow-up protocols.

6.16 Conclusion

Hypoglossal nerve stimulation is now a well-supported surgical option for patients with moderate-to-severe OSA who cannot tolerate CPAP. The evidence base from the STAR trial and subsequent real-world registries demonstrates sustained AHI reduction and quality-of-life benefit over five or more years, with a low rate of serious adverse events. Careful patient selection, particularly DISE-confirmed absence of complete concentric collapse and BMI within device-specific limits remains the principal determinant of treatment success [1–6].

References

1. Strollo PJ Jr, Soose RJ, Maurer JT, et al. STAR Trial Group. Upper-airway stimulation for obstructive sleep apnea. N Engl J Med. 2014;370(2):139–49.
2. Woodson BT, Soose RJ, Gillespie MB, et al. STAR Trial Investigators. Three-year outcomes of cranial nerve stimulation for obstructive sleep apnea: the STAR trial. Otolaryngol Head Neck Surg. 2016;154(1):181–8.
3. Boon M, Huntley C, Steffen A, et al. Upper airway stimulation for obstructive sleep apnea: results from the ADHERE registry. Otolaryngol Head Neck Surg. 2018;159(2):379–85.
4. Heiser C, Steffen A, Boon M, et al. ADHERE registry investigators. Post-approval upper airway stimulation predictors of treatment effectiveness in the ADHERE registry. Eur Respir J. 2019;53(1):1801405.
5. Eastwood PR, Barnes M, MacKay SG, Wheatley JR, Hillman DR, Nguyên XL, Lewis R, Campbell MC, Pételle B, Walsh JH, Jones AC, Palme CE, Bizon A, Meslier N, Bertolus C, Maddison KJ, Laccourreye L, Raux G, Denoncin K, Attali V, Gagnadoux F, Launois SH. Bilateral hypoglossal nerve stimulation for treatment of adult obstructive sleep apnoea. Eur Respir J. 2020;55(1):1901320.
6. Jacobowitz O, Schwartz AR, Lovett EG, Ranuzzi G, Malhotra A. Design and rationale for the treating Obstructive Sleep Apnea using Targeted Hypoglossal Nerve Stimulation (OSPREY) trial. Contemp Clin Trials. 2022;119:106804.
7. Olson MD, Junna MR. Hypoglossal nerve stimulation therapy for the treatment of obstructive sleep apnea. Neurotherapeutics. 2021;18(1):91–9.
8. Eastwood PR, Barnes M, Walsh JH, et al. Treating obstructive sleep apnea with hypoglossal nerve stimulation. Sleep. 2011;34(11):1479–86.
9. Kent DT, Soose RJ, Woodson BT, et al. Upper airway stimulation for OSA: early adherence and outcome patterns. Otolaryngol Head Neck Surg. 2016;155(1):188–93.
10. Heiser C, Edenharter G, Bas M, Wirth M, Hofauer B. Palatoglossus coupling in selective upper airway stimulation. Laryngoscope. 2017;127(10):E378–83.

Chapter 7
Bony Surgery for Obstructive Sleep Apnea

May Nak Lau, Muhammad Kamil Hassan, and Firdaus Hariri

7.1 Lateral Cephalometric Assessment

May Nak Lau

7.1.1 Introduction

A lateral cephalogram is a standardized, lateral-view radiographic image of the skull that provides a two-dimensional representation of craniofacial structures and the soft tissue profile. It allows for reproducible linear and angular measurements to assess sagittal and vertical relationships of the maxilla, mandible, and surrounding soft tissues, including the tongue and soft palate.

In patients with obstructive sleep apnea (OSA), lateral cephalometry serves as an adjuctive tool for evaluating structural risk factors for airway compromise and complements functional assessments such as polysomnography and dynamic evaluations such as drug-induced sleep endoscopy (DISE). While sleep studies quantify disease severity and DISE enables dynamic assessment of the anatomical site, level, degree, and pattern of upper airway collapse, cephalometry identifies underlying skeletal and soft-tissue features associated with airway obstruction,

M. N. Lau (✉)
Department of Orthodontics, Paediatric and Special Care Dentistry, Faculty of Dentistry, Universiti Malaya, Kuala Lumpur, Malaysia
e-mail: minalau@um.edu.my

M. K. Hassan (✉) · F. Hariri
Department of Oral & Maxillofacial Clinical Sciences, Faculty of Dentistry, Universiti Malaya, Kuala Lumpur, Malaysia
e-mail: kamil.hassank@um.edu.my; firdaushariri@um.edu.my

L. C. Goh, S. T. Toh (eds.), *Sleep Surgery in a Nutshell*,
https://doi.org/10.1007/978-981-95-9749-9_7

including retrognathia, inferior positioning of the hyoid bone, increased soft palate length, and reduced posterior airway space. Although limited by its two-dimensional nature, cephalometric analysis provides useful structural insights that contribute to the identification of potential anatomical targets for intervention, particularly in bony surgical procedures.

Beyond its role in structural assessment, cephalometry plays an important role in treatment planning and outcome monitoring. It can establish a baseline before orthodontic or orthognathic interventions, and allows for objective posttreatment comparison. For instance, in patients undergoing maxillomandibular advancement surgery, cephalometry demonstrates forward repositioning of the facial skeleton and corresponding enlargement of the airway space, providing a radiographic correlate of clinical improvement. Similarly, subtle changes following palatal or tongue base procedures can be monitored to assess their structural impact over time.

In addition to clinical utility, cephalometric analysis frameworks, such as the Eastman analysis, provide a systematic method for interpreting craniofacial measurements in patients with OSA. This stepwise approach enhances reproducibility and enables correlation of anatomical findings with functional outcomes. Although advanced imaging modalities like cone-beam computed tomography (CBCT) and three-dimensional airway modeling have emerged, lateral cephalometry remains a valuable, cost-effective, and low-radiation tool, particularly in resource-limited settings.

7.1.2 Radiograph Acquisition

For accurate cephalometric analysis, proper radiograph acquisition is essential. A standardized lateral cephalogram should be obtained with the patient in a natural head position to ensure accurate and reproducible measurements for clinical assessment and reliable comparison with normative values and follow-up images. The teeth are typically maintained in centric occlusion, and the lips are kept gently relaxed to avoid distortion of the soft-tissue profile. Consistent positioning minimizes measurement error and enhances measurement reliability. High-quality radiographs with adequate contrast and resolution are critical for precise identification of skeletal and soft-tissue landmarks, including the maxilla, mandible, hyoid bone, and posterior airway space. Proper technique not only enhances diagnostic accuracy but also ensures that subtle craniofacial and airway changes—whether due to growth, orthodontic intervention, or surgical treatment—can be objectively evaluated over time.

7.1.3 Key Landmarks and Reference Planes

- Landmarks

Landmark	Name	Definition
S	Sella	The midpoint of the Sella turcica (pituitary fossa)
N	Nasion	The most anterior point on the frontonasal suture
Po	Porion	The upper- and outermost point on the external auditory meatus
Or	Orbitale	The most inferior and anterior point of the orbital margin
Cd	Condylion	The most posterior and superior point on the mandibular condyle
ANS	Anterior nasal sSpine	The tip of the bony anterior nasal spine in the midline
PNS	Posterior nasal spine	The tip of the posterior nasal spine in the midline (located as a continuation of the base of the pterygopalatine fossa when it intersects with the nasal floor)
PtM	Pterygo-maxillare	The point at the inferoposterior aspect of the pterygomaxillary fissure, where it meets the posterior nasal spine
A	A/subspinale	The deepest point on the curved profile of the maxilla between the anterior nasal spine and alveolar crest
B	B/supramentale	The deepest point on the curved profile of the mandible between the chin and alveolar crest
Pog	Pogonion	The most anterior point on the bony chin
Me	Menton	The most inferior point of the mandibular symphysis in the midline
Gn	Gnathion	The most anterior and inferior point on the bony chin
Go	Gonion	The most posterior and inferior point on the angle of the mandible
U	Uvula tip	The tip of soft palate
AH	Anterior hyoid	The most anterosuperior point on the body of the hyoid bone
V	Vallecula	Intersection of the epiglottis and the base of the tongue/the most posteroinferior point on the base of the tongue
Et	Epiglottic tip	The most superior (or uppermost) point on the contour of the epiglottis
Cb	Base of epiglottis	The most inferior and anterior point on the contour of the epiglottis
TB	Base of tongue	This point is located where the line extending from the B to the Go intersects with the dorsal (back) surface of the tongue base
C3	3rd cervical vertebrae	The most anteroinferior point on the 3rd cervical vertebrae

- Reference planes

Plane	Name
Cranial base	S–N
Frankfort horizontal (FH)	Or–Po
Maxillary/palatal plane (MxPl)	ANS–PNS
Mandibular plane (MnPl)	Go–Me or Go–Gn
Cervical vertebrae (CV)	The line overlying the anterior surface of the 2nd and 3rd cervical vertebrae
Posterior pharyngeal wall (PPW)	Line contouring the posterior wall of the pharynx

The craniofacial landmarks and reference planes used in cephalometric analysis are well established in the literature [1–6] and serve as references for various angular and linear measurements, such as the cranial base (S-N) for SNA/SNB angles, and the mandibular plane for MP-H, FMPA/MMPA, among others (Fig. 7.1).

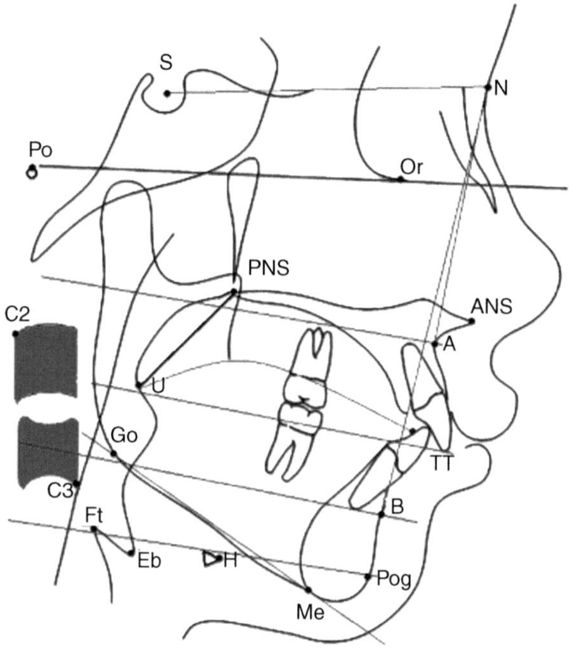

Fig. 7.1 Common landmarks and reference planes. (Adapted from Mohamed et al. [3])

7.1.4 Measurements

Measurement	Definition	Norm	Uses	Implications
Skeletal angular (sagittal)				
SNA (°)	Angle S–N–A	Malay: 84 ± 3 Chinese: 83 ± 4 Indian: 82 ± 3	Assess maxillary position relative to cranial base	Low SNA (maxillary retrognathia) may contribute to airway obstruction and OSA. Consider maxillary advancement surgery
SNB (°)	Angle S–N–B	Malay: 81 ± 4 Chinese: 80 ± 4 Indian: 79 ± 3	Assess mandibular position relative to cranial base	Low SNB (mandibular retrognathia) contributes to airway obstruction and is common in OSA patients. Consider mandibular advancement surgery, with or without advancement genioplasty
ANB (°)	Angle A–N–B (or SNA minus SNB)	Malay, Chinese, or Indian: 3 ± 2	Assess sagittal skeletal relationship	High ANB with ANB >4° (Class II skeletal relationship) is common in OSA patients
Skeletal angular (vertical)				
Mandibular plane angle (MPA) (°)	SN–GoGn Frankfort (Or–Po)–GoMe or maxillary (ANS–PNS)–GoMe/maxillary mandibular plane angle (MMPA)	MMPA: Malay: 26 ± 5 Chinese: 26 ± 5 Indian: 28 ± 5	Assess vertical skeletal relationship	High MPA indicates a steep (clockwise-rotated) mandibular plane, which is often exhibited by OSA patients
Lower anterior facial height (LAFH) (%)	Me perpendicular to ANS–PNS	55 ± 2	Assess vertical skeletal relationship	OSA patients typically have an increased LAFH (inferior displacement of the mandible), especially when the MPA is high with a normal or reduced posterior facial height
Skeletal linear				
Maxillary length (mm)	S–PNS or Co–ANS Co–A	Co–A: Chinese adult: 87.5 ± 4.8 (male) 92.0 ± 5.3 (female)	Assess maxillary length	A shorter maxillary length has been related to OSA, as a reduced maxillary length may narrow the nasopharynx

Measurement	Definition	Norm	Uses	Implications
Mandibular length (mm)	Co–Gn, Go–Gn, or Go–Me	Co–Gn Chinese adult: 125.4 ± 7.1 (male) 119.4 ± 6.2 (female)	Assess mandibular length	A shorter mandibular length has been related to OSA, as a shorter mandible (especially ramus height) reduces airway space
Pharyngeal length (mm)	PNS–Cb	–	Assess length of the pharyngeal airway, along the posterior border	A longer pharyngeal length has been associated with higher pharyngeal collapsibility and a higher AHI
Soft tissue and airway				
Soft palate length (mm)	PNS–U or PtM–U	Chinese: 31.3 ± 4.6	Assess length of soft palate/uvula	A longer palate can fold/block airway. Many OSA patients have an elongated uvula/palate. Consider palatal surgery, e.g., uvulopalatopharyngoplasty, to widen retropalatal airway
Soft palate thickness (mm)	Measured at the thickest part of velum (soft palate)	–	Assess thickness of soft palate/uvula	Increased thickness may narrow airway. Some OSA patients show thicker palate. Consider palatal surgery, e.g., uvulopalatopharyngoplasty, to widen retropalatal airway
Position of hyoid bone in horizontal plane (mm)	AH–CV (parallel to FH)	–	Assess position of hyoid bone in horizontal plane	A more posteriorly displaced hyoid narrow the retroglossal and hypopharyngeal airway spaces, contributing to or exacerbating airway collapse
Position of hyoid bone in vertical plane (mm)	AH–FH (perpendicular to FH) or AH–MnPl (perpendicular to MnPl)	–	Assess position of hyoid bone in vertical plane	Inferiorly placed hyoid (large H–FH/H–MnPl) correlates with more collapsible airway Consider hyoid suspension or geniohyoid advancement in addition to mandibular advancement surgery
Hyoid–mandibular plane angle (°)	AH–C3 to MnPl	–	Assess position of hyoid bone in vertical plane	Inferiorly placed hyoid (small H–C3 to MnPl) correlates with more collapsible airway. Consider hyoid suspension or geniohyoid advancement in addition to mandibular advancement surgery

Measurement	Definition	Norm	Uses	Implications
Nasopharyngeal airway space (mm)	PNS–upper pharyngeal wall (UPW) or PtM–UPW	–	Assess nasopharyngeal airway space	This measurement defines the anteroposterior dimension of the airway behind the nasal cavity and above the soft palate. A reduced nasopharyngeal airway space indicates potential obstruction in the upper pharynx
Depth of oropharyngeal airway space (mm)	U–middle pharyngeal wall (MPW)	–	Assess depth of oropharyngeal airway space	This measures the anteroposterior dimension of the airway directly behind the oral cavity. A decreased depth is often due to a large tongue or a retrognathic mandible
Minimum of Pharyngeal Airway spaces (PASmin) (mm)	TB perpendicular to posterior pharyngeal wall (PPW)	–	Assess retroglossal oropharyngeal airway space	PASmin represents the narrowest anteroposterior dimension along the entire pharyngeal airway. It is a critical indicator of the most likely site of collapse
Depth of hypopharyngeal airway space (mm)	V–lower pharyngeal wall (LPW)	–	Assess depth of hypopharyngeal airway space	This measures the anteroposterior dimension of the lowest part of the pharyngeal airway, located behind the epiglottis and above the larynx. A reduced depth in this region suggests potential obstruction near the laryngeal inlet
Position of vallecula in horizontal plane (mm)	V–CV (parallel to FH)	–	Assess position of vallecula in horizontal plane	This measures the horizontal placement of the vallecula (the space between the tongue base and epiglottis). A more posterior position indicates greater backward displacement of the tongue base and epiglottis, contributing to hypopharyngeal narrowing
Position of vallecula in vertical plane (mm)	V–FH (perpendicular to FH)	–	Assess position of vallecula in vertical plane	This measures the vertical placement of the vallecula. An inferiorly displaced vallecula can be associated with a downwardly positioned hyoid bone and increased pharyngeal tissue laxity

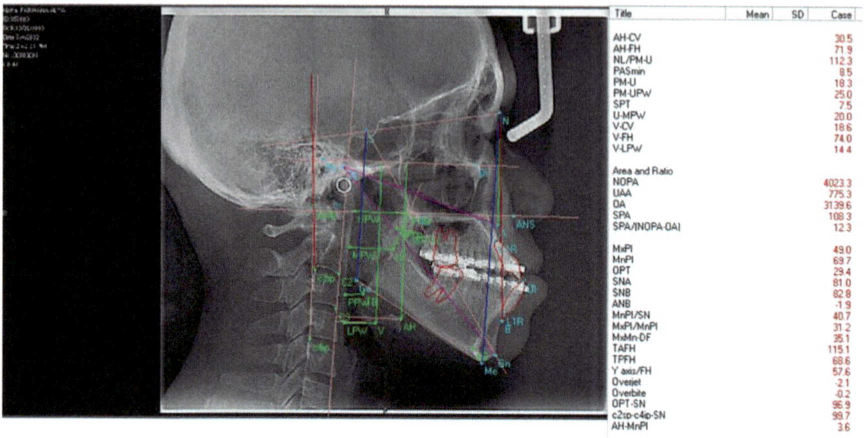

Fig. 7.2 Lateral cephalometric analysis using Winceph

While conventional linear and angular measurements derived from lateral cephalograms offer valuable insights into craniofacial and airway morphology, a more comprehensive assessment of pharyngeal airway dimensions may require area measurements. These complex calculations provide a two-dimensional representation of airway are and are most reliably performed using digital cephalometric measurement tools, such as specialized software (e.g., Winceph, Dolphin Imaging) or increasingly prevalent AI-driven web-based platforms such as WebCeph (Fig. 7.2).

Measurement	Definition
Airway area	
Naso-oropharyngeal area (NOPA) (mm^2)	The computed total area of the pharyngeal airway, extending from the nasopharynx through the oropharynx to the hypopharynx. It is typically bounded posteriorly by the posterior pharyngeal wall (defined by points such as PtM, UPW, LPW, and V) and anteriorly by the dorsal outline of the tongue including the SPA
Upper airway area (UAA) (mm^2)	The computed area within the pharyngeal space, specifically defined by its boundaries. Posteriorly, it is delimited by the PPW. Its superior extent is established by the line connecting PtM to the UPW. Anteriorly, the boundary follows the posterior contour of the soft palate, extending from the U to Cb, and continues along the residual part of the tongue base, from TB to V. Finally, the inferior boundary is defined by the line connecting the LPW to V
Oral area (OA) (mm^2)	The computed area encompassing the oral cavity. It includes the entire tongue area and extends superiorly to the outline of the soft and hard palates
Soft palate area (SPA) (mm^2)	The computed area defined by its outline. This outline includes the anterior and posterior contours of the soft palate. Its superior border is defined by a line passing through PtM perpendicular to the PtM–U line
SPA/(NOPA-OA) (mm^2)	The ratio of the SPA to the difference between NOPA and OA. The denominator, NOPA–OA, specifically refers to the computed pharyngeal airway area (excluding the oral cavity)

7.1.5 *Beyond Lateral Cephalometry: Imaging Modalities for Craniofacial and Airway Assessment in OSA*

While lateral cephalometry remains a useful, low-dose screening tool, contemporary evaluation of craniofacial structure and the bony framework in OSA increasingly relies on three-dimensional and dynamic imaging. These modalities offer volumetric measurements, multiplanar views, and—importantly—context on how skeletal form interacts with the airway and surrounding soft tissues.

7.1.5.1 Cone-Beam Computed Tomography

Cone-beam computed tomography (CBCT) provides high-resolution, three-dimensional assessment of the maxilla, mandible, hyoid position, and upper-airway lumen, with relatively lower radiation exposure compared with conventional CT. It enables volumetric analysis (e.g., oropharyngeal volume and minimal cross-sectional area), as well as evaluation of transverse maxillary deficiency, mandibular retrognathia, and posterior airway space. CBCT is widely available in dental and surgical practices. Systematic reviews highlight its value in quantifying airway dimensions in adults with OSA [7–9], while also noting variability in segmentation protocols and the need for standardized analysis pipelines to ensure reproducibility. Overall, CBCT is a powerful tool for assessing static skeletal and airway geometry, although such measurements may not reliably predict dynamic airway collapsibility.

7.1.5.2 Multidetector Computed Tomography

Conventional computed tomography (CT) remains a robust option when broader sinonasal or craniofacial evaluation is needed (e.g., complex deformity, syndromic anatomy, and surgical planning). With fast gantry speeds, CT can also be applied in dynamic or time-resolved (4D) protocols to visualize airway motion and change in airway calibre during respiration or simulated sleep, thereby complementing structural measurements with rudimentary functional insight. Dynamic upper airway CT has been shown to identify patterns of retropalatal and retroglossal narrowing and may be useful in complex, revision, or research settings, although its use must be balanced against radiation exposure and accessibility considerations [10, 11].

7.1.5.3 Magnetic Resonance Imaging

Magnetic Resonance Imaging (MRI) excels at depicting soft tissues together with the bony framework without ionizing radiation. Static MRI characterizes tongue volume, soft palate length and thickness, lateral pharyngeal walls, parapharyngeal fat pads, and their relationship to skeletal boundaries (maxilla, mandible, and cranial base). Cine (dynamic) MRI further extends this capability by capturing airway motion during natural or sedated sleep, demonstrating how anatomic relationships translate into patterns of airway collapse. Dynamic MRI provides insight into multi-level airway collapse, including contributions from the retropalatal, retroglossal, and lateral pharyngeal walls, which may influence surgical planning and highlight the limitations of single-level approaches [12, 13].

7.1.5.4 Three-Dimensional Facial Imaging

Three-dimensional (3D) facial imaging provides rapid, radiation-free acquisition of external craniofacial morphology, including facial width, mandibular projection, and facial convexity, which may reflect underlying skeletal patterning. Studies suggest that selected facial metrics can contribute OSA risk stratification and reflect craniofacial skeletal relationships, although performance varies across population and age groups; in pediatric cohorts, standalone predictive value has been inconsistent. As a complement to CBCT or MRI, 3D facial imaging can document pre- and post-treatment changes in facial form and aid phenotypic characterisation without additional radiation [14, 15].

Beyond stereophotogrammetry, other optical surface-scanning techniques are emerging for craniofacial and upper airway evaluation. Infrared-based scanning utilizes structured light or depth sensors to capture three-dimensional facial morphology in real time. These devices are increasingly portable, low-cost, and non-ionizing, enabling point-of-care acquisition without radiation exposure. Preliminary studies suggest that infrared scanning can quantify facial width, mandibular angle, and midface retrusion, with potential applications in OSA risk stratification and surgical follow-up [16].

Blue-light scanning (structured blue-light surface imaging) offers higher resolution than infrared-based systems, particularly for fine surface topography, and has been validated against stereophotogrammetry for the accuracy of facial measurements [17]. In OSA, blue-light systems have been used to document external craniofacial morphology and to monitor changes following orthognathic or maxillomandibular advancement surgical procedures. Their strengths include high reproducibility, short acquisition time, and suitability for longitudinal studies, although current limitations include cost and limited integration into sleep-specific workflows [18].

7.2 Skeletal Surgery for Obstructive Sleep Apnea

Muhammad Kamil Hassan and Firdaus Hariri

7.2.1 Introduction

Maxillomandibular advancement (MMA) is a skeletal surgical procedure that involves advancing the *maxilla and mandible* to enlarge the upper airway, particularly in patients with *moderate to severe obstructive sleep apnea (OSA)*. MMA is recognized as an effective surgical intervention for OSA, particularly in patients who are intolerant to CPAP or have failed other surgical treatments [19, 20].

The MMA procedure involves a combination of:

- *Le Fort I osteotomy* of the maxilla
- *Bilateral sagittal split osteotomy (BSSO)* of the mandible [19, 20]
- Optional *sliding genioplasty* for further airway improvement [24]

The surgical principles of MMA include the following [19, 20]:

1. Maxillary advancement (with posterior downgraft or disimpaction, with or without anterior impaction). This movement rotates the maxillary occlusal plane in a counterclockwise vector. This movement stretches the palatal and pharyngeal soft tissues, thus preventing collapse at the velum level of the upper airway.
2. Mandibular advancement via bilateral sagittal split osteotomy allows forward placement of the tongue and suprahyoid muscles, thus reducing retrolingual collapse [21–23].
3. Genioplasty advancement complements mandibular advancement and helps to anchor the tongue anteriorly and prevent retrolingual collapse [24].

The surgery aims to *advance the facial skeleton*—and therefore the pharyngeal soft tissues—*in a counterclockwise vector*, reducing pharyngeal collapse and increasing retrolingual and retropalatal airway dimensions (Fig. 7.3).

Among surgical options, maxillomandibular advancement (MMA) is regarded as the most effective skeletal framework surgery for moderate to severe OSA. MMA involves Le Fort I maxillary advancement combined with bilateral sagittal split osteotomy of the mandible, typically with counterclockwise rotation of the occlusal plane. By repositioning the maxillomandibular complex anteriorly, MMA enlarges the retropalatal and retrolingual airway, reduces pharyngeal collapsibility, and stabilizes the tongue base and suprahyoid structures. Adjunctive genioplasty can further augment tongue-base stabilization.

Multiple systematic reviews and meta-analyses demonstrate that MMA achieves the highest success and cure rates among all OSA surgeries, with mean reductions in Apnea–Hypopnea Index (AHI) exceeding 80% and long-term durability beyond 5–10 years. Compared to soft tissue surgeries such as uvulopalatopharyngoplasty (UPPP), MMA addresses the multilevel pathophysiology of OSA, making it particularly valuable for patients with severe disease, craniofacial abnormalities, or failed prior procedures. Careful patient selection, virtual surgical planning, and multidisciplinary perioperative management have further improved safety, predictability, and patient-reported outcomes [19, 20].

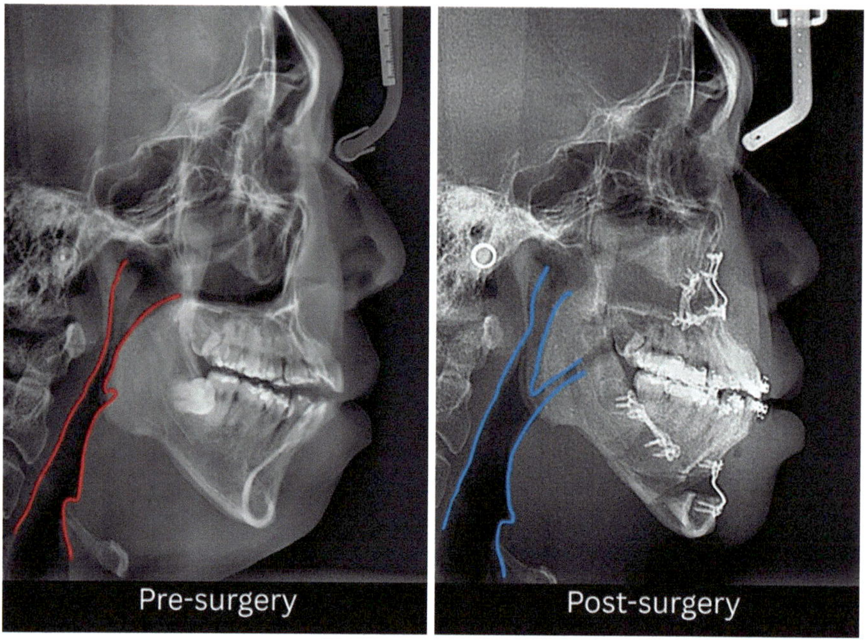

Fig. 7.3 Lateral Cephalogram showing pre and post surgery outcomes of Maxillomandibular advancement (MMA) [19, 20]

7.2.2 Le Fort I Osteotomy (Maxilla)

7.2.2.1 Surgical Approach

The maxillary bone is accessed via a *transoral* approach, using cheek retractors. Infiltrate local anesthetic around the maxillary vestibule, from the region of 1st molar to contralateral 1st molar.

Incision

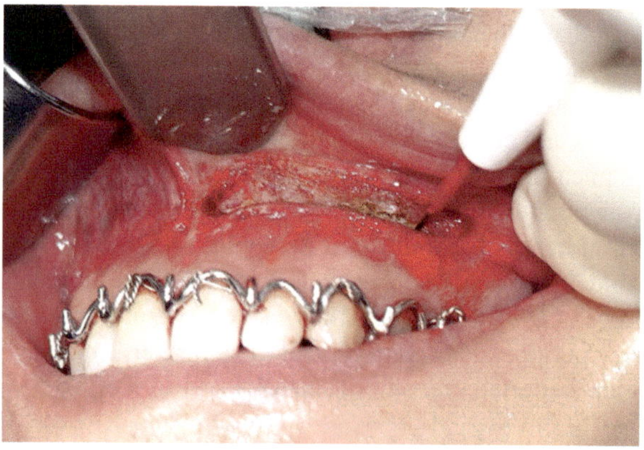

Make a vestibular incision ~5 mm above the mucogingival junction from right to left 1st molar. Incision is made through full thickness of the mucoperiosteum, either using a no. 15 scalpel blade or diathermy instrument. Care is made to not incise too posteriorly to avoid injury to the *parotid duct* near the 2nd molars.

Flap Elevation

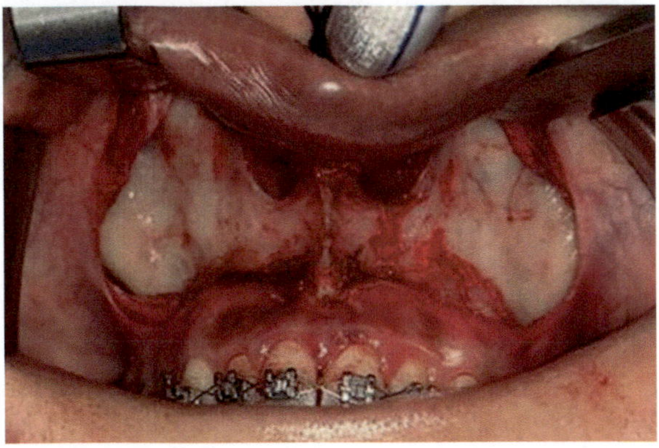

Elevate *full thickness mucoperiosteal flap* using Howarth's, Molt, or Obwegeser elevators. The following regions are exposed:

- Pyriform aperture and lateral nasal rims
- Anterior nasal spine and detach septum if needed
- Infraorbital nerve
- Zygomaticomaxillary buttress, anterior and posterior maxillary sinus walls

Osteotomy Design

Osteotomy line is made ≥*5 mm above the maxillary teeth apices*, from lateral nasal rim to posterior maxillary sinus. Various pre-osteotomy measurements can be done prior to osteotomy. The measurements are either bone-borne or dental-bone-borne or dental-soft tissue borne. They serve the purpose of ensuring the planned position of the Le Fort I segment is achieved. This is not necessary when using virtual surgical planning with cutting guides.

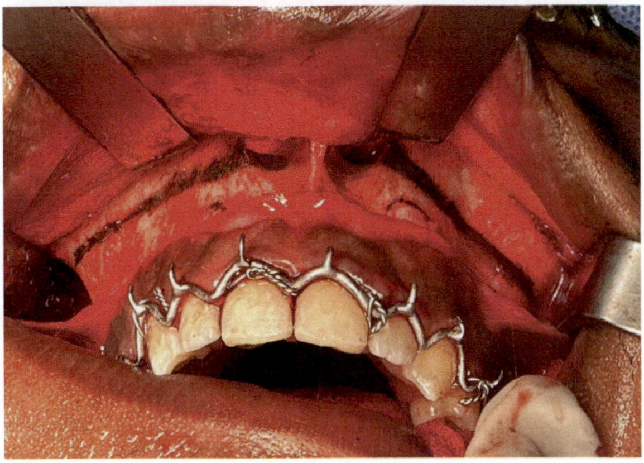

Osteotomy

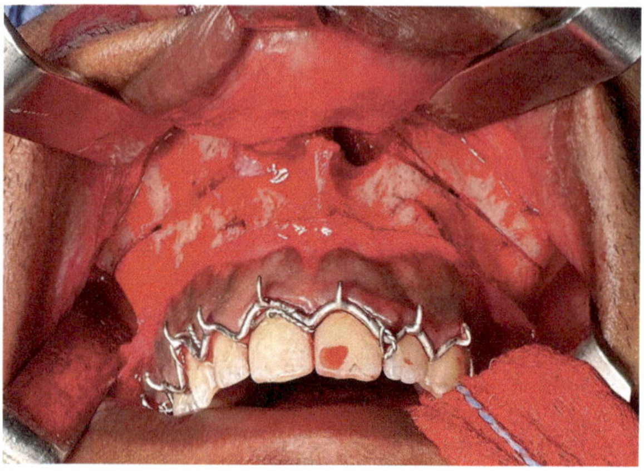

The osteotomy is done using either a reciprocating saw, piezosurgery, or bur. Osteotomy is done in either direction from posterior to anterior or vice versa, while protecting the nasal mucosa, ensuring a full cut. Following this, osteotomies are manually completed using chisels and osteotomes at:

- Nasal septum using nasal septum osteotome
- Lateral nasal walls
- Posterior sinus wall/maxillary buttress
- *Pterygoid disjunction* (curve osteotome or tuberosity cut)

Downfracture

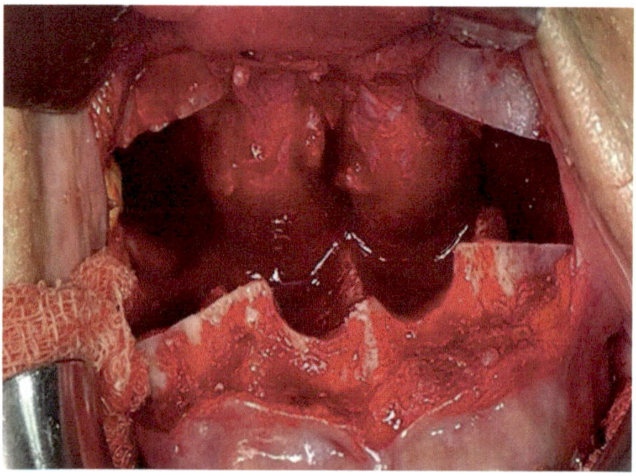

The osteotomized segments is initially separated either with digital pressure or using bone spreaders. Rowe's disimpaction forceps is then used to further mobilize the maxilla. Any bony interferences are removed, and any soft tissue tears are repaired.

Positioning and Fixation

The new planned position of the Le Fort I segment is guided by a *prefabricated occlusal splint, or 3D-printed patient-specific implant.* Conventionally, the maxilla is fixed with *two L-shaped miniplates and screws* on each side.

Adjunct Measures

There are other adjunct procedures involved with the Le Fort I osteotomy. These include the following:

- *Septoplasty* (to avoid septal deviation)
- *Turbinectomy* (to avoid obstruction and reduction of nasal cavity volume in impaction cases)
- *Alar cinch suture* (to prevent nostril flaring)
- *V-Y mucosal closure* (to preserve lip length)

Once all procedures are complete, the incision closure is made with resorbable sutures, such as 4-0 Vicryl.

7.2.3 *Bilateral Sagittal Split Osteotomy, BSSO (Mandible) [21–23]*

7.2.3.1 Approach

The incision is done *transorally* via the posterior buccal vestibule. Infiltrate local anesthesia at the posterior buccal vestibule and medial ramus region.

7.2.3.2 Incision

Incision is made 5 mm below mucogingival junction from distal 2nd premolar to the external oblique ridge. Incision is made through mucosa, submucosa, and periosteum. Care is made not to incise too buccally as it may involve more muscular tissue (i.e., buccinator muscle) and enhance bleeding.

7.2.3.3 Flap Elevation

A full thickness mucoperiosteal flap is elevated buccally, anteriorly, and inferiorly to the lower border of mandible. It is not necessarily needed to identify the mental foramen and *mental nerve. However, the nerve is protected when encountered.* The flap is further raised by exposing the *coronoid process and detaching the temporalis muscle tendon.* Following this, the medial ramus is exposed to identify the lingula and sigmoid notch, an important landmark for the medial osteotomy.

7.2.3.4 Osteotomy Design

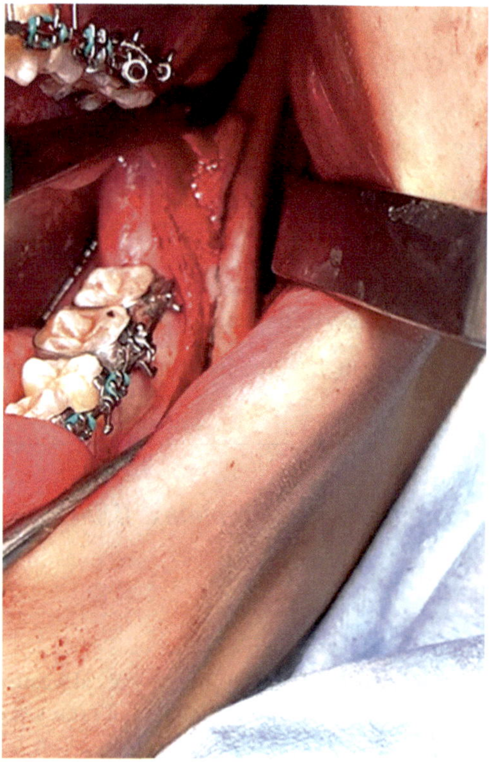

The sagittal split osteotomy comprises of four connected osteotomies, namely the medial, sagittal, vertical or lateral, and inferior border osteotomies. The medial osteotomy is at the level of the lingula, parallel to the occlusal plane, and below the sigmoid notch. This is then connected to the sagittal osteotomy that runs sagitally between the buccal cortex of the ramus/body and roots of the molar teeth. The endpoint of the sagittal cut usually locates at the 2nd or 1st molar and connects with the vertical/lateral osteotomy, which then runs through the whole length of the mandibular body. Finally the vertical/lateral osteotomy connects with the inferior border of the mandible.

7.2.3.5 Osteotomy Execution

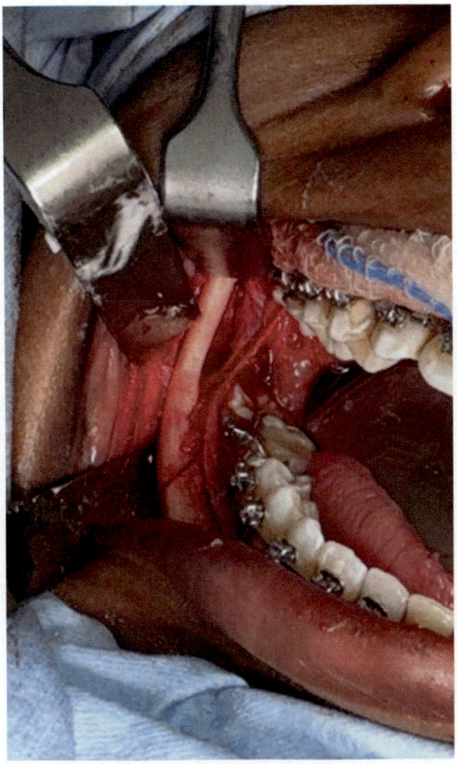

The osteotomies are made using either a reciprocating saw, piezosurgery tip, or surgical burs. The common order of osteotomies starts from the medial, sagittal, vertical, and finally inferior. An important note for sagittal split osteotomy is that the cuts are made through single cortices only, except for the inferior border cut, which must be made bicortically.

7.2.3.6 Mandibular Split

The sagittal split is initiated with osteotomes at various regions of the osteotomy, mainly at the angle and vertical osteotomy sites. Osteotomes help to initiate and propagate the split in a controlled manner. This is then followed by completion of split using a bone spreader such as Smith spreaders. Bone spreaders help to gradually split the mandible while allowing the surgeon to assess the split pattern and inferior alveolar nerve pathway. If the nerve is crossing the proximal segment, it can be released at this stage and prevents severance. A good split will result in a proximal segment that comprises of the ramus and condyle, and a distal segment that bears the teeth. Both segments should be allowed to move independently.

The same steps are repeated for the contralateral side.

7.2.3.7 Fixation

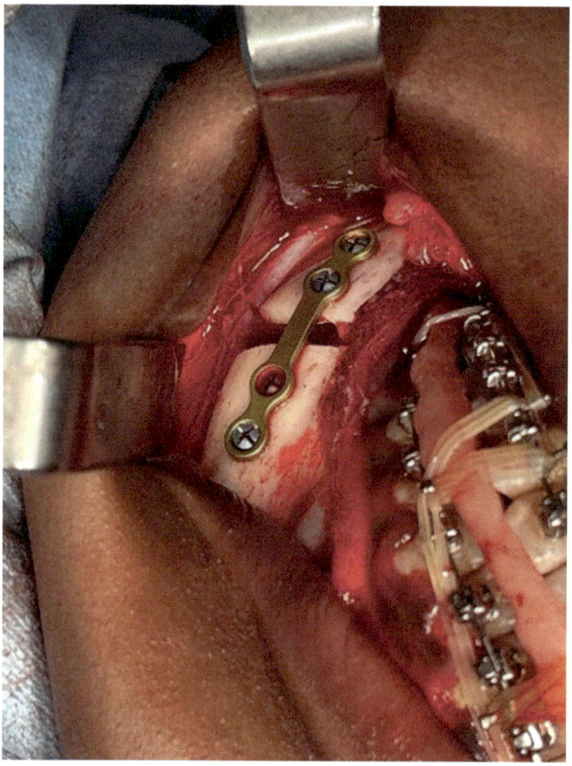

Once both sides of the mandible are split, the new position of the distal segment is fixed in the preplanned position using the final occlusal splint. The splint is fixed between the upper and lower teeth and secured using wires and/or elastics. The proximal and distal segments of the sagittal split are then fixed using 2.0 mm miniplates and screws on each side. The proximal segment should be fixed passively and condyles seated in the fossa.

7.2.3.8 Occlusion Check

An important part of the whole procedure is to ensure occlusion is stable and correct as planned. Once the plates are fixed, the intermaxillary fixation is released and the occlusion is checked. In cases whereby the occlusion is wrong or not as planned, the mandibular position is readjusted and refixed.

7.2.3.9 Wound Closure

All incision wounds are closed with resorbable sutures such as 4-0 Vicryl.

7.2.4 Sliding Genioplasty [24]

7.2.4.1 Approach

A transoral approach is done for the sliding genioplasty procedure. Local anesthesia infiltration is done around the lower labial vestibule [24].

7.2.4.2 Incision

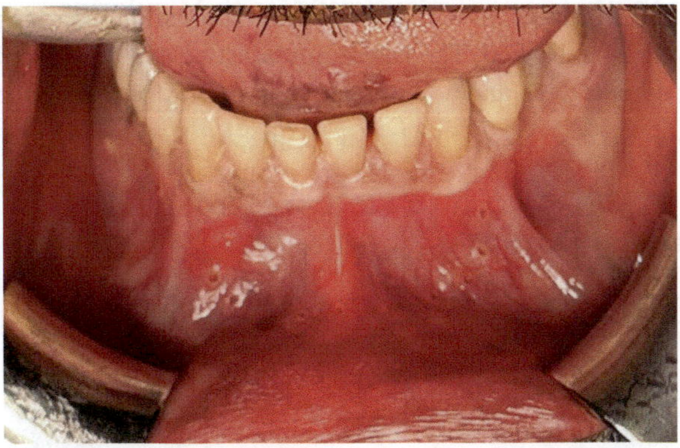

The incision typically runs from canine to canine: 5 mm below the mucogingival junction and approximately 10 mm in the incisal regions. This is to allow incorporation of the mentalis muscle for resuspension during wound closure. The incision may be extended further posteriorly or at times connected with the BSSO incisions. This is to allow better visualization of the mental nerves, especially for protection.

7.2.4.3 Dissection

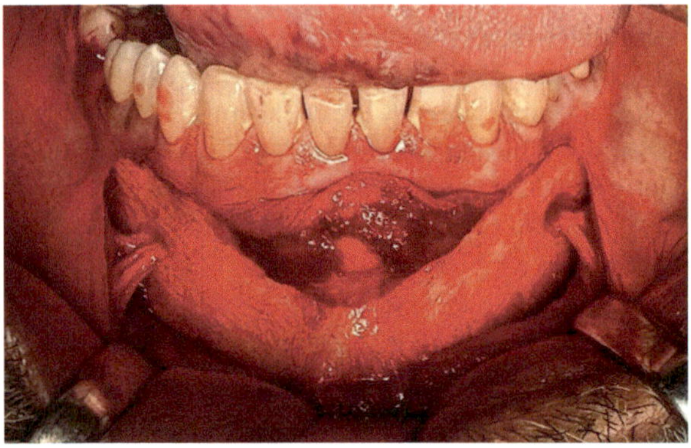

A full thickness mucoperiosteal flap is elevated, exposing the symphysis and inferior border. In cases whereby the planned sliding genioplasty runs below the mental nerve, the dissection is extended to expose the nerve and surround regions. The mental nerve may or may not be skeletonized.

7.2.4.4 Osteotomy Design

In order to ensure symmetry of the chin position to the facial midline, the midpoint of the chin and lower incisors is marked. Other vertical landmarks such as canine positions may also be marked. The osteotomy must be at least 5 mm below the apices of the mandibular teeth and 6–7 mm away from the circumference of the mental foramen.

7.2.4.5 Osteotomy Execution

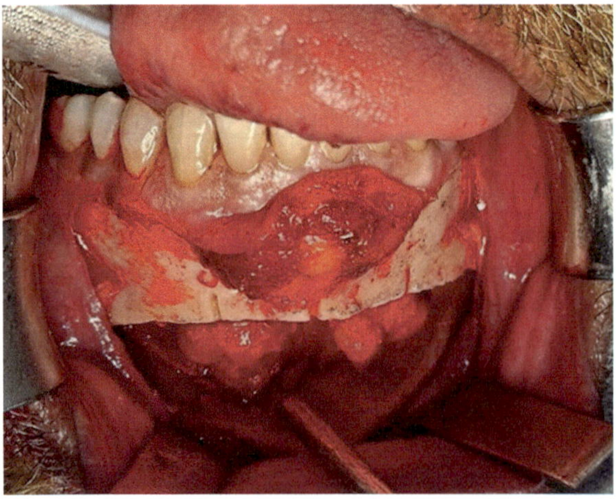

Osteotomy is done using reciprocating saw, piezo, or surgical burs. Osteotomy is made through both cortices. It is important to ensure the *genial tubercle with genioglossus attachment* is preserved or transferred to the chin segment.

7.2.4.6 Positioning and Fixation

The new chin position is fixed with a prebent chin plate that comes in various advancement lengths. The plate is fixed with screws.

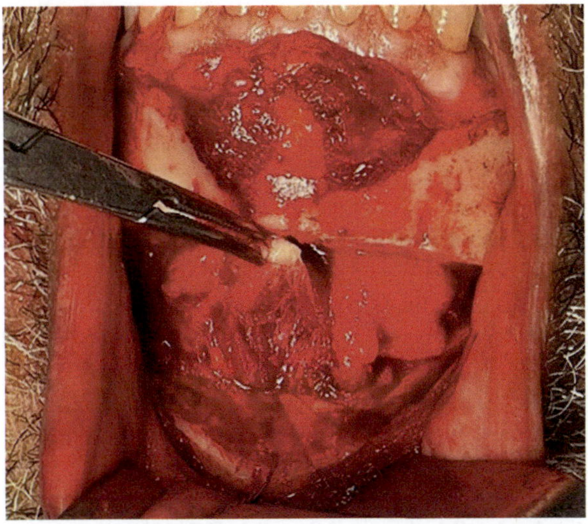

7.2.4.7 Closure

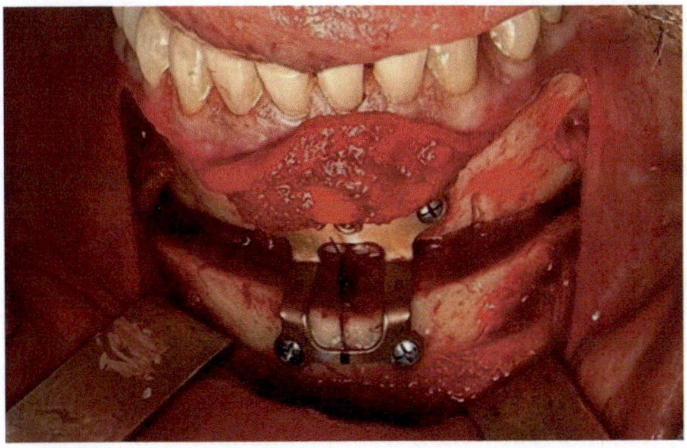

The mentalis muscle is resuspended to avoid chin ptosis. The mucosa later is closed with resorbable 4-0 Vicryl sutures.

7.2.5 *Postoperative Considerations [26]*

Meticulous postoperative management after maxillomandibular advancement (MMA) is essential to ensure surgical success, prevent complications, and support functional recovery of mastication, speech, and airway patency.

7.2.5.1 Airway and Immediate Monitoring

- *Airway vigilance:* Patients should be closely monitored for airway compromise in the early postoperative period, as facial swelling, hematoma, or bleeding may exacerbate obstruction.
- *ICU/high-dependency monitoring* is considered for patients with severe OSA, obesity hypoventilation, or significant comorbidities.

7.2.5.2 Intermaxillary Fixation (IMF) and Occlusion Management

- *Duration:* Intermaxillary fixation or guiding elastics are typically maintained for 1–2 weeks depending on occlusal stability. In many centers, rigid fixation allows early mobilization with elastics rather than complete IMF.
- *Occlusion checks:* Early follow-up is critical to identify malocclusion, open bite, or premature contact. Adjustments by the maxillofacial team may be required.

7.2.5.3 Analgesia, Antibiotics, and Steroids [27–29]

- *Analgesia:* A multimodal regimen (acetaminophen ± NSAIDs, with opioids reserved for breakthrough pain) is preferred to limit sedation and respiratory depression.
- *Antibiotics:* Short perioperative coverage (24–48 h) is common, though some surgeons extend coverage for 5–7 days to reduce the risk of hardware infection.
- *Steroids:* Perioperative corticosteroids may reduce edema, trismus, and postoperative discomfort.

7.2.5.4 Diet and Nutrition

- *Initial diet:* Clear liquids advancing to soft/pureed diet for at least 2–4 weeks.
- *Nutritional support:* Patients often have reduced oral intake due to IMF; dietitian referral may help prevent weight loss and malnutrition.
- *Hydration:* Close attention to fluid intake is essential, especially in the first week.

7.2.5.5 Oral Hygiene and Wound Care

- *Oral rinses:* Chlorhexidine or saline rinses are recommended to maintain hygiene around intraoral incisions and prevent infection.
- *Tooth brushing:* Gentle brushing with a soft-bristled toothbrush is encouraged once tolerated, avoiding trauma to surgical sites.

7.2.5.6 Monitoring and Complications

- *Infection:* Watch for fever, wound breakdown, purulent discharge, or localized swelling.
- *Nerve function:* Inferior alveolar and infraorbital nerve paresthesia is common postoperatively; recovery may take months. Early documentation and reassurance are important [25].
- *Malocclusion or relapse:* Requires orthodontic review and possible adjustment of elastics or splints.
- *Hardware issues:* Rarely, loosening or exposure of plates/screws may necessitate revision.

7.2.5.7 Functional Recovery and Rehabilitation

- *Jaw mobility:* Progressive jaw opening exercises are usually started once fixation is released.
- *Speech and swallowing:* Temporary speech changes are common; speech therapy may be considered if persistent.
- *Return to work/activities:* Light activity can resume in 2 weeks, but heavy exertion should be avoided for 6 weeks. Contact sports are restricted for at least 3 months.

7.2.5.8 Long-Term Follow-up

- *OSA reassessment:* Repeat polysomnography is generally performed after 3–6 months to assess efficacy.
- *Orthodontic follow-up:* Continuous coordination between the surgeon and orthodontist is required for occlusal stability.
- *Psychosocial support:* Patients may experience changes in facial appearance; psychological support or counseling may help adjustment.

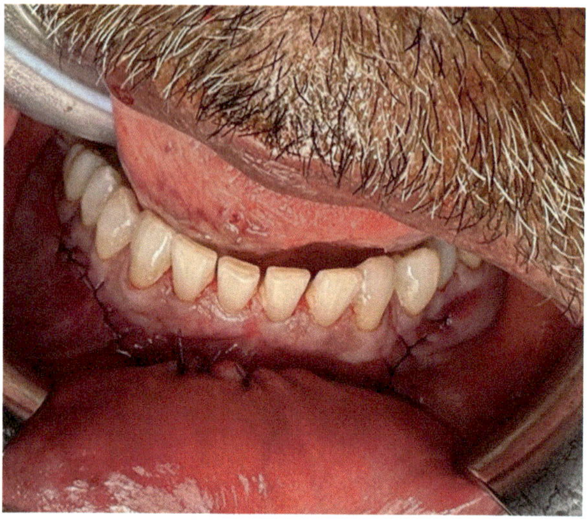

7.2.6 *Complications*

1. *Neurosensory disturbance (inferior alveolar/lingual/infraorbital)*
   (a) Very common immediately; a smaller subset persists ≥6–12 months. Risk rises with older age, large movements, close mandibular canal proximity, unfavorable (high-lingual) splits.
   (b) *Prevention*: careful split design, avoid high lingual fracture, consider piezo-assisted corticotomy.
   (c) *Management*: reassurance and serial neurosensory exams; neuropathic pain is uncommon—treat with standard orofacial pain protocols and refer when persistent.
2. *Unfavorable ("bad") splits and ramus/condylar fractures (BSSO)*
   (a) Pooled "bad-split" incidence ≈2–3%. Third molars in situ and reduced ramus width increase risk.
   (b) *Prevention*: remove 3rd molars well before BSSO; meticulous osteotomy technique.
   (c) *Management*: intra-op stabilization (recontouring, rigid fixation) ± staged repair if condylar injury.
3. *Hemorrhage and delayed epistaxis (Le Fort I)* [32]
   (a) Intra-op bleeding is usually controllable; rare delayed epistaxis (often 1–2 weeks post-op) may reflect pseudoaneurysm (descending palatine/internal maxillary) [33, 34].

   (b) *Management*: stepwise—anterior/posterior packing—endoscopic control; low threshold for urgent angiography and selective embolization. Warn patients about "red flag" bleeding after discharge.

4. *Surgical-site infection (SSI)/hardware irritation*

   (a) Overall risk is low single-digit. Longer prophylaxis (2–7 days) reduces SSI versus single-day regimens, but balance against stewardship; a single pre-op dose alone is least protective.
   (b) *Management*: local care, culture-directed antibiotics; consider plate/screw removal if chronic.

5. *Sinonasal issues after Le Fort I*

   (a) Radiologic mucosal thickening/inflammation on CBCT is not uncommon; symptomatic rhinosinusitis is less frequent [35, 36].
   (b) *Management*: saline irrigations, short antibiotic courses when indicated; ENT referral and endoscopic sinus surgery for persistent disease or obstructed ostiomeatal complex.

6. *Temporomandibular joint (TMJ) symptoms* [37, 38]

   (a) Many patients with preexisting TMD improve after orthognathic surgery; a smaller group without prior TMD may develop new symptoms.
   (b) *Management*: soft diet, NSAIDs, early physiotherapy; escalate to splints and specialty care if pain/dysfunction persists. Avoid excessive counterclockwise rotation in at-risk joints.

7. *Condylar resorption (CR) and skeletal relapse* [30, 31]

   (a) Uncommon but clinically important; risk factors include female sex, high mandibular plane angle, large advancements, and counterclockwise rotations. Surveillance with serial imaging (CBCT) at 6–12 months.
   (b) Management ranges from orthodontic/occlusal splints and anti-inflammatories to revision surgery or TMJ reconstruction in progressive cases.

8. *Nonunion/malunion (less common)*

   (a) Occurs infrequently with modern rigid fixation; presents with segmental mobility, pain, or infection.
   (b) *Management*: debridement, re-osteosynthesis, and bone grafting when indicated. Risk may rise with extensive segmentations or large maxillary displacements.

References

1. Gu M, McGrath CPJ, Wong RWK, Hägg U, Yang Y (2014) Cephalometric norms for the upper airway of 12-year-old Chinese children. Head Face Med. 10:38.
2. Gu Y, McNamara JA Jr, Sigler LM, Baccetti T. Comparison of craniofacial characteristics of typical Chinese and Caucasian young adults. Eur J Orthod. 2011;33(2):205–11.
3. Mohamed AM, Chen Y, Wafaie K, Al-Balaa M, Abusafia B, Mohammed OM, Yang Y, Qiao Y. Cephalometric evaluation of posterior airway space in Chinese and Egyptian races. APOS. 2023;13:205–14.
4. Samman N, Mohammadi H, Xia J. Cephalometric norms for the upper airway in a healthy Hong Kong Chinese population. Hong Kong Med J. 2003;9(1):25–30.
5. Savoldia F, Xinyueb G, McGrath CPJ, Yang Y, Chow SC, Tsoif JKH, Gu M. Reliability of lateral cephalometric radiographs in the assessment of the upper airway in children: a retrospective study. Angle Orthod. 2019;80(5):766–72. https://doi.org/10.2319/082009-456.1.
6. Zakaria NN, Kamarudin Y, Ong KS, Koo ZQ. Lower incisor changes following non-extraction orthodontic decompensation in Class III surgical cases. Ann Dent Univ Malaya. 2021;28:15–22.
7. Gurgel ML, Magalhães B, Flores-Mir C, Paranhos LR. Methods for upper airway assessment using cone-beam computed tomography in adults with obstructive sleep apnea: a systematic review. Sleep Breath. 2023;27(1):9–22.
8. Momany SM, Al Jassim A, Cisneros GJ, et al. Upper airway analysis in obstructive sleep apnea patients using cone beam computed tomography compared with control subjects. Am J Med Sci. 2016;352(4):376–85.
9. Thereza-Bussolaro C, de Oliveira L, Bombardelli P, et al. Some challenges and potential issues regarding cone beam computed tomography of the upper airway. J Dent Sleep Med. 2021;8(2).
10. Fleck RJ, Shott SR, Mahmoud M, Amin RS, Donnelly LF. Dynamic volumetric imaging of the upper airway in children during sleep: initial experience with drug-induced sleep CT. J Clin Sleep Med. 2017;13(2):201–10.
11. Whyte A, Gibson D. Imaging of adult obstructive sleep apnoea. Eur J Radiol. 2018;102:176–87.
12. Volner K, Schwab RJ. Dynamic sleep MRI in obstructive sleep apnea: state of the art. J Magn Reson Imaging. 2021;53(5):1381–97.
13. Schwab RJ, Pasirstein M, Pierson R, et al. Identification of upper airway anatomic risk factors for obstructive sleep apnea with volumetric MRI. Am J Respir Crit Care Med. 2003;168(5):522–30.
14. Eastwood PR, Malhotra A, Palmer LJ, et al. Facial structure and obesity as risk factors for sleep apnea. J Clin Sleep Med. 2020;16(12):2013–24.
15. Lee RWW, Petocz P, Prvan T, Chan ASL, Grunstein RR, Cistulli PA. Prediction of obstructive sleep apnea with craniofacial photographic analysis. Sleep. 2009;32(1):46–52.
16. Schimmel M, Christou P, Houstis O, Herrmann FR, Kiliaridis S, Müller F. Distances between facial landmarks can be measured accurately with a new digital 3-dimensional video system. Am J Orthod Dentofacial Orthop. 2010;137(5):580.e1–580.e10; discussion 580–1.
17. Knoops PG, Beaumont CA, Borghi A, Rodriguez-Florez N, Breakey RW, Rodgers W, Angullia F, Jeelani NU, Schievano S, Dunaway DJ. Comparison of three-dimensional scanner systems for craniomaxillofacial imaging. J Plast Reconstr Aesthet Surg. 2017;70(4):441–9.
18. Chin EW, Goh LC, Lau MN, Abu Bakar MZ. Handheld blue light three-dimensional (3D) scanner versus lateral cephalometry for facial morphology assessment in obstructive sleep apnoea participants. Sleep Breath. 2025;29(1):118.
19. Holty JE, Guilleminault C. Maxillomandibular advancement for obstructive sleep apnea: a systematic review and meta-analysis. Sleep Med Rev. 2010;14(5):287–97.
20. Zaghi S, Holty JE, Certal V, et al. Maxillomandibular advancement for treatment of obstructive sleep apnea: a meta-analysis. JAMA Otolaryngol Head Neck Surg. 2016;142(1):58–66.

21. Steenen SA, van Wijk AJ, Becking AG. Bad splits in bilateral sagittal split osteotomy: systematic review and meta-analysis of reported risk factors. Int J Oral Maxillofac Surg. 2016;45:971–9.
22. Verweij JP, Houppermans PN, Gooris P, Mensink G, van Merkesteyn JP. Risk factors for common complications associated with bilateral sagittal split osteotomy: a literature review and meta-analysis. J Craniomaxillofac Surg. 2016;44(9):1170–80.
23. Verweij JP, Mensink G, Fiocco M, van Merkesteyn JP. Presence of mandibular third molars during bilateral sagittal split osteotomy increases the possibility of bad split but not the risk of other post-operative complications. J Craniomaxillofac Surg. 2014;42(7):e359–63.
24. Song SA, Chang ET, Certal V, et al. Genial tubercle advancement and genioplasty for obstructive sleep apnea: a systematic review and meta-analysis. Laryngoscope. 2017;127(4):984–92.
25. Agbaje JO, Salem AS, Lambrichts I, Jacobs R, Politis C. Systematic review of the incidence of inferior alveolar nerve injury in bilateral sagittal split osteotomy and the assessment of neurosensory disturbances. Int J Oral Maxillofac Surg. 2015;44(4):447–51.
26. Kim YK, Park JY, Kim SG. Complications associated with orthognathic surgery. J Korean Assoc Oral Maxillofac Surg. 2017;43(1):3–15.
27. Danda AK, Ravi P. Effectiveness of postoperative antibiotics in orthognathic surgery: a meta-analysis. J Oral Maxillofac Surg. 2011;69(10):2650–6.
28. Brignardello-Petersen R, Guyatt GH, Lytvyn L, et al. Antibiotic prophylaxis for preventing infectious complications in orthognathic surgery. Cochrane Database Syst Rev. 2015;(1):CD010266.
29. Tang X, Wen K, Yang Y. Impact of long-term vs. short-term and single day vs. single dose of antibiotic prophylaxis in reducing infection rates after orthognathic surgery: a systematic review and meta-analysis. Med Oral Patol Oral Cir Bucal. 2024;29(3):e380–9.
30. Catherine Z, Breton P, Bouletreau P. Condylar resorption after orthognathic surgery: a systematic review. Rev Stomatol Chir Maxillofac Chir Orale. 2016;117(1):3–10.
31. Barone S, Cosentini G, Bennardo F, Antonelli A, Giudice A. Incidence and management of condylar resorption after orthognathic surgery: an overview. Korean J Orthod. 2022;52(1):29–41.
32. Kramer FJ, Baethge C, Swennen G, Teltzrow T, Schulze M, Dempf R. Intra- and perioperative complications of the LeFort I osteotomy: a prospective evaluation of 1000 patients. J Craniofac Surg. 2004;15(6):971–9.
33. Lanigan DT, Hey JH, West RA. Major vascular complications of orthognathic surgery: hemorrhage associated with Le Fort I osteotomies. J Oral Maxillofac Surg. 1990;48(6):561–73.
34. Chepla KJ, Totonchi A, Hsu DP, Gosain AK. Maxillary artery pseudoaneurysm after Le Fort I osteotomy: treatment using transcatheter arterial embolization. J Craniofac Surg. 2010;21(4):1079–81.
35. Nocini PF, Trevisiol L, Bertossi D, et al. Is Le Fort I osteotomy associated with maxillary sinusitis? J Oral Maxillofac Surg. 2016;74(2):400.e1–400.e12.
36. Pereira-Filho VA, Gabrielli MF, Gabrielli MA, et al. Incidence of maxillary sinusitis following Le Fort I osteotomy. J Oral Maxillofac Surg. 2011;69(2):346–51.
37. Al-Moraissi EA, Perez D, Ellis E III. Does orthognathic surgery cause or cure temporomandibular disorders? A systematic review and meta-analysis. J Oral Maxillofac Surg. 2017;75(9):1835–47.
38. Jung HD, Kim SY, Park HS, Jung YS. Orthognathic surgery and temporomandibular joint symptoms. Maxillofac Plast Reconstr Surg. 2015;37:14.

Index

L. C. Goh, S. T. Toh (eds.), *Sleep Surgery in a Nutshell*,
https://doi.org/10.1007/978-981-95-9749-9

GPSR Compliance

The European Union's (EU) General Product Safety Regulation (GPSR) is a set of rules that requires consumer products to be safe and our obligations to ensure this.

If you have any concerns about our products, you can contact us on ProductSafety@springernature.com

In case Publisher is established outside the EU, the EU authorized representative is:

Springer Nature Customer Service Center GmbH
Europaplatz 3
69115 Heidelberg, Germany

Batch number: 10732090

Printed by Printforce, the Netherlands